Respiratory Drug Delivery

Editor

Peter R. Byron, Ph.D.

Associate Professor
Department of Pharmacy and Pharmaceutics
Medical College of Virginia/Virginia Commonwealth University
Richmond, Virginia

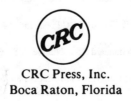

CRC Press, Inc.
Boca Raton, Florida

Library of Congress Cataloging-in-Publication Data

Respiratory drug delivery / editor, Peter R. Byron.
   p.   cm.
   Based on a symposium on respiratory drug delivery held in May 1988 at the University of Kentucky.
   Includes bibliographies and index.
   ISBN 0-8493-5344-0
   1. Respiratory therapy--Congresses. 2. Respiratory agents--Administration--Congresses.
   [DNLM: 1. Administration, Inhalation--congresses. 2. Respiration Disorders--drug therapy--congresses.
   WF 145 R4343 1988]
RM161.R448   1990
615.8'.36—dc20   89-24018 CIP
DNLM/DLC
for Library of Congress

Direct all inquires to CRC Press, Inc., 2000 Corporate Blvd., N.W., Boca Raton, Florida, 33431.

© 1990 by CRC Press, Inc.

International Standard Book Number 0-8493-5344-0

Library of Congress Card Number 89-24018
Printed in the United States

PREFACE

While bronchodilators, steroids, and antiallergic compounds have been administered as aerosols for some years, recent advances in respiratory physiology, immunology, and biotechnology have substantially increased the number of new drug candidates for delivery to the lung. Compounds requiring aerosol administration may be intended for local or systemic activity and to enable the nonparenteral administration of new generation peptides and protein requies that alternative routes are explored for all compounds with substantial first-pass metabolism and/or breakdown in other sites of administration. While some routes of drug delivery have been explored in detail, this cannot be said of the respiratory tract. Drug delivery to the lung can be difficult to accomplish and expertise in the area is spread across several academic disciplines.

The present text, which is focused on subjects embracing the topic of drug delivery to the lung itself, has been created by a group of scientists who assembled at The University of Kentucky to present the subject material at a symposium on respiratory drug delivery held in May 1988. This text, and the symposium from which it was created, was designed to span the relevant subject areas from aerosol deposition through pharmaceutical chemistry and formulation, to the final clinical evaluation of pharmaceutical products. The authors, who are recognized authorities in their subject areas, were asked to present and apply their topics through the current state of the art as it affects drug delivery to the lung. Thus, toxicology is considered from the point of view of drugs and the pharmaceutical excipients used in aerosols. Metabolism of drugs in the respiratory tract is addressed prior to considerations of pharmaceutical chemistry, where pro-drug approaches are introduced as a means of improving molecular targeting to the lung. The simultaneous kinetic processes of particulate clearance, dissolution, and absorption are considered with specific regard to answering questions concerning drug longevity in the lung. Later chapters consider the formulation of drugs as metered and nonmetered aerosol dosage forms. An appendix to the chapter on formulation of MDIs reviews the importance of trace quantities of water to the stability of suspension formulations. Chapter 8 in the text reviews the current practices employed in the clinical testing of aerosol products alongside a number of issues which are currently undergoing debate between clinical scientists and regulatory authorities in the U.S. and other countries. As editor, I extend my thanks to all those who have contributed material for this book, to Michael Shannon who made the symposium at Kentucky possible, to numerous colleagues in the pharmaceutical industry, and to my graduate students who continued to provide data up to the last minute.

Peter R. Byron

THE EDITOR

Peter R. Byron, Ph.D. is Associate Professor of Physical Pharmacy, Department of Pharmacy and Pharmaceutics, Medical College of Virginia/Virginia Commonwealth University School of Pharmacy, Richmond, VA.

He graduated in 1970 from the University of Manchester, England, with a B.Sc. in Pharmacy (Honors in Pharmaceutics) and obtained his Ph.D. from the same institution in 1973. He performed postdoctoral research in the U.K. (University of Aston) and the U.S. (Ohio State University) between 1974 and 1977. Between 1975 and 1984 he held the position of Lecturer in Pharmaceutics at Aston University, Birmingham, England. He joined the faculty at the University of Kentucky College of Pharmacy in July 1984. He moved to Richmond to his present position in June 1988.

Dr. Byron is a registered pharmacist in the U.K. and Charter Member of the American Association of Pharmaceutical Scientists in the U.S. He has received several awards and recognition for research and has made numerous invited presentations within the pharmaceutical industry and academic institutions in Europe and the U.S.

He has published over 40 research articles, received research funding from local, federal, and industrial institutions and acted as advisor and major professor for a number of graduate students and postdoctorals. His current research is focused on inhalation aerosol science where he is attempting optimized drug delivery to the respiratory tract and investigating physicochemical and formulation factors controlling aerosol generation, deposition, release, and absorption via the lung.

ACKNOWLEDGMENTS

The Continuing Education Office at the University of Kentucky is most pleased to have participated in the organization and delivery of the symposium on respiratory drug delivery which resulted in the publication of this text. We are grateful to two companies for support of our endeavors in this respect. These are 3M Company, St. Paul, MN and ATI Pharmaceuticals, New Canaan, CT. We thank Catherine Kriske and H. R. Shepherd in particular and also colleagues at the University of Kentucky and staff of the Continuing Education Office for their assistance in bringing events to such a successful conclusion. This marked a beginning for us in the area of scientific program development. It is our belief that symposia, such as this one, provide a much needed and extremely useful forum for the dissemination of scientific knowledge, the teasing out of innovative ideas among colleagues, and the cross-fertilization of the scientific enterprise. From such interactions come new and creative approaches to solving the problems faced by any science, collaborative research efforts, and the opportunity to develop a growing collegiality among like-minded scientists.

Michael C. Shannon, Ph.D.
Director, Continuing Pharmacy Education
College of Pharmacy
University of Kentucky
Lexington, Kentucky

Peter R. Byron, Ph.D.
Associate Professor
School of Pharmacy
Virginia Commonwealth University
Richmond, Virginia

CONTRIBUTORS

Tahir Ahmed, M.D.
Associate Professor of Medicine
Pulmonary Division/Department of
  Medicine
Mount Sinai Medical Center
Miami Beach, Florida

Peter R. Byron, Ph.D.
Associate Professor
Department of Pharmacy
Medical College of Virginia/Virginia
  Commonwealth University
Richmond, Virginia

Peter A. Crooks, Ph.D.
The Southern Research Institute
Birmingham, Alabama

L. A. Damani, Ph.D.
Professor and Head
Chelsea Department of Pharmacy
Kings College London
London, England

Timothy R. Gerrity, Ph.D.
Chief, Aerobiology Section
Clinical Research Branch
EPA
Research Triangle Park, North Carolina

Harry B. Kostenbauder, Ph.D.
Professor, Associate Dean for Research
College of Pharmacy
University of Kentucky
Lexington, Kentucky

Nicholas C. Miller
Pharmaceuticals Division
3M Company
St. Paul, Minnesota

Elaine M. Phillips
Research Assistant
Department of Pharmacy and
  Pharmaceutics
Medical College of Virginia/Virginia
  Commonwealth University
Richmond, Virginia

Steven Slonecker
Department of Pharmacy
University of Kentucky
Lexington, Kentucky

David J. Velasquez, Ph.D.
Research Specialist
Biosciences Laboratory
3M Company
St. Paul, Minnesota

TABLE OF CONTENTS

Chapter 1

PATHOPHYSIOLOGICAL AND DISEASE CONSTRAINTS ON AEROSOL DELIVERY*

Timothy R. Gerrity

TABLE OF CONTENTS

*   This chapter has been reviewed by the Health Effects Research Laboratory, U.S. Environmental Protection Agency,
    and was approved for publication. Mention of trade names or commercial products does not constitute endorsement
    or recommendation for use.

I. INTRODUCTION

The use of inhaled therapeutic aerosols is a common method for the treatment of various lung diseases such as asthma and irreversible chronic obstructive lung disease. Among these drugs are bronchodilators such as β-agonists and anticholinergics, mast cell stabilizers such as sodium cromoglycate, corticosteroids, mucolytics, and antimicrobials.

Despite the widespread use of these drugs there are still many problems associated with their use. Aerosolized β-agonists often result in untoward side effects such as palpitations, tachycardia, and nervousness. Mucolytics and antimicrobials have been largely ineffective for their intended purposes. Problems such as these may, in part, be related to the pattern of aerosol deposition within the respiratory tract. For example, deposition of an inhaled bronchodialator may lead to systemic side effects because the drug is deposited in the mouth and then swallowed. An understanding of the dynamics of aerosol deposition within the respiratory tract may help in the design of better therapeutic aerosol particles and better delivery systems.

The efficacy of inhaled therapeutic aerosols depends upon several factors related to the particles comprising the aerosol:

1.   The aerosol must be capable of reaching desired tissue sites within the respiratory tract.
2.   Therapeutic concentrations of the drug must be deliverable within a relatively few number of breaths to be practical for most patient uses.
3.   The aerosol particles, once having deposited upon the airway lumen, must be capable of releasing the pharmaceutic compound in sufficient time before the particles (and thus the drug) are transported away from the deposition site by various clearance mechanisms.

This chapter focuses upon the mechanisms by which aerosols deposit in the respiratory tract, and how these mechanisms can influence the dose of an inhaled therapeutic aerosol. Both the experimental determination of respiratory tract deposition of aerosols and mathematical models of aerosol deposition are presented. For clarity, nonhygroscopic aerosol behavior will be emphasized, but hygroscopic aerosol behavior and how it affects aerosol deposition is also discussed. Since therapeutic aerosols are most frequently used by patients with altered lung function, the effect of pathologic states of the lung on the deposition of aerosols is presented. Finally, particle transport mechanisms associated with lung defense mechanisms are discussed briefly in terms of how they can affect the delivery of a therapeutic agent.

Before aerosol deposition within the human respiratory tract is discussed, some basic principles of aerosols and their dynamic behavior are reviewed followed by a discussion of respiratory tract structure and function and respiratory tract morphometry.

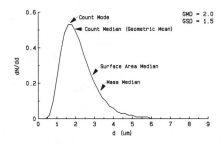

FIGURE 1. An example of a log-normal distribution of aerosol particle sizes plotted linearly against particle size. The vertical axis is the fraction of particles per unit particle diameter.

II. AEROSOLS

An aerosol is a relatively stable suspension of solid or liquid particles in a gas. For all of our considerations here the gas will be air. Typically, the size range of aerosols extends from around a diameter of 0.001 µm to a diameter of 100 µm.[1] Particles at the lower end of the spectrum are approaching the size of individual molecules and are therefore not appropriately described as comprising aerosols; those at the upper end approach sizes where the rate of settling in quiet air is too rapid to be considered stable.

The dynamic behavior of aerosol particles is governed by the interactions of the particles with the surrounding air molecules. Generally, the behavior of aerosol particles is described by the processes of inertial impaction, sedimentation, and diffusion. The first two of these processes are functions of the macroscopic interactions of the particles with air; the last is a function of microscopic interactions with air molecules.

Aerosols can come in a variety of shapes as well as sizes. Aerosol particles can be perfectly spherical, fibrous (such as asbestos fibers), or complex aggregates of smaller particles with a highly irregular shape. Because of this variey of shapes it is sometimes difficult to describe an aerosol particle by a single number such as diameter. One way of describing the size of a particle is by its settling velocity in still air. Such a description is the aerodynamic equivalent diameter. Aerodynamic equivalent diameter (d_{ae}) is the diamete r of a perfect sphere of unit density (1 g/cm^3) that has the same settling velocity in still air as the particle which we are describing. A more precise definition of d_{ae} is given shortly.

In real life, aerosols are not composed of particles with all the same size. Rather, they are composed of particles with a distribution of sizes. Thus, to describe adequately an aerosol we will need two numbers: one to describe the typical size of an aerosol particle and the other to describe the shape of the distribution.

Suppose a sample of spherical particles were collected on a filter and examined under a microscope with some sort of optical device for measuring particle diameter. A frequency distribution of the particle diameters can be plotted by counting the number of particles that have diameters that fall within equally spaced bins. For most aerosols, when their size distribution is plotted in this manner, the distribution is asymmetric as is shown in the example of Figure 1. A model for size distribution which describes well many spherical aerosols is the log-normal distribution. If particle size is log-normally distributed, a frequency distribution plotted with respect to the log of particle diameter will result in the symmetric distribution shown in Figure 2.

For a log-normally distributed aerosol, the geometric mean diameter (GMD) and the geometric standard deviation (GSD) are parameters most frequently used to describe the distribution. It can be shown that the GMD for a log-normally distributed aerosol equals the count median diameter (CMD), the particle diameter for which 50% of all the particles have a larger diameter.[2]

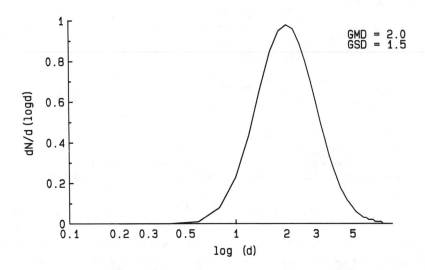

FIGURE 2.   The particle distribution shown in Figure 1 replotted as a function of the logarithm of particle size. The vertical axis is the fraction of particles per unit increment of the logarithm of particle diameter.

There are other diameters that can also be used to characterize the aerosol distribution. For example, the particle diameter above which 50% of the aerosol mass is contained is frequently used. This parameter is called the mass median diameter (MMD). Similarly the distribution can be described by the diameter above which 50% of the aerosol surface area is contained. This parameter is called the area median diameter (AMD). Which parameter is used depends upon the particular property of the aerosol that is of greatest interest. For example, in inhalation toxicology, if the total mass of a particle contributes to the toxic effect, the MMD probably best describes the aerosol. However, it may occur that the toxic components are contained upon the particle surface, in which case AMD may best describe the aerosol. The importance of these distinctions is demonstrated in Figure 1 where the various parameters used to describe the log-normal distribution are given. Clearly, MMD and AMD are numerically different, though they describe the same distribution.

If an aerosol distribution is log-normal, MMD and AMD can be derived from GMD and GSD:

$$\text{Log}_{10}(\text{AMD}) = \text{Log}_{10}(\text{GMD}) + 4.6(\text{Log}_{10}\text{GSD})^2 \tag{1}$$

and

$$\text{Log}_{10}(\text{MMD}) = \text{Log}_{10}(\text{GMD}) + 6.9(\text{Log}_{10}\text{GSD})^2 \tag{2}$$

These equations were first derived by Hatch and Choate.[3]

III. AEROSOL DYNAMICS

As was stated earlier, aerosol particles can have a wide range of sizes. These sizes can be smaller or greater than the mean free molecular path of air molecules. For particles larger than the mean free path, the behavior of an aerosol in air is governed by the bulk drag forces exerted on the particles by air. Particles with zero initial velocity in still air will settle by the force of gravity, reaching a terminal settling velocity. Particles entering still air with non-zero initial velocity will be decelerated by the viscous forces of the surrounding air.

Particles with diameters smaller than the molecular mean free path are constantly bombarded by air molecules which transfer enough momentum to affect particle motion. This type of motion is called Brownian motion and it is described by a diffusion equation. The dynamics of air-particle interactions are next examined in more detail.

A. SEDIMENTATION

When a particle greater than approximately 1 μm in diameter is allowed to fall in still air, the magnitude of the force, F, exerted on the particle by aerodynamic drag is given by the Stokes' law:[1]

$$F = 3\pi\eta vd \tag{3}$$

where η is the viscosity of air, v is the particle velocity in the direction of fall, and d is the particle diameter. When the force of gravity (mg, where m is the particle mass and g is the acceleration due to gravity) and the drag force are equal, the particle has reached its terminal settling velocity given by:

$$v_t = \rho d^2/18\eta \tag{4}$$

where ρ is the particle density. Equation 4 is only valid for the following conditions:[1]

$$Re = \text{Particle Reynold's number} = \rho dv/\eta \ < 0.1 \tag{5}$$

$$Kn = \text{Knudsen number} = 2\lambda/d \ < 0.01 \tag{6}$$

where λ is the molecular mean free path.

B. PARTICLE STOPPING DISTANCE

Similar to Equation 4, the distance (x) that it takes to stop a particle, with an initial velocity, v, in still air is given by:

$$x = \rho d^2 v/18\eta \tag{7}$$

This equation is also valid only under the conditions given by Equations 5 and 6.

C. STOKES-CUNNINGHAM SLIP CORRECTION FACTOR

When the diameter of a particle is small, approaching the size of the mean free path of air molecules, Stokes' law, and consequently Equations 4 and 7, are no longer strictly valid because air can no longer be treated in a bulk manner. This problem has been overcome by the application of a correction factor to Stokes' law[1] known as the Stokes-Cunningham slip correction factor. The correction is based upon experiments conducted by Millikan and others. There have been several forms developed for this correction factor, but the one we use here is given by:

$$C = 1 + 2 \times 10^{-5}\left(0.82 + 0.264e^{-8.3d}\right)\!/d \tag{8}$$

where d is the particle diameter in microns. For particles satisfying the criterion of Equation 6, C is very nearly unity. For smaller particles, C > 1. The form of Stokes' law, taking slippage into account, then becomes:

$$F = 3\pi\eta vd/C \qquad (9)$$

and terminal settling velocity becomes:

$$v = \rho d^2 Cg/18\eta \qquad (10)$$

and the stopping distance becomes:

$$x = \rho d^2 Cv/18\eta \qquad (11)$$

D. AERODYNAMIC EQUIVALENT DIAMETER

The form of Equation 10 is suggestive of a way in which spherical particle diameters can be expressed that is independent of the density of the particle leading to a description of the inertial behavior of particles that does not depend upon particle density. From Equation 10 a particle of diameter d, density ρ, and slip correction factor C will settle with a velocity equal to that of another particle with diameter d_{ae}, slip correction factor C_0, and density ρ_0 equal to 1 g/cm^3 provided:

$$d_{ae} = \left(\rho/\rho_0\right)^{1/2}\left(C/C_0\right)^{1/2}d \qquad (12)$$

d_{ae} is referred to as the aerodynamic equivalent diameter. This is a more precise definition of d_{ae} than was given earlier. The value of $(C/C_0)^{1/2}$ is usually so close to unity that Equation 12 is most often expressed as:

$$d_{ae} = \left(\rho/\rho_0\right)^{1/2}d \qquad (13)$$

By expressing particle diameter as d_{ae}, comparisons of inertial behavior between particles of different densities are facilitated.

E. DIFFUSION

When the size of aerosol particles is on the order of the mean free path of air molecules, they can undergo a significant amount of random motion due to the bombardment and transfer of energy from air molecules. This motion is referred to as Brownian motion. The theory of Brownian diffusion was worked out many years ago by Einstein.[4] Because the motion is random, particles under this influence will tend, like gas molecules, to diffuse from regions of high particle concentration to regions of low particle concentration. A formulation of particle diffusion and deposition by diffusion is deferred for the present discussion.

IV. STRUCTURE AND FUNCTION OF THE HUMAN RESPIRATORY TRACT

The human respiratory tract is broadly composed of three distinct units. The upper respiratory tract extends from the lips or nares to the top of the trachea. The tracheobronchial or conducting airways extend from the top of the trachea through the terminal bronchioles. The alveolar or pulmonary region of the respiratory tract extends from the respiratory bronchioles to the distal alveolar sacs. The combination of the conducting airways and pulmonary region is often referred to as the lower respiratory tract. In simplistic terms the upper respiratory tract and tracheobronchial airways conduct inspired air by bulk flow to the alveoli where gas exchange occurs by diffusion. However, each region of the respiratory tract possesses many specialized functions that affect the deposition and fate of inhaled aerosols.

A. UPPER RESPIRATORY TRACT

The upper respiratory tract consists of the nose, mouth, nasopharynx, oropharynx, and larynx. These structures serve several functions such as air conditioning (raising the temperature and relative humidity of the inspired air), defense against airborne contaminants, olfaction, and phonation.[5] The upper respiratory tract has a volume of approximately 50 ml. The oral and nasal paths to the lower respiratory tract are extremely tortuous in nature. This is particularly true of the nasal path.

The entrance to the nasal passage has a cross-sectional area of approximately 500 mm^2 that then narrows rapidly to approximately 30 mm^2 on each side upon entry into the nasal turbinates.[5] This region of the nose is a complex passage composed of a flat side along the nasal septum and curved projections passing laterally. The width of this passage varies from a fraction of 1 to as much as 5 mm.[5] The posterior nasal turbinates open into the nasopharynx which is, at this point, a single airway with an average cross-sectional area of approximately 700 mm^2. The shape of the passage from this point depends in large part on the contraction of muscles such as the soft palate, tongue, pharynx, and larynx.

The epithelium of the nose consists in large part of ciliated columnar epithelial cells that contain mucus secreting glands. Only the vocal cords, epiglottis, oropharynx, olfactory areas, and the space between the nares and anterior turbinates lack ciliated epithelial cells.[5] The serous fluid and mucus lining this epithelium, along with the rich vascular bed of the nose, provide much of the humidification of inspired air.

The larynx is the final structure through which inspired air passes. During quiet breathing the glottis opens approximately 13 mm.[6] It has been speculated that upon exiting the glottis, air entering the trachea is in the form of a jet with relatively high linear velocities.[7] This phenomenon may enhance deposition of aerosols at the top of the trachea.

Taking into account the varying cross-sectional area of the upper airways the linear velocity of inspired air can vary dramatically. For a normal inspiratory flow of 500 ml/s, the average velocity through the upper airway is approximately 200 cm/s.

As can be seen, the structures of the upper airways have a complex geometry. As discussed later, this complexity has a marked effect on the amount of aerosol that can penetrate into the lower airways.

B. CONDUCTING AIRWAYS

The conducting, or tracheobronchial, airways form an essentially asymmetric dichotomously branching structure. The number of airway branches that are traversed between the trachea and an acinus (terminal gas exchange unit) can range between 8 and 32.[8] The conducting airways are composed of an outer layer of smooth muscle and cartilage. Moving inward from the smooth muscle toward the airway lumen the submucosa is encountered. The submucosa contains the bronchial vasculature, nerves, and the secretory portions of the mucous and serous secreting units. Further inward is the elastic lamina propria which also contains nervous and vascular networks as well as lymphocytes. Adjacent to the lamina propria is the basement membrane and the epithelium of the airway lumen.[9]

The bronchial ephithelium[10] consists of pseudostratified ciliated columnar cells and mucus secreting goblet cells. The latter comprise approximately 25% of the number of differentiated cells in the large conducting airways. The proportion of goblet cells decreases toward the distal bronchioles. In addition to the ciliated cells and goblet cells, the bronchial epithelium also contains basal cells, mucous and serous fluid glands, and scattered "brush" cells and mast cells.

At the level of the terminal and respiratory bronchioles (the airways most proximal to the alveolar spaces of the lung) goblet cells are almost entirely absent and there is a sparse distribution of ciliated cells. The goblet cells are replaced by Clara cells in which secretory granules have been identified. The actual role of Clara cells is not entirely determined, though it has been suggested that secretions from them may contribute to the surfactant layer. Finally,

8   *Respiratory Drug Delivery*

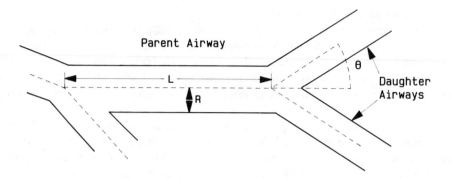

FIGURE 3. Schematic showing a symmetric dichotomous branching of a parent airway into two daughter airways. L is the length of the parent airway, and R is the radius. θ is the branching angle between parent and daughter airway. For symmetric branching, the branching angles of the daughter airways are equal.

there are "Kultschitzky-like" cells that cluster in neuroepithelial bodies throughout the conducting airways. These cells may be involved in coordination of ventilation and perfusion.

C. ALVEOLAR AIRSPACES

The terminal bronchioles lead into the respiratory bronchioles which have small outcroppings of alveoli. The respiratory bronchioles then lead into the alveolar ducts which are almost completely alveolated. Each alveolus has an epithelial lining consisting of granular pneumocytes and membranous pneumocytes. The granular pneumocytes are responsible for the secretion of surfactant phospholipids. The membranous pneumocytes are involved in gas exchange. The alveolar epithelial cells are connected by "tight" junctions that prevent fluid from the circulation leaking into the alveoli. The epithelium is like a sieve with a pore size of between 0.5 and 0.6 nm. In addition to these epithelial cells, there are also alveolar macrophages that orginate in the bone marrow and act as scavengers of inhaled particles as well as cellular debris.[10]

V. MORPHOMETIC DESCRIPTIONS OF THE RESPIRATORY TRACT

The previous discussion of the structure and function of the respiratory tract is important to understand the biological framework within which pharmaceutical aerosol deposition will be discussed. However, a physical framework within which to apply the principles of aerosol behavior that were previously discussed is needed. This need can be satisfied by resorting to a number of morphological models of the respiratory tract. Morphological models describe the geometric properties of the respiratory tract in a systematic fashion. Such modeling, however, has been restricted to the lower respiratory tract since the inherently irregular structure of the upper respiratory tract does not lend itself to systematic descriptions. Therefore, discussion in this section is devoted to models of the lower respiratory tract.

For the purpose of aerosol deposition considerations, the conducting airways are usually viewed as an array of rigid tubes with specific diameters, lengths, and branching angles. Figure 3 shows a generalized diagram of a set of dichotomously branching airways with the various parameters associated with such a set. A dichotomous branching pattern is one in which a "parent" airway bifurcates into exactly two "daughter" airways. When the physical properties of aerosol behavior are applied to a model of the respiratory tract, the geometric parameters of Figure 3 will play important roles.

Findeisen[11] first modeled the lower respiratory tract and divided it into ten symmetric compartments, of which the conducting airways comprised six. This picture of the airways has

TABLE 1
Airway Lengths and Diameters from the
Morphological Model of Weibel[12]

Generation	Length (cm)	Diameter (cm)
0	12.000	1.800
1	4.760	1.220
2	1.900	0.830
3	0.760	0.560
4	1.270	0.450
5	1.070	0.350
6	0.900	0.280
7	0.760	0.230
8	0.640	0.186
9	0.540	0.154
10	0.460	0.130
11	0.390	0.109
12	0.330	0.095
13	0.270	0.082
14	0.230	0.074
15	0.200	0.066
16	1.165	0.060
17	0.141	0.054
18	0.117	0.050
19	0.099	0.047
20	0.083	0.045
21	0.070	0.043
22	0.059	0.041
23	0.050	0.041

proved to be inadequate. Weibel[12] developed a more detailed anatomical model with his Model A. In this model the conducting airways are comprised of 16 generations of symmetric (i.e., daughters of a parent airway are identical to each other), dichotomously branching airways extending from the trachea (labeled as airway generation 0) through the terminal bronchioles (generation 15). The Weibel Model A also extends into the pulmonary region from generation 16 (the respiratory bronchioles) through the alveolar ducts and terminating at generation 23. The pulmonary region of this model lacks, however, a morphological description of the alveoli that bud off from the alveolar ducts. In the Weibel A model, neither individual branching angles nor angle of inclination of airways with respect to the horizontal are given. Table 1 gives the lengths and diameters associated with the Weibel A lung model.

The Weibel A anatomical lung model has proved over the years to be very useful in modeling airflow, gas diffusion, and aerosol deposition. One drawback of the Weibel lung model is its lack of asymmetry. Though relative to other animal species the human lung is remarkably symmetric, in reality there is a great degree of asymmetry associated with the human lung. This asymmetry can have an influence upon the distribution of both gases and particles within the lung. In addition to the influence of geometric asymmetry, the upright nature of humans can also affect the distribution of aerosol within the lungs. Due to the weight of the lungs, alveoli in the lower lobes of tidally ventilated lungs in upright humans tend to be more collapsed compared with alveoli in upper lobes. Consequently, during an inspiration alveoli in the lower lobes have a greater capacity to expand. Thus a greater proportion of the inspired air goes to lower lobes.

To overcome some of the disadvantages of the pure symmetry of the Weibel Model A, Horsfield and Cummings[8] and Yeh and Schum[13] have attempted to describe morphometry of the human lung in more realistic terms that take into account its inherent asymmetry. The drawback of these models is in their complexity and the difficulty with which they are adaptable to models

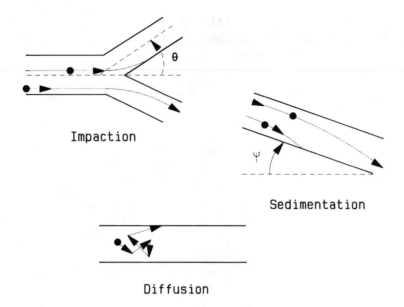

Impaction

Sedimentation

Diffusion

FIGURE 4.   Schematic illustrating the three primary mechanisms of deposition within the human respiratory tract. ψ is the angle of inclination of an airway with respect to the horizontal.

of aerosol deposition. Since the Weibel Model A has provided a good reference within which to describe deposition in the past,[14] deposition predictions will be considered primarily within the framework of this model. Since the Weibel model lacks a description of alveolar spaces, it is necessary to add this information based upon other measurements. Hansen and Ampaya[15] made extensive morphometric measurements of the human acinar region. For the purpose of this chapter, the Weibel lung model is augmented by the addition of a mophometric description of the human acinus based on the work of Hansen and Ampaya.

VI. AEROSOL DEPOSITION WITHIN THE LOWER RESPIRATORY TRACT

A. INERTIAL IMPACTION

When a particle is moving in a stream of air toward a bifurcation, such as in Figure 4, its inertia will tend to carry it toward the inside wall of one of the daughter branches. Countering this is the drag force exerted by the airstream as it bends at the bifurcation. The question is whether the particle will impact on the daughter airway or continue to the next bifurcation. To answer this question it is clear that Stokes' law will play a role. However, its application is complicated by three issues: (1) the position of the particle in the airstream of the parent branch, (2) the angle of bifurcation (θ), and (3) the fact that the velocity of the particle depends upon its position in the airstream. The problem is further complicated by the fact that an aerosol can be composed of as many as 1 million particles per cubic centimeter distributed across the whole cross-section of the parent airway. Landahl[16] perceived that the solution was best framed in a stochastic or probabilistic framework. Landahl's original work was framed in the context of the lung morphology described by Findeisen.[11] Gerrity et al.[17] later applied Landahl's approach to the Weibel[12] morphometry. This latter formulation provides the basis of the current discussion.

Landahl originally derived an equation expressing the probability of deposition of particles in an aerosol stream moving with velocity $v_{\alpha-1}$ in a parent airway, on the walls of a daughter airway, α. This probability is expressed as:

$$I_\alpha = \text{Stk}_{\alpha-1}\sin\left(\theta_\alpha\right)\big/\left(1+\text{Stk}_{\alpha-1}\sin\left(\theta_\alpha\right)\right) \qquad (14)$$

where $\text{Stk}_{\alpha-1}$ is the Stokes number of the parent airway and is given by:

$$\text{Stk}_{\alpha-1} = d_{ae}^2 v_{\alpha-1}\big/18\eta R_\alpha \qquad (15)$$

θ_α is the bifurcation angle between parent and daughter airways and R_α is the radius of the daughter airway. Since Weibel's lung model does not specify bifurcation angles, it is assumed that θ_α equals 30°. Landahl's impaction probability equation has some drawbacks to it. For one, its use for all airway generations assumes that the velocity profile of air has the same shape at all bifurcations within the lung. Indeed, this has been shown not to be the case.[18] At each bifurcation the flow profile is altered, thus presenting an aerosol with a different distribution of velocities at each airway bifurcation. Thus, the analytic expression of impaction probability would clearly have to differ at different airway generations. Since the work of Landahl, other investigators have derived different empirical equations for the impaction deposition probability. These equations were reviewed by Agnew et al.[19] Based upon experimental evidence, Agnew found little overall justification for the abandonment of Landahl's original equation in favor of the other equations. Thus, for the purpose of this review Landahl's original equation is used.

Equation 14 is written for the inspiratory phase. For the expiratory phase the same expression is used, but the Stokes' number is for the daughter airways with the velocity being the average air velocity in the daughter airway and the airway diameter being that of the parent airway. The assumption of an identical formulation for impaction probability upon expiration depends upon the velocity profiles being the same on expiration as upon inspiration. This is probably an incorrect assumption, but as is seen later this assumption is not likely to induce a significant amount of error in the overall prediction of deposition.

B. SEDIMENTATION

As particles traverse an airway, they also fall under the influence of gravity, as demonstrated in Figure 4. The question is whether a particle that enters an airway at one end will make it to the other before it strikes the airway wall. Again, the answer to this question will depend upon the viscous forces acting on the particle in the vertical direction; where the particle is located radially when it enters the airway; its longitudinal velocity, v, through the airway (which will depend upon its radial location); the diameter of the airway; and the angle of inclination of the airway with respect to the horizontal. Again, Landahl[16] derived an equation describing the probability of deposition by sedimentation in an airway labeled α given by

$$S_\alpha = 1 - e^{-0.8v_t t_\alpha \cos(\psi_\alpha)/R_\alpha} \qquad (16)$$

where v_t is the terminal settling velocity given by Equation 4, ψ_α is the angle of inclination of the airway with respect to the horizontal, t_α is the transit time of the particle across airway α, and R_α is the airway radius. As with bifurcation angle, the angles of inclination of airways in the Weibel model is not specified. Thus, it is assumed that all airways have randomly distributed inclination angles with an average of 45°.

As with impaction, the sedimentation equation is a stochastic equation with all of the drawbacks discussed for the impaction equation. However, as with the impaction equation it has worked well and we use it here.

During a breath pause t_α is replaced by the breath pause time t_p.

During expiration, the same deposition probability for sedimentation is assumed to hold. This is probably a better assumption than the one made for impaction probability upon expiration, since it will be somewhat less dependent upon the different velocity profiles that occur on inspiration and expiration.

C. DIFFUSION

Landahl also derived an equation for the probability of deposition in an airway by diffusion. This equation is given by:

$$D_\alpha 1 - e^{-4\times10^{-2}\sqrt{Ct_\alpha/d/R_\alpha}}$$ (17)

where t_α is the transit time of the particle across airway α (or the time of a breath pause), and C is the Stokes-Cunningham slip correction factor. The deposition probability by diffusional processes is assumed to be the same upon expiration.

Equation 17 was derived by Landahl assuming a uniform concentration distribution throughout the cross-section of an airway. Gormley and Kennedy[20] derived a diffusion probability equation under the assumption of laminar flow and nonuniform concentration distribution. Martin and Jacobi[21] compared experimentally these two formulations using physical models of the lung, and found that the Landahl equation predicts more accurately diffusional deposition than the Gormley and Kennedy formulation. This is probably due to the fact that pure laminar flow only occurs in straight tubes. In the human lung, airway bifurcations tend to disrupt flow, causing mixing of the aerosol, thus making the assumptions of Landahl closer to reality. Martin and Jacobi[21] also compared diffusional deposition between inspiration and expiration and found that they were virtually identical except at unphysiologically low flow rates.

D. OTHER MECHANISMS OF DEPOSITION

Besides impaction, sedimentation, and diffusion, there are other mechanisms by which particles can be removed from an inspired airstream. These include interception, electrostatic interactions with image charges in airway walls, and thermophoresis. Interception occurs when the physical dimension of a particle is sufficient to bring it in contact with a surface. Since the particles that are important for pulmonary deposition are significantly smaller than the dimensions of human airspaces, interception is not an important factor. (An exception to this would be for fiber aerosols that may be very large in the long dimension of the fiber, but small in the short dimension. Since this chapter is primarily concerned with deposition of spherical particles, this is not an issue). Likewise, electrostatic forces and thermophoretic processes, though they are present, contribute much less to pulmonary deposition than the three primary mechanisms of impaction, sedimentation, and diffusion. The discussions in this paper are, therefore, restricted to the three primary mechanisms.

E. JOINT DEPOSITION PROBABILITY

Since all three deposition mechanisms act simultaneously, a joint deposition probability equation must be derived from the three separate ones. For deposition in an airway α during inspiration or expiration, this is given by:

$$P_\alpha = I_\alpha + S_\alpha + D_\alpha - I_\alpha S_\alpha - I_\alpha D_\alpha - S_\alpha D_\alpha + I_\alpha S_\alpha D_\alpha$$ (18)

The cross terms take into account the fact that once particles deposited by one mechanism are removed from the stream they are no longer available for deposition by another mechanism. During a breath pause $I_\alpha = 0$ and Equation 18 is altered accordingly.

F. CALCULATION OF LOWER RESPIRATORY TRACT DEPOSITION

In this section the deposition probability equations from the above discussion are applied to the problem of deposition of an aerosol entering the lower respiratory tract. A discussion of deposition in the upper respiratory tract is reserved until later in the chapter.

To formulate expressions for the deposition fractions, the probability that upon inspiration a particle entering the trachea (generation 0) reaches generation α is derived. Given the joint probability for deposition on inspiration in any airway generation P_α^{ins} is given by Equation 16, the probability of penetration to α is given by:

$$f_\alpha = \prod_{\gamma=0}^{\alpha-1}\left(1 - P_\gamma^{ins}\right) \tag{19}$$

Not all air containing aerosol reaches down to generation α. Thus, the probability of penetrating to airway generation α must be weighted by the fraction of tidal volume (V_t) that passes generation α, given by:

$$F_\alpha = \sum_{\beta=\alpha}^{\delta} V_\beta / V_t \tag{20}$$

where V_β is the volume of generation β. The upper limit δ on the sum represents the most distal generation to which the tidal volume penetrates. This generation is determined under the assumption of a blunt flow profile and symmetric filling of the lung. Finally, the deposition fraction in generation α is obtained by multiplying Equations 19 and 20 and the probability of deposition in generation α together. Thus, the deposition fraction during inspiration in generation α is given by:

$$R_\alpha^{ins} = f_\alpha F_\alpha P_\alpha^{ins} \tag{21}$$

At the end of inspiration, there may be a breath pause. Particles that deposit in airway generation α during the breath pause will come from particles that have not deposited within that generation during inspiration, and they will be primarily under the influence of sedimentation and diffusion processes, but not impaction because the air is still. The deposition fraction during breath pause is therefore given by:

$$R_\alpha^p = f_\alpha\left(1 - P_\alpha^{ins}\right)P_\alpha^p V_\alpha / V_t = f_{\alpha+1} P_\alpha^p V_\alpha / V_t \tag{22}$$

Upon expiration, particles that have not deposited either during inspiration or during the breath pause will be available for deposition. The equation expressing this fraction is given by:

$$R_\alpha^{ex} = R_{\alpha+1}^p / P_{\alpha+1}^p (1 - P_{\alpha+1}^p)P_\alpha^{ex} + \sum_{\beta=\alpha+1}^{\delta} (R_\beta^p / P_\beta^p (1 - P_\beta^p)) \prod_{\gamma=\alpha+1}^{\beta-1} (1 - P_\gamma^{ex})P_\alpha^{ex} \tag{23}$$

The total fraction of particles entering the trachea that deposit in the lower respiratory tract is then given by:

$$R_T = \sum_{\alpha}^{\delta} \left(R_\alpha^{ins} + R_\alpha^p + R_\alpha^{ex}\right) \tag{24}$$

G. PREDICTIONS OF LOWER RESPIRATORY TRACT DEPOSITION

In this section the above equations for lower respiratory tract deposition are used to examine the dependence of inhaled particle deposition on particle size and breathing pattern and thereby come to some understanding of how particle deposition patterns can be manipulated.

First, the fractional deposition per airway generation for a monodisperse, unit density aerosol of 5 µm diameter, inhaled with V_t equal to 700 ml is examined. Inspiratory and expiratory flow are assumed to be equal at 500 ml/s. Figure 5 shows the fraction of particles entering the trachea that deposit in each generation. There are two peaks of deposition, one occurring at generation 4 (subsegmental bronchi) and one at generation 18 (proximal alveoli). The peak at generation 4 is due primarily to inertial impaction since linear velocities are still relatively high in these airways. Deposition falls off as the aerosol penetrates more distally because the impaction probability falls with declining linear velocity, and because the airway diameters are still

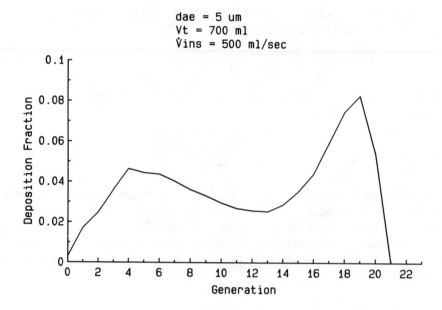

FIGURE 5.   Plot of the predicted fraction of particles entering the trachea that deposit in each airway generation for fixed particle size and breathing pattern.

sufficiently large to minimize deposition by sedimentation. As the aerosol moves deeper into the lung, the linear velocities decline further and the airway diameters continue to get smaller. As this occurs, the probability of deposition by sedimentation increases, thus accounting for the rise again in deposition fraction around generation 18. Deposition fraction falls off again because the aerosol concentration has been reduced by deposition in more central airways. Deposition by diffusion is virtually nonexistent for this particle size. It only becomes effective when particle size is approximately 0.5 μm or smaller.

Particle deposition within the lower respiratory tract is a function of particle size, inspiratory and expiratory flow, breath pause time, and tidal volume. The effects of these factors are now examined independently.

Figure 6 shows the deposition by airway generation of unit density particles from 1 to 10 μm inhaled (and exhaled) with a flow of 500 ml/s and a tidal volume of 700 ml. For particles smaller than approximately 5 μm inertial impaction is not very efficient in the large airways. Thus, particles deposit primarily by sedimentation in the periphery of the lung. As the particle size increases, impaction becomes more efficient. The fraction of particles depositing by impaction increases with increasing particle size. Despite the fact that larger particles deposit more efficiently by sedimentation, the contribution to the deposited fraction by sedimentation actually decreases with increasing particle size because fewer particles can penetrate deeply into the lung. Furthermore, as particle size increases the efficiency of deposition by sedimentation increases for larger and larger airways. Thus the peak of the distribution in the small airways shifts toward larger airways.

Figure 7 shows the distribution of particles for a unit density aerosol of 5 μm diameter inhaled with a tidal volume of 700 ml and with inspiratory (and expiratory) flows from 200 ml/s to 1000 ml/s. The greater the inspiratory flow the greater the particle inertia, and thus the greater the fraction of particles deposited in the large airways. At the same time, as flow increases, the residence time of particles in peripheral airspaces decreases, thus reducing the probability of deposition by sedimentation. Therefore, the effect of increasing flow is to drive up deposition in the large airways and significantly reduce deposition in the peripheral airways and alveoli.

Vt = 700 ml

V̇ins = 500 ml/sec

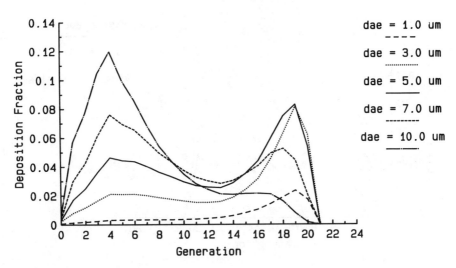

FIGURE 6. Plots of predicted fraction of particles entering the trachea that deposit in each airway generation for various particle sizes.

The shorter residence times that occur with increasing flow tend to push the peak in the small airways to smaller airways.

Figure 8 shows the distribution of particles for a unit density aerosol of 1 μm diameter inhaled with a tidal volume of 700 ml and with inspiratory and expiratory flow of 500 ml/s. Between inspiration and expiration there are varying breath pauses ranging from 0 to 10 s. The effect of these breath pauses is primarily to increase deposition in the peripheral airways. Though there is some sedimentation of particles in the large airways, the smaller diameters of the peripheral airways and alveoli favor greater deposition in them. Indeed, for breath pauses as long as 10 s, there is virutally no change in deposition as a function of breath pause time out to generation 8 because the sedimentation distances in the large airways are so large. Most of the large airway deposition in this figure is from impaction.

Finally, Figure 9 shows the effect of tidal volume on the distribution of particles in the lower respiratory tract. The aerosol is again composed of unit density particles with 5 μm diameter, inhaled and exhaled with a flow of 500 ml/s, but with tidal volume varied between 500 and 1500 ml. The effect of increasing tidal volume is to push the aerosol deeper into the lung where linear velocities are lower and airway diameters are smaller. These two factors enhance deposition by sedimentation and thereby increase the size of the small airway deposition peak and cause it to shift to a more peripheral location.

Up to this point the deposition efficiency of the lower respiratory tract has been examined. The upper respiratory tract, however, plays a major role in determining the amount of aerosol that enters the trachea, and in turn the amount of aerosol that can deposit on lower respiratory tract surfaces. The next section examines deposition efficiency in the upper respiratory tract.

VII. UPPER RESPIRATORY TRACT DEPOSITION

As was observed earlier, the structure of the upper respiratory tract has a complexity which is not amenable to morphologic modeling. Consequently, models of aerosol deposition

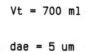

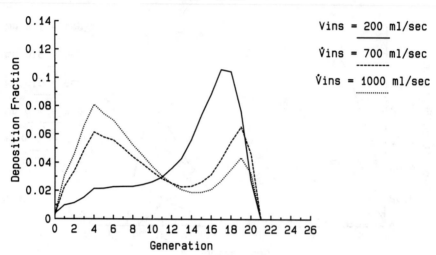

FIGURE 7. Plots of predicted fraction of particles entering the trachea that deposit in each airway generation for various inspiratory flow rates.

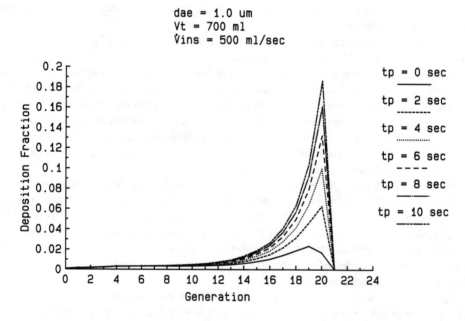

FIGURE 8. Plots of predicted fraction of particles entering the trachea that deposit in each airway generation for various breath pause times.

fashioned in a manner similar to those for the lower respiratory tract are not possible. Investigators have had to resort to empirical formulations derived directly from data on upper respiratory tract deposition. There are, however, some qualitative speculations that can be made before examining the data. The structure of the upper respiratory tract is such that spherical particle deposition should be dominated by its inertial properties. It seems reasonable to assume

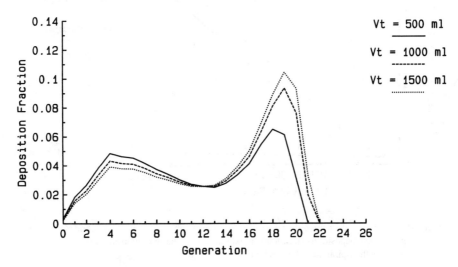

FIGURE 9. Plots of predicted fraction of particles entering the trachea that deposit in each airway generation for various tidal volumes.

that deposition probability should be some function of the Stokes' stopping distance given in Equation 11. With this in mind, deposition in the mouth and nose, and later deposition in the larynx, is examined.

A. DEPOSITION IN THE MOUTH AND NOSE

Yu and Soong[22] have done the most extensive empirical modeling of deposition in the nose and mouth. They collected virtually all the available data on nose and mouth during inspiration and expiration. Each of these sets of data was plotted against what Yu and Soong[22] call "impaction parameter" equal to $d_{ae}^2 V$, where V is either the average inspiratory flow (V_{ins}) or average expiratory flow (V_{ex}). When plotted in this manner, all of the data appear to collapse to a single function of impaction parameter. Since impaction parameter is proportional to the Stokes' stopping distance this is not at all surprising.

For deposition upon inspiration in the nose the best fit to the data was given by a "broken stick" log-linear regression against impaction parameter. The regression equations are given by:

$$R_{nose} = -0.014 + 0.0231 \log(d_{ae}^2 \dot{V}_{ins})(d_{ae}^2 \dot{V}_{ins} < 337 \text{ g}\mu\text{m}^2/\text{s}) \quad (25)$$

and

$$R_{nose} = -0.959 + 0.3971 \log(d_{ae}^2 \dot{V}_{ins})(d_{ae}^2 \dot{V}_{ins} > 337 \text{ g}\mu\text{m}^2/\text{s}) \quad (26)$$

For deposition in the nose upon expiration, the equations are given by:

$$R_{nose} = 0.033 + 0.0031 \log(d_{ae}^2 \dot{V}_{ex})(d_{ae}^2 \dot{V}_{ex} < 215 \text{ g}\mu\text{m}^2/\text{s}) \quad (27)$$

and

$$R_{nose} = -0.851 + 0.3991 \log(d_{ae}^2 \dot{V}_{ex})(d_{ae}^2 \dot{V}_{ex} > 215 \text{ g}\mu\text{m}^2/\text{s}) \quad (28)$$

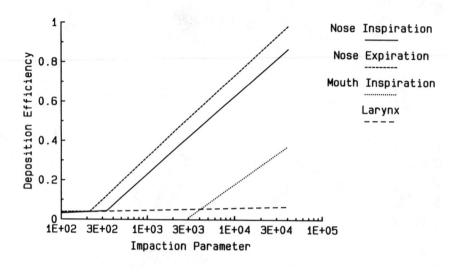

FIGURE 10.   Particle deposition efficiencies for the nose, mouth, and larynx as a function of impaction parameter (see text). Deposition in the mouth on expiration is 0. The deposition efficiency for the larynx is the same for both inspiration and expiration.

For deposition in the mouth on inspiration they give:

$$R_{mouth} = -1.117 + 0.3241 \log(d_{ae}^2 \dot{V}_{ins})(d_{ae}^2 \dot{V}_{ins} > 3000 \text{ g}\mu\text{m}^2/\text{s}) \tag{29}$$

For expiration and for $d_{ae}^2 V_{ins} < 3000$ gμm^2/s, mouth deposition is effectively 0.

Figure 10 shows these equations so that we can see the relative contributions from each of these. Clearly, the nose is a much more efficient impactor than the mouth. Furthermore, the deposition efficiency of the nose on expiration is higher than upon inspiration, which may be related to changes in nasopharyngeal configuration.

To give a better idea of the meaning of these equations, deposition efficiencies of the mouth and nose for fixed particle size as a function of flow and for fixed flow as a function of particle size are shown in Figure 11.

B. DEPOSITION IN THE LARYNX

Deposition in the larynx is probably the most difficult to accurately model. First, like the mouth and nose, its structure does not allow for the development of a model based upon physical principles. Second, unlike the mouth and nose, data on particle deposition in the larynx are virtually nonexistent because the larynx cannot be studied in isolation in the same manner as the nose and mouth. Martonen and Lowe[23] have attempted to overcome this problem by studying aerosol deposition in casts of human larynxes. The relationship they found that best fit their data is given by:

$$R_{larynx} = 0.035 + 3.9Stk \tag{30}$$

where Stk is the Stokes' number for the larynx assuming a laryngeal radius of 1.65 cm. This equation applies for both inspiration and expiration. However, since it was derived from a fixed cast, this equation does not take into account the different laryngeal configurations between inspiration and expiration. The contribution from the larynx to deposition is small compared to the mouth and nose, as is shown in Figures 10 and 11. However, since the surface area of the larynx is small, surface concentrations of deposited particles may be high.

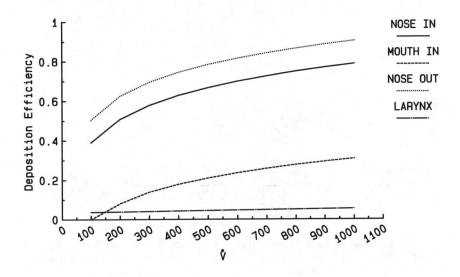

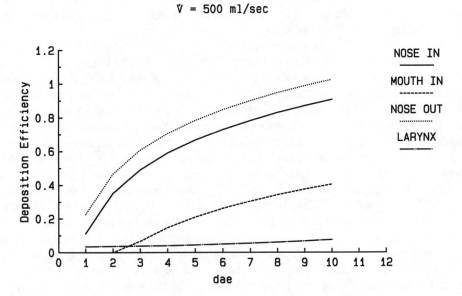

FIGURE 11. Particle deposition efficiencies for the nose, mouth, and larynx as a function of (A) flow for fixed particle diameter and (B) aerodynamic diameter for fixed flow.

VIII. DEPOSITION WITHIN THE ENTIRE RESPIRATORY TRACT AND COMPARISONS WITH DATA

Models of aerosol deposition in the respiratory tract are only as good as their ability to predict measured deposition. The problem in this respect is that measurements of deposition have been

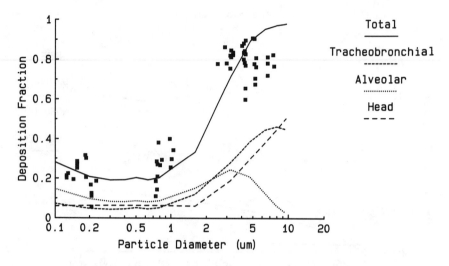

FIGURE 12.   Prediction of total deposition fraction in the respiratory tract as a function of particle diameter compared with the data of Chan and Lippmann.[35] Diameters above 0.5 μm are aerodynamic whereas those below are true physical diameters.

restricted to measurements of total respiratory tract deposition,[24-34] alveolar desposition,[35-37] and, as discussed previously, nasal and oral deposition.[25,28-29,38-44] Data reflecting deposition on an individual airway basis are nonexistent for humans. Thus, the accuracy of predictions of deposition within individual airways can only be inferred from the quality of agreement between models and data of the above three types.

Deposition of aerosols in the total respiratory tract (referred to as total deposition) has almost exclusively been measured using photometric techniques whereby the mass of an aerosol inhaled is compared with the mass exhaled. An example of total deposition in the human respiratory tract as a function of particle size is shown in Figure 12. The data were gathered by Chan and Lippmann[35] in subjects who inhaled the aerosols while mouth breathing with an average inspiratory flow of 766 ml/s and a tidal volume of 1000 ml. The prediction of deposition equations presented here for this breathing pattern is also shown with the various contributions from the head (mouth and larynx), tracheobronchial region (generations 0 through 16), and alveolar region (generations 17 and above). For particle sizes less than 1 μm, each region contributes a similar amount to total deposition. The minimum in deposition that occurs in the vicinity of 0.5 μm particles is due to the fact that at that particle size deposition by sedimentation and diffusion contribute equally with sedimentation decreasing with decreasing particle size and diffusion increasing. Between 1 and 4 μm, deposition in the tracheobronchial and alveolar zones dominate. Above 4 μm, with the domination of the mechanism of impaction, deposition in the head and tracheobronchial zone begins to dominate. Above 10 μm, it appears as though head deposition takes over almost entirely. The extent to which this is true, however, has not been definitely established. Figure 13 shows a comparison of predictions with the data of Stahlhofen et al.[36] These data respresent deposition of an insoluble aerosol inhaled by mouth with a tidal volume of 1000 ml and a variety of flows and particle sizes. Agreement between model predictions and data here are good at flows below 500 ml/s. At and above this flow rate, the model overestimates deposition. Other data, collected by other investigators, are also available and show similar behavior as has been shown here.[24-34] It is important to note, however, that the model equations do yield relatively good agreement with total deposition data except when flow rates become unphysiologically high.

When the equations for deposition probabilities were presented earlier, it was assumed that they were equally valid for inspiration and expiration. Although this is probably a reasonable

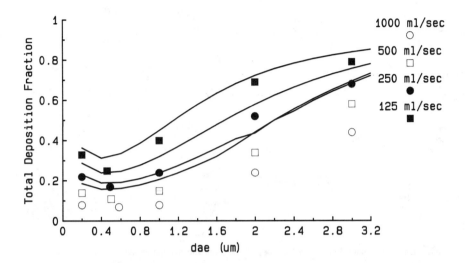

FIGURE 13.   Predictions of total deposition fraction in the respiratory tract as a function of aerodynamic diameter compared with the data of Stahlhofen et al.[36]

assumption for sedimentation, it is not likely to be the case for impaction. On expiration, the
bifurcation angle that is encountered is the same as on inspiration, but the velocity profiles are
likely to be quite different. This potential difference has been ignored, but the importance of this
assumption is now addressed. Figure 14 shows the predicted contributions to deposition as a
function of particle size for the head, tracheobronchial zone, and alveolar zone for inspiration
and expiration. As can be seen, expiration contributes on a level comparable to inspiration only
for small particles less than about 1 μm and this contribution comes from sedimentation. When
impaction is an important mechanism of deposition on inspiration, the amount that contributes
on expiration is small. Therefore, the weakness of the assumption of the same functional form
for deposition on expiration appears to have little impact on the overall predictions.

Deposition of particles within the alveolar zone of the human lung is measured in a derivative
fashion using radiolabeled aerosols. Immediately after an insoluble aerosol is inhaled, particles
deposited in the tracheobronchial zone begin cephalad movement by mucus transport.[45] Most
particles deposited in the tracheobronchial zone disappear from the lung in a matter of hours.
Particles deposited in alveoli, however, disappear from the lung at a much slower rate, taking
from days to months to completely disappear.[36-46] Investigators have taken advantage of this
dichotomy of clearance rates to measure alveolar deposition. By measuring the retention of
radioactivity 24 h after an aerosol is deposited, and comparing this with the amount of
radioactivity measured immediately following deposition, the fraction of particles initially
deposited in alveoli is determined. Figure 15 shows an example of alveolar deposition data
obtained by Lippmann and Chan[35] as a function of particle size. The model predictions have been
plotted along with the data by summing airway deposition fractions distal to generation 16. The
model equations underestimate measured alveolar deposition except for particles above 4 μm
in diameter. Figure 16 shows alveolar deposition data from Stahlhofen et al.[36] as a function of
particle size. In contrast to the alveolar deposition measurements of Chan and Lippmann,[35]
Stahlhofen et al.[36] measured alveolar deposition fraction by extrapolating the slow alveolar
clearance phase back to the time of deposition. In this figure, alveolar deposition is expressed
as a fraction of the total amount deposited in the lower respiratory tract, thus accounting for the

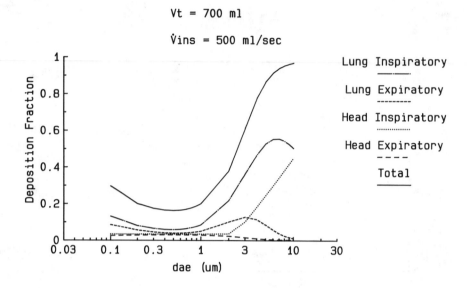

FIGURE 14.   The contributions to total deposition from the inspiratory and expiratory phases of breathing.

qualitative difference between these data and that of Chan and Lippmann.[35] As with the data of Chan and Lippmann,[35] the model equations predict a lower alveolar deposition fraction than the data indicate. The discrepancy between the predictions and the data of Stahlhofen et al.[36] may be due to a number of factors. First, of course, the model predictions could be wrong. Second, the definition of alveolar deposition could be wrong. With respect to the latter possibility, it may be that particles deposited in the tracheobronchial zone are not completely cleared by mucus transport in as short a time as has been traditionally thought. Thus, using retention measurements 24 h after deposition may include particles still present in the tracheobronchial zone. Indeed, the better agreement with the data of Chan and Lippmann[35] may be due to the fact that the extrapolation to the time of deposition, done by Stahlhofen et al.,[36] includes more of these particles than does using the retention measurement at 24 h. There is further indirect evidence that particles are retained for long periods of time in the tracheobronchial zone, but definitive evidence has yet to be established.

For the present, it will suffice to say that though the absolute accuracy of deposition models has yet to be established, they can be used with some confidence, especially if the intent is to use them to learn about the factors that control the sites of deposition. Since this is the main goal of this chapter, their validity is assumed.

IX. HYGROSCOPIC AEROSOL BEHAVIOR

Up until now deposition of stable nonhygroscopic aerosols has been the main focus. However, many pharmacologic agents that are delivered in aerosol form are water soluble and therefore hygroscopic. The hygroscopic nature of an aerosol means that it will interact with its environment, in particular the water content of the air. Depending upon the dewpoint of the surrounding air, an aerosol that is composed of a water droplet with some solute will either grow or shrink due to condensation and evaporation, respectively, of water. Since the environment of the respiratory tract tends to be warm and humid, a hygroscopic aerosol that is delivered to the mouth at relatively low temperature and humidity would be expected to increase in size as it transits the airways. Because of what is known of the dynamics of deposition of nonhygroscopic aerosols, an increase in aerosol size above the initial size at the entry into the mouth should affect

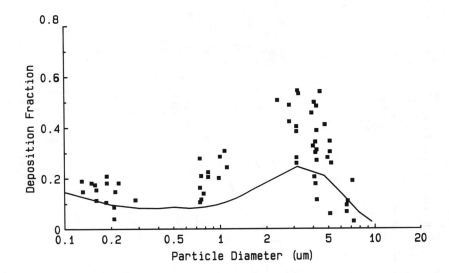

FIGURE 15.   Predicted alveolar deposition as a function of particle diameter compared with the data of Chan and Lippmann.[35] The alveolar deposition fraction is normalized to the amount of aerosol inhaled. Diameters above 0.5 μm are aerodynamic whereas those below are true physical diameters.

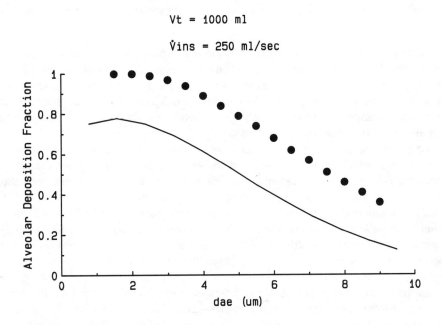

FIGURE 16.   Predicted alveolar deposition as a function of aerodynamic diameter compared with the data of Stahlhofen et al.[36] The alveolar deposition fraction is normalized to the total amount of aerosol deposited in the lower respiratory tract.

the amount and distribution of the aerosol within the respiratory tract. The key question that must be answered in order to quantitatively predict hygroscopic aerosol deposition is how much does an aerosol grow?

A detailed review of the physics involved in aerosol growth is beyond the scope of this chapter and the interested reader is invited to read Morrow.[46] In this section some of the main features of particle growth are examined as well as some of the experiments and models of particle growth that are most relevant to the present discussion.

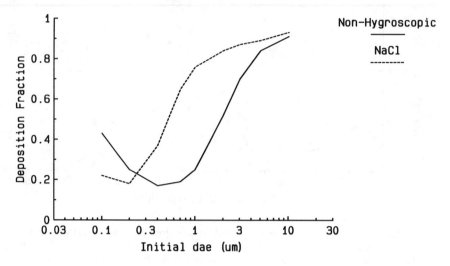

FIGURE 17.   Predicted total deposition fraction of a dry NaCl aerosol as a function of initial particle aerodynamic diameter compared with the prediction for a nonhygroscopic aerosol (curves adapted from Ferron et al.[61]).

To determine how much an aerosol grows in the respiratory tract is experimentally very difficult. The particle size of an aerosol can only be measured as it enters and as it leaves the respiratory tract. The final size of an aerosol upon expiration is not of much help since the aerosol may both grow during inspiration and then begin to shrink as it returns water to the respiratory tract upon expiration. Therefore, modeling of aqueous aerosol growth is very important to understanding aqueous aerosol deposition.

It is known that the growth (or shrinkage) of a hygroscopic aerosol depends upon several factors, chief of which are the osmolarity of the solute of the aerosol, the temperature of the surrounding air, and the water content of the surrounding air. There have been several attempts at modeling aerosol size behavior in controlled environments[47-50] that have been tested with controlled experiments.[51-57] A limiting factor in the development of good models of hygroscopic aerosol behavior in the human respiratory tract has been the limited knowledge of the precise temperature and humidity profiles within the respiratory tract. Morrow[46] has reviewed these experiments in detail. Briefly, though, it is generally believed that during mouth breathing the temperature of the inspired air (starting at about 22°C) increases to about 32°C by the time it reaches the trachea and rises to core body temperature of 37°C by the time it reaches the segmental bronchi. Upon expiration, the temperature at these locations is higher, being about 36°C at the trachea and falling to about 32°C at the mouth. If the air at the mouth at the start of inspiration has a relative humidity of about 50%, it rises to about 95% relative humidity at the trachea, and reaches near saturation by the mainstem bronchi. The term "near saturation" is used because it still has yet to be firmly established whether the humidity in the deep lung is saturated at 100% relative humidity, or is around 99.5%. During expiration, the relative humidity at these locations is also somewhat higher than on inspiration, being near saturation at the pharynx and about 85% at the mouth.[58]

Ferron et al.[59-61] has done extensive modeling of aerosol growth and deposition in the human respiratory tract. He has computed the growth and deposition of initially dry NaCl and histamine aerosols in the human respiratory tract. The predictions for NaCl deposition are shown in Figure

17 as a function of the aerodynamic diameter of the dry aerosol. Predictions for nonhygroscopic aerosols are shown for comparison. As can be seen, the hygroscopic aerosol deposition curve as a function of diameter is shifted to the left relative to the stable aerosol curve. Compared to a nonhygroscopic aerosol, there is not much predicted difference between NaCl and histamine deposition. The predictions of Ferron et al.[61] agree reasonably well with measurements of NaCl particle deposition made by Blanchard and Willeke.[62]

The primary effect of the growth of therapeutic aerosols is to enhance deposition since most of these aerosols have initial particle sizes greater than 0.3 μm. Ferron et al.[61] have predicted that for initial sizes between 0.7 and 10 μm, total deposition of hygroscopic aerosols increases by a factor of 2. As can be seen from Figure 17, this is not the case for nonhygroscopic aerosols. Over this size range, nonhygroscopic aerosol deposition increases by about a factor of 5. The question is, where is deposition most enhanced? This depends upon the initial dry particle size. For initial particle sizes less than approximately 0.3 μm, deposition actually decreases. For initial particle sizes between 0.3 and 1.0 μm, pulmonary deposition is enhanced due to increased sedimentation as the particle grows. For initial particle size greater than about 1.0 μm, tracheobronchial deposition is enhanced since now particles are growing into a size where impaction is important.

It is important to note that though hygroscopic particles grow, and thus alter deposition from that of nonhygroscopic particles, virtually all dynamic considerations remain valid. The only difference is that the particle size domains over which the various deposition mechanisms are important change with the growth behavior of the aerosol of interest. Much more work needs to be done on hygroscopic aerosol behavior in the human respiratory tract before a complete picture can be formed.

X. SURFACE CONCENTRATION OF DEPOSITED PARTICLES

A question of importance in considering therapeutic aerosol delivery is that of the appropriate way to express delivered dose of particles. Should dose be expressed as the mass of drug per unit tissue surface area, mass of drug per unit tissue mass, or some other measure? If the appropriate expression is the mass of drug per unit tissue surface area, the surface area of tissue within the lung can work against the efficient delivery of a therapeutic dose.

Figure 18 shows lung surface area as a function of airway generation for the Weibel lung. As can be seen the lung surface area increases by nearly four orders of magnitude between the trachea and the most peripheral alveoli, with a surface area minimum occurring at generation 4. If calculated deposition fractions are divided by surface area it can be seen that surface area drives the distribution of dose when expressed on a unit surface area basis. Figure 19 shows the deposited fraction per unit surface area for 1, 5, and 10 μm aerosols inhaled by mouth with a tidal volume of 700 ml and average inspiratory flow of 500 ml/s. If a therapeutic aerosol is targeted to the small airways beyond, say, generation 10, it can be seen that the greatest surface concentrations occur in much larger airways almost regardless of the size particle that is used. Decreasing particle size still results in high concentrations in the large airways. If the large airways are the target, then the news is good, as it is easy to achieve high concentrations while minimizing the concentrations in other regions of the lung.

Although for many applications it may not matter that drug dose is high in areas that are not targeted, this could be an important issue for some drugs. For example, suppose it is desired to deliver a drug to the small airways. If at effective therapeutic concentrations the drug has irritant properties that can stimulate cough, the receptors of which are located in the large airways, effective use of the drug in inhaled form may be prevented.

The initial surface concentration of drug particles is only one consideration of many that are discussed herein that needs to be examined when evaluating aerosolized pharmaceutical agents.

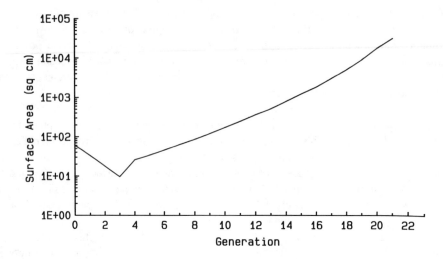

FIGURE 18.   Airway surface area for each airway generation of the Weibel A lung model.[12]

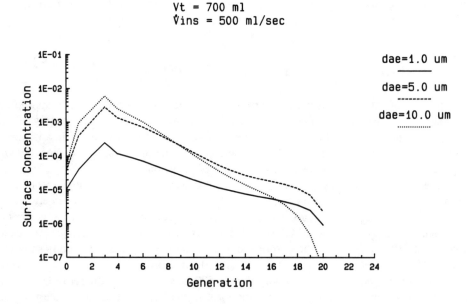

FIGURE 19.   Predicted airway surface concentrations of inhaled particles for various particle sizes. The surface concentration is expressed as a fraction per unit square centimeter of surface, where the fraction is normalized to the number of particles inhaled.

XI. PATHOLOGICAL CONSTRAINTS ON AEROSOL DEPOSITION

Until now deposition within the normal respiratory tract has been the focus of this chapter. However, in most instances where a therapeutic aerosol is indicated, the respiratory tract is far from normal. Diseases of the lung that affect the flow of air within the lung are likely to affect the pattern of deposition of inhaled aerosols. Thus, the diseases that are desirable to treat with aerosols may affect the delivery of therapeutic agent by aerosol. In this section the manner by which lung pathologies may affect aerosol deposition is considered.

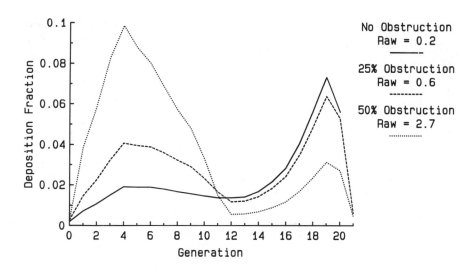

FIGURE 20. Predicted airway deposition fractions for various degrees of central obstruction. The predicted airways resistances are in units of cm-H$_2$O/l/s.

There are two pathologic conditions that primarily affect aerosol deposition: obstructive defects and defects in lung compliance. Furthermore, these defects could be focal in nature, i.e., isolated within particular regions of the lung, or diffuse, i.e., spread throughout large regions of the lung. Examples of obstructive defects include chronic bronchitis, asthma, and cystic fibrosis. Examples of lung diseases involving compliance defects include emphysema, pulmonary fibrosis, and bronchiectasis. Frequently, obstructive defects and compliance defects occur simultaneously. Irreversible chronic obstructive lung disease, secondary to cigarette smoking, is usually a mixture of chronic bronchitis and emphysema. The potential effects of lung pathology on aerosol deposition inferable from considerations of aerosol dynamics are examined first. Experimental evidence supporting these observations is then presented.

The effect of diffuse obstruction on deposition, insofar as flow is altered thereby affecting deposition by impaction and sedimentation, is examined first. Figure 20 shows the predicted patterns of deposition per airway generation for a 3-μm unit density aerosol when airway generations 0 through 11 (trachea down to the 4 mm diameter airways) are narrowed by 25 and 50%. Using the Weibel A lung model the airways resistance (R_{aw}) of the normal lung and the obstructed lung assuming Poiseuelle flow for each case has been calculated. The calculated unobstructed airways resistance is low compared to what is measured in normal humans (approximately 0.5 to 2 cm-H$_2$0/l/s), however, this calculation does not include the head which may contribute significantly to R_{aw} in normal humans. There is a marked shift of aerosol deposition from the lung periphery to the central airways. Between the normal lung and the 50% obstructed lung there is a predicted 10-fold increase in particle deposition.

The effect of peripheral obstruction (i.e., obstruction of airways beyond generation 11) induced by the same percentage decreases in lung airway diameters is shown in Figure 21. Less of an effect on both R_{aw} and deposition is predicted compared with central obstruction. The apparent increase in deposition by sedimentation in the airways around generation 11 may or may not represent what actually occurs in the peripheral obstructed human lung.

Obstruction of airways usually is not uniform throughout the lung. One airway may be more obstructed than its anatomical equivalent elsewhere in the lung. The focal nature of obstruction can have two effects: (1) it can alter the bulk flow properties of air in the lung and (2) it can alter the mechanical time constants of different lung regions, thus affecting aerosol mixing between tidal air and reserve air (the air within the lung prior to a tidal inspiration). The effect of focal

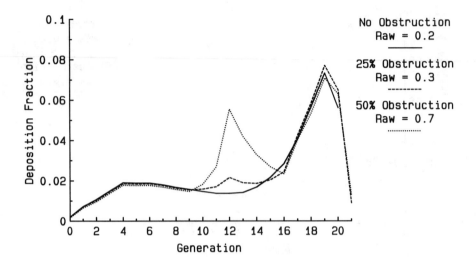

FIGURE 21.   Predicted airway deposition fractions for various degrees of peripheral obstruction. The predicted airways resistances are in units of cm-H$_2$O/l/s.

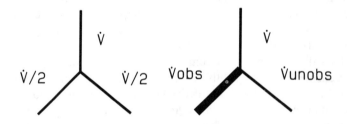

FIGURE 22.   Diagram illustrating the focal obstruction of an otherwise symmetric branching of airways. All other things being equal, flow divides equally between the two unobstructed daughter branches shown on the left.

obstruction on bulk flow properties is examined first. Suppose, in a healthy lung, there is a symmetric branching of a parent airway into two identical daughter airways, as shown in Figure 22. Furthermore, for simplicity, assume that flow divides equally down the two daughter branches. Now suppose that one of the daughters is obstructed by the reduction of airway diameter by a fraction f. Figure 23 shows the effect of obstruction in one of the daughters on the ratio of flow between the obstructed and unobstructed daughter flow as a function of f. The more obstructed the one daughter, the greater the flow in the unobstructed daughter and the lower the flow in the obstructed daughter. Figure 24 shows how this type of obstruction affects the transit time of air across each of the daughters. As the obstruction increases the transit time across the obstructed daughter increases dramatically, with little effect on transit time across the unobstructed daughter.

If this type of obstruction occurs in large airways where impaction dominates, the effect is to increase the amount of aerosol deposited away from the site of obstruction due to the greater velocities through the unobstructed daughter and from the greater volumetric flow of aerosol through the unobstructed path. This phenomenon has been experimentally observed.[63] If the obstruction were to represent the site of a lesion to be treated, clearly this situation would prevent effective delivery of a drug to the site. If this type of obstruction were to occur in more peripheral regions of the lung where sedimentation dominates, the longer transit times across the obstructed

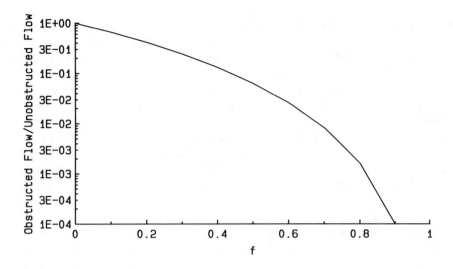

FIGURE 23. Predicted ratio of flow in the obstructed branch to the flow in unobstructed branch as a function of the fraction of obstruction. f = 0 corresponds to unobstructed flow and f = 1 corresponds to total obstruction.

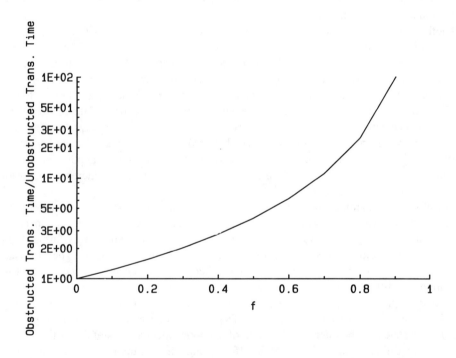

FIGURE 24. Predicted ratio of particle transit time across the obstructed branch to the transit time across the unobstructed branch as a function of the fraction of obstruction. f = 0 corresponds to unobstructed flow and f = 1 corresponds to total obstruction.

path would help facilitate deposition in this region. However, the greater bulk flow through the unobstructed airway would still be working against delivery of aerosol to the affected airway.

Compliance defects alter bulk flow patterns as do obstructive defects. Defects in lung compliance usually result in lungs that are stiff or noncompliant. A region of the lung that encompasses alveoli that have lost compliance has different pressure-volume characteristics than a normal region. It may, depending on the pressure-volume curve, result in greater or lesser flow rates into the diseased region of the lung. Thus, depending on the detailed pressure-volume characteristic associated with a compliance defect, aerosol may preferentially deposit in the vicinity of the defect, or away from the defect.

Besides the effects obstructive and compliance defects have on flow velocities and transit times across airways, these defects can have another effect on aerosol deposition. If any region of the lung is considered as an isolated mechanical system, it has an equivalent compliance and an equivalent resistance to air flow. In qualitative terms, the product of resistance and compliance provides a characteristic time constant for the filling and emptying of that region. In the normal lung, all anatomically equivalent regions of the lung have very similar time constants, thus to a first approximation these regions fill and empty in relative synchrony during a normal breathing cycle. In diseased lungs the combination of resistance and compliance defects in various lung regions can lead to mismatched time constants. The consequence of this mismatching of time constants is that during a breathing cycle, some regions may be emptying while others are still filling. Thus, particles of an aerosol that started out in one portion of a tidal breath may end up, if they have not deposited during inspiration, being shuttled into another region of the lung during expiration, where they may have further opportunity to deposit. This phenomenon of air flowing from one lung region into another parallel region has sometimes been referred to as "pendeluft". The implications of this phenomenon for aerosol therapy are not clear, but some investigators, as shall be seen momentarily, attribute some alterations in aerosol deposition in diseased lungs to this phenomenon.

Another phenomenon which could affect the deposition of particles within the lung is the presence of highly localized constrictions. The types of obstructions considered earlier were uniform in the sense that the diameters of airways were narrowed along their entire length. However, a more highly localized airway constriction could occur, for example, in the vicinity of a tumor or in a region of excess mucus secretions. Air flowing through such constrictions can develop turbulent eddies downstream of them and thereby cause enhanced deposition. Kim et al.[64] investigated the effect of this type of constriction in glass models of airways. From empirical equations derived from these experiments, Kim has predicted that a constriction in a generation 3 airway, sufficient to increase airway resistance by 119%, would increase deposition of a 3-μm aerosol by 54%, assuming a tracheal flow of 500 ml/s, with most of the increased deposition occurring downstream of the constriction.

Kim et al.[64] also examined the effect of two-phase flow on deposition in airway models. Two-phase flow occurs when air flowing over a liquid surface causes the liquid to move. Kim and co-workers[64] hypothesized that two-phase flow interactions between air and airway surface liquid, such as mucus, could cause surface irregularities that enhance deposition. They measured aerosol deposition in dry glass tubes and tubes lined with human mucus. They found that deposition of a 3-μm aerosol in the mucus-lined tubes increased by 85%.

All of these phenomena are likely to play a role to some extent in altering patterns of aerosol deposition within the human respiratory tract. Deposition experiments in humans with various lung disease states can be interpreted in light of the above mechanisms of deposition.

Several investigators have examined the effect of lung disease upon aerosol deposition and the distribution of inhaled aerosols within the lung. Love and Muir[65] studied total deposition in a population of 58 coal miners. Of this population, 42 were cigarette smokers. The majority of subjects had chronic cough. These investigators found that there was a correlation between lung function in these subjects and the total deposition fraction of a 1-μm nonhygroscopic aerosol that was tidally breathed. They found the strongest correlation between deposition and forced expiratory flow betwen 50 and 75% of vital capacity (MEF50-75%). The lower the expiratory flow, the greater the deposition. Low MEF50-75% is considered to be a reflection of small airway obstruction. Their observation has two possible explanations. One is that increased flow turbulence in the large airways in obstructed subjects enhanced deposition distal to these airways. The other is that focal obstructions in the small airways altered the patterns of mixing of tidal air with reserve air, thereby increasing the retention and thus deposition of particles from reserve air. Simple enhancement of deposition by impaction in the large airways is unlikely since the small particle size combined with the mild disease in these subjects would obviate against these mechanisms. Since these investigators were only able to measure total deposition fractions, precise assessment of the possible mechanism was not possible.

Lourenco et al.[66] studied the deposition and clearance of a 2-μm radiolabeled aerosol in 14 patients with bronchiectasis, a disease noted for marked retention of secretions in the lung. They studied these subjects with a gamma camera that allowed two-dimensional visualization of the distribution of the inhaled radiolabeled particles. Of the 14 subjects, 6 had relatively normal, diffuse deposition patterns when compared with normal subjects. The remaining 8 subjects demonstrated more central patterns of aerosol deposition, i.e., greater amounts of aerosol deposited in large airways. At 24 h following inhalation, those subjects with diffuse patterns of deposition retained 44.7% of the deposited particles, whereas those with central deposition patterns retained only 13%. The severity of obstruction in these patients appeared to correspond with the degree to which particles were deposited centrally. Of greatest interest here is the fact that those patients who had the greatest sputum production also had the most central patterns of deposition. Despite the presence of obstructed airways, possibly due to mucus hypersecretion, bronchiectatic patients also have significant loss of lung tissue due to tissue damage in small airways. Mucus hypersecretion combined with tissue losses may account for the fact that in this study aerosol deposited primarily in regions contralateral to the bronchiectatic lesions.

Asthma is characterized by reversible smooth muscle contraction, mucus hypersecretion, and in severe cases mucus plugging of small airways. In mild asthma, the disease is probably diffuse with a moderate effect upon deposition of inhaled aerosols. Agnew et al.[67] studied the deposition of a 5-μm aerosol in patients with mild asthma compared with normal volunteers. They found that the ability of the aerosol to penetrate to small airways was related to the degree to which mid-maximal expiratory flow rates (MMFR) were impaired (i.e., the smaller the MMFR the less the aerosol penetrated). Since only large airway deposition by impaction is capable of reducing penetration of an aerosol, it is surprising that they would find this relationship since MMFR is obstensibly a measure of small airways function. However, the decline in aerosol penetration may also have been caused by the development of asynchronous ventilation due to airway closure in the base of the lung at the beginning of inspiration.[67]

Weiss et al.[68] studied the distribution of a highly heterodisperse radioaerosol in more seriously obstructed patients with chronic obstructive lung disease. Using a gamma camera they found, qualitatively, that the two-dimensional images showed more areas of localized concentrations of aerosol than would be found in normal subjects. They also found quantitatively that the variance of activity among different lung regions was much greater in the diseased population compared with a normal population. Linn and Goodwin[69] found that in bronchitic patients the retention of particles 24 h after inhalation (a measure of penetration into the alveoli) was directly related to the ratio of forced expired volume in 1 s (FEV1) to forced vital capacity (FVC) and to MMFR. This observation is probably related more to the large airway obstruction reflected in FEV1/FVC ratio. Garrard et al.,[70] when studying the initial distribution of particles as analyzed from a gamma camera scintigram, found that MMFR was predictive of aerosol distribution even in a population of healthy volunteers. This indicates that even very mild airway obstruction that might occur within an otherwise healthy population, can affect aerosol penetration.

There have been virtually no experimental studies that relate specific changes in airway or lung function with changes in either total deposition or regional deposition of aerosols. This is not surprising though, since most tests of lung function are incapable of clearly defining the region of the lung responsible for any change. One exception to this has been the work of Svartengren et al.[71] They challenged the airways of normal volunteers with methacholine to induce bronchoconstriction. The amount of methacholine administered was sufficient to reduce peak expiratory flow by 20%. They measured the retention of 4 µm radiolabeled teflon particles inhaled either before or after bronchial challenge. They then plotted 24 h percent retention against airways resistance. As would be expected from theoretical considerations, the retention at 24 h was lower in subjects when methacholine was administered before teflon particle inhalation. When Svartengren et al.[71] performed theoretical deposition calculations with the Weibel A lung model, they found that constriction of all airway diameters by 60% produced 24 h percent retention values and airways resistance values consistent with their experimental data. This would suggest, though far from proven, that methacholine induced bronchoconstriction occurs throughout the conducting airways composed of smooth muscle.

The fact that relationships between specific mechanical changes in lung function and classical measurements of lung function, such as forced expiratory maneuvers and body plethysmography, do not exist has in part limited the interpretation of changes in aerosol deposition in diseased states. However, because the behavior of inhaled particles differs from that of gases, there have been attempts to use aerosols directly as measurements of lung function. Various investigators[72-78] have used the sedimentation properties of inhaled aerosols as a method of sizing airways. As was seen in Figure 8, when a 1-µm aerosol is inhaled, a breath pause is predicted to increase deposition in the distal conducting airways and alveoli. As the breath pause time is increased, only the deposition in distal airways and alveoli is predicted to increase. By varying the depth of the aerosol (i.e., the tidal volume) different distal airspace dimensions can be explored. By examining the recovered fraction of aerosol on expiration, model-dependent estimates of distal small airway and alveolar caliber can be made. Rosenthal[79] developed a more detailed model of sedimentation than given in this chapter with the specific goal of estimating airspace dimensions from breath pause data. Using his model in conjunction with aerosol recovery data of Palmes et al.,[73] he calculated diameters of respiratory bronchioles, alveolar ducts, and alveoli in six human subjects. The calculated values for these diameters agreed well with the diameters measured by Weibel.[12]

Another area of promise for the use of aerosols as a measure of lung function is that of bolus dispersion.[80-83] In studies such as these, an aerosol bolus, of finite volume ranging between 50 to 250 ml, is inhaled in different parts of a tidal volume. The aerosol size is between 0.5 and 1.0 µm. By examining the shape of the concentration profile of the exhaled bolus, compared to the shape upon inhalation, inferences about the convective mixing behavior of the distal lung can be made. These studies exploit the fact that aerosols in this size range behave as a diffusionless gas.

XII. EFFECT OF LUNG CLEARANCE OF INHALED PARTICLES ON DOSE

Although this topic is discussed in more detail in a later chapter, it is worthwhile to consider the effect of lung clearance of particles on delivered dose in the current context. As has already been mentioned, when insoluble particles deposit on bronchial epithelium, they are swept away toward the larynx by mucociliary transport. Mucociliary transport can clear almost all particles deposited on bronchial epithelium within a matter of several hours. Though this picture may not be completely correct, as was discussed earlier, for the present discussion it will suffice. Particles that deposit beyond the conducting bronchial airways, in alveoli, clear by much slower mechanisms, taking from days to weeks to even months to complete the process. Since pharmaceutical agents are in general short acting, mucociliary clearance mechanisms will be focused upon since they are most likely to affect drug delivery to tissue.

When a therapeutic agent is delivered in aerosol form to the lung, it must dissolve and release its constituents. The constituents must then reach the target lesion. There are two factors related to mucociliary transport that can obviate against this process: (1) the particles may be swept away from the site of the lesion by the time the particles sufficiently dissolve and (2) the mucus and periciliary fluid lining the conducting airways serve as barriers across which the drug, once dissolved, must diffuse to reach a target lesion (unless, of course, the drug is meant to directly affect the mucus, as would be the case with mucolytics).

Mucociliary clearance of inhaled particles has been studied by many investigators in both health and disease. It is well known that the rate of mucociliary clearance of particles depends both on the efficiency of transport of mucus within individual airways of the lung and upon the pattern of aerosol deposition within the lung. If the mucociliary clearance process is pictured as a conveyor belt, it can be seen that particles that land on bronchial epithelium have two distinct opportunities to deliver their consitituents. First, at the site of deposition, and secondly, at sites farther up in the airways that the particles pass during the process of transport out of the lung.

To help gain insight into the effect of mucociliary clearance on the delivery of dose, a kinetic model of mucociliary clearance developed by Lee et al.[84] is used. This model utilizes the initial deposition fractions of particles in airway generations of the Weibel A lung model, calculated using equations such as those presented in this chapter. The clearance model also depends on the transport rate of mucus in each airway generation. In humans, mucus transport rates have only been measured in trachea[85] and mainstem bronchi.[86] To overcome this deficit, the model assumes that transport rates scale in inverse proportion to total circumference of an airway generation. Thus, using 5 mm/min as the transport rate of mucus in the trachea,[84] the transport rates in distal airways can be estimated. Figure 25 shows the calculated clearance curve using this model for an insoluble 3 μm aerosol inhaled with a tidal volume of 700 ml and average inspiratory flow of 500 ml/s. The clearance curve is normalized to 1 at a time of deposition. In Figure 26 the relative amount of particles in each airway generation as a function of time is shown. This figure shows the relative number of particles that would be available to an airway as a function of time provided that the particles did not dissolve. Reductions of 50% in peak retention can occur at times ranging from about 30 min in the trachea to about 8 h in the distal conducting airways. Obviously, a dissolution component needs to be added to this model so that relative mass release in each generation as a function of time can be computed as well. What is clear from this demonstration, though, is that if a drug in particulate form does not release its constituents relatively rapidly, then the therapeutic benefit may be lost. Furthermore, it shows that there may be some potential for the use of transport mechanisms to deliver a drug deposited initially more deeply.

XIII. SUMMARY

The effectiveness of an inhaled therapeutic aerosol depends, in part, upon distribution of the deposited particles within the respiratory tract. The distribution depends upon the physical characteristics of the particles comprising the aerosol, and upon the pattern with which it is inhaled. Over the past decades there has been a considerable amount of experimental research done on the distribution of inhaled nonhygroscopic aerosols in the healthy human respiratory tract. Within the constraints of research conducted in humans, models of aerosol deposition and distribution within the respiratory tract have been largely successful in predicting the behavior of inhaled aerosols, especially when the questions are confined to total respiratory tract deposition. Uncertainties still exist with respect to precise regional behavior of inhaled aerosols within the respiratory tract. For small particles (<2 μm) and high inspiratory flow rates, there appears to be a lack of general agreement between model predictions and experimental data with respect to deposition within the alveolar and tracheobronchial regions of the respiratory tract. Though this may be a failing of the models, the measurement techniques themselves may be in error since measurement of alveolar deposition fractions depends upon a simplistic definition of the slow phase of particle clearance, i.e., the slow phase of clearance arises entirely from particles deposited in alveolar spaces. Improved investigational techniques that can better define

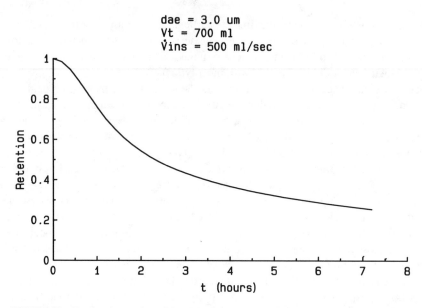

FIGURE 25.   Predicted retention of insoluble particles in the tracheobronchial airways as a function of time after deposition. Prediction based on the model of Lee et al.[84]

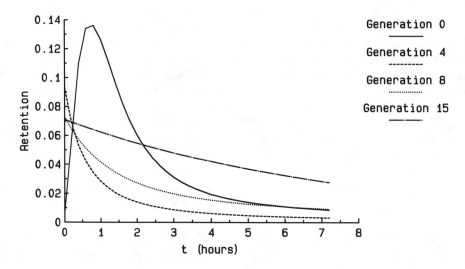

FIGURE 26.   Predicted retention of insoluble particles in various airways in the tracheobronchial zone as a function of time after deposition. Prediction based on the model of Lee et al.[84]

alveolar vs. tracheobronchial deposition are needed before more progress in the use of predictive deposition models can be made.

The knowledge of respiratory tract deposition of hygroscopic aerosols is less well known than that of nonhygroscopic aerosols. This has been primarily due to the fact that hygroscopic aerosols grow and shrink as they pass through environments with varying temperature and humidity profiles, such as the human respiratory tract. As aqueous aerosol particles traverse the respiratory tract, their sizes change continuously, thus imposing continuous changes upon deposition efficiency. Predicting these changes is highly dependent upon detailed information on the temperature and humidity profiles within the respiratory tract. This information has been difficult to obtain experimentally and is still subject to considerable uncertainty. The only validating data in humans on hygroscopic aerosol deposition are measurements of total respiratory tract deposition, leaving problems of regional deposition open to question.

The patterns of respiratory tract deposition seem to favor high particle surface concentrations in the large tracheobronchial airways. This phenomenon is largely due to the relatively low surface area contained in these airways. Consequently, if particle surface concentration is an important dosimetric measure for therapeutic effect, the ability to achieve adequate dosing of smaller airways may be confounded by the presence of significantly higher doses to the large airways. This latter issue could potentially pose problems with a therapeutic aerosol if application to the conducting airways is undesirable.

Much of the data on the dependence of aerosol deposition on lung pathology is more qualitative than quantitative. Examples include observations of "hot spots" on two-dimensional scintigrams of the lung that are attributable to regional obstructions, and more "central" deposition patterns, i.e., a greater amount of aerosol deposited in the tracheobronchial airways compared to the alveoli. The use of mathematical and physical models of aerosol deposition have been useful in identifying more clearly the potential impact of lung pathology on aerosol deposition. Diffuse obstruction and compliance loss appears to be responsible for the centralization of aerosol deposition, whereas more focal obstructive and compliance defects appear to be responsible for so-called "hot spots". However, the effect of focal defects may be to divert aerosol away from the sites of the defects, thus impairing the ability of therapeutic aerosols to reach their desired target.

Finally, the delivery of therapeutic dose may depend upon the translocation rate of the aerosol particles after they have deposited. Mucociliary clearance, and to a lesser extent alveolar clearance, may cause particles to move from their initial deposition sites before they release their constituent material for uptake by surrounding tissue. Thus, when considering the effectiveness of an inhaled therapeutic agent, the dissolution rate of the agent in particulate form must be sufficiently rapid to release its contents before being cleared from the lung. A corollary to this is that though aerosol particles may deposit initially at sites peripheral to the targeted lesion, they may still be effective if the release of their contents occurs in larger airways as a result of mucociliary transport.

REFERENCES

1. **Hidy, G. M.,** *Aerosols: An Industrial and Environmental Science,* Academic Press, Orlando, FL, 1984.
2. **Fuchs, S. K.,** *The Mechanics of Aerosols,* Macmillan, New York, 1964.
3. **Hatch, T. F. and Choate, S. J. J.,** *Franklin Inst.,* 207, 369, 1933.
4. **Einstein, A.,** *Investigations on the Theory of Brownian Motion,* Dover, New York, republished 1955.
5. **Proctor, D. F.,** Physiology of the upper airway, in *Handbook of Physiology,* Vol. 3, Sect. 1, Fenn, W. O. and Rahn, H., Eds., American Physiological Society, Washington, D.C., 1964, 309.
6. **Negus, V. E.,** Certain anatomical and physiological considerations in paralysis of the larynx, *Proc. R. Soc. Med.,* 40, 849, 1947.
7. **Simone, A. F. and Ultman, J. S.,** Longitudinal mixing by the human larynx, *Resp. Physiol.,* 49, 187, 1982.
8. **Horsfield, K. and Cummings, G.,** Morphology of the bronchial tree in man, *J. Appl. Physiol.,* 24, 373, 1968.
9. **Krahl, V. E.** Anatomy of the mammalian lung, in *Handbook of Physiology,* Vol. 3., Sect. 1, Fenn, W. O. and Rahn, H., Eds. American Physiological Society, Washington, D.C., 1964, 213.
10. **Robertson, B.,** Basic morphology of the pulmonary defense system, *Eur. J. Res. Dis.,* 61 (Suppl. 107), 21, 1980.
11. **Findeisen, W.,** Uber das absetzen Kleiner, in der luft Suspendierten tielchen in der Menschilichen lunge bei der Atmung, *Pflueger's Arch. Ges. Physiol.,* 236, 367, 1935.
12. **Weibel, E. R.,** *Morphometry of the Human Lung,* Springer-Verlag, Berlin, 1963.
13. **Yeh, H. and Schum, G. M.,** Models of human lung airways and their application to inhaled particle deposition, *Bull. Math. Biol.,* 42, 461, 1980.

14. **Yu, C. P. and Diu, C. K.,** A comparative study of aerosol deposition in different lung models, *Am. Ind. Hyg. Assoc. J.,* 43, 54, 1982.

15. **Hansen, J. E. and Ampaya, E. P.,** Human air space shapes, sizes, area, and volumes, *J. Appl. Physiol.,* 38, 990, 1975.

16. **Landahl, H. D.,** On the removal of air-borne droplets by the human respiratory tract I. The lung, *Bull. Math. Biophys.,* 12, 43, 1950.

17. **Gerrity, T. R., Lee, P. S., Hass, F. J., Marinelli, A., Werner, P., and Lourenco, R. V.,** Calculated deposition of inhaled particles in the airway generations of normal subjects, *J. Appl. Physiol.,* 47, 867, 1979.

18. **Schroter, R. C. and Sudlow, M. F.,** Flow patterns in models of the human bronchial airways, *Resp. Physiol.,* 7, 341, 1969.

19. **Agnew, J. E., Pavia, D., and Clarke, S. W.,** Aerosol particle impaction in the conducting airways, *Phys. Med. Biol.,* 29, 767, 1984.

20. **Gormley, P. G. and Kennedy, M.,** Diffusion from a stream flowing through a cylinder, *Proc. R. Ir. Acad.,* A52, 163, 1949.

21. **Martin, D. and Jacobi, W.,** Diffusion deposition of small-sized particles in the bronchial tree, *Health Phys.,* 23, 23, 1972.

22. **Yu, C. P. and Soong, T. T.,** Statistical analysis of aerosol deposition in the nose and mouth, *Am. Ind. Hyg. Assoc. J.,* 42, 726, 1981.

23. **Martonen, T. and Lowe, J.,** Assessment of aerosol deposition patterns in human respiratory, in *Aerosols in the Mining and Industrial Work Environment,* Vol. 1, Marple, V. A. and Liu, B. Y. H., Eds., Ann Arbor Science, Ann Arbor, MI, 1983, 151.

24. **Davies, C. N.,** The deposition of aerosol in the human lung, in *Aerosole in Physik, Medizin und Technik,* Gesselschaft fur Aerosolforschung, Bad Sonen, West Germany, 1973, 90.

25. **Lippmann, M.,** Regional deposition of particles in the human respiratory tract, in *Handbook of Physiology,* Vol. 3, Sect. 9, American Physiological Society, Bethesda, MD, 1977, 213.

26. **Landahl, H. D., Tracewell, T. N., and Lassen, W. H.,** *Arch. Ind. Hyg. Occup. Med.,* 3, 359, 1951.

27. **Altshuler, B., Yarmus, L., Palmes, E. D., and Nelson, N.** Aerosol deposition in the human respiratory tract, *Arch. Ind. Health,* 15, 293, 1957.

28. **Giacomelli-Maltoni, G., Melandri, C., Prodi, V., and Tarroni, G.,** Deposition efficiency of monodisperse particles in human respiratory tract, *Am. Ind. Hyg. Assoc. J.,* 33, 603, 1972.

29. **Martens, A. and Jacobi, W.,** Die *in vivo* bestimmung der aerosolteilchendeposition im Atemtrakt bei mund- bzw. Nasenatmung, in *Aerosole in Physik, Medizin und Technik,* Gesellschaft fur Aerosolforschung, Bad Sonen, West German, 1973, 117.

30. **Foord, N., Black, A., and Walsh, M.,** Regional deposition of 2.5-7.5 μm diameter particles in healthy male non-smokers, *J. Aerosol Sci.,* 9, 343, 1978.

31. **Muir, D. C. F. and Davies, C. N.,** The deposition of 0.5 μm diameter aerosols in the lungs of man, *Ann. Occup. Hyg.,* 10, 161, 1967.

32. **Heyder, J., Gebhart, J., Heigwer, G., Roth, C., and Stahlhofen, W.,** Experimental studies of the total deposition of aerosol particles in the human respiratory tract, *J. Aerosol Sci.,* 4, 191, 1973.

33. **Heyder, J., Armbruster, L., Gebhart, J., and Stahlhofen, W.,** in *Aerosole in Physik, Medizin, und Technik,* Gesellschaft fur Aerosolforschung, Bad Sonen, West Germany, 1973, 122.

34. **Heyder, J., Gebhart, J., Roth, C., Stahlhofen, W., Stuck, B., Tarroni, G., DeZaiacomo, T., Formignani, M., and Melandri, C.,** Intercomparison of lung deposition data for aerosol particles, *J. Aerosol Sci.,* 9, 147, 1978.

35. **Chan, T. L. and Lippmann, M.,** Experimental measurements and empirical modelling of the regional deposition of inhaled particles in humans, *Am. Ind. Hyg. Assoc. J.,* 41, 399, 1980.

36. **Stahlhofen, W., Gebhart, J., and Heyder, J.** Experimental determination of the regional deposition of aerosol particles in the human respiratory tract, *Am. Ind. Hyg. Assoc. J.,* 41, 385, 1980.

37. **Lippmann, M. and Altshuler, B.,** Regional deposition of aerosols, in *Air Pollution and the Lung,* Aharonson, E. F., Ben-David, A., and Klingberg, M. A., Eds., Halsted Press-John Wiley, Jerusalem, 1976, 25.

38. **Landahl, H. D. and Black, S.,** Penetration of airborne particulates through the human nose, *J. Ind. Hyg. Toxicol.,* 29, 269, 1947.

39. **Landahl, H. D. and Tracewell, T.,** Penetration of airborne particulates through the human nose. II., *J. Ind. Hyg. Toxicol.,* 31, 55, 1949.

40. **Pattle, R. E.,** The retention of gases and particles in the human nose, in *Inhaled Particles and Vapours,* Davies, C. N., Ed., Pergamon Press, Oxford, 1961, 301.

41. **Hounam, R. F., Black, A., and Walsh, M.,** Deposition of aerosol particles in the nasopharyngeal region of the human respiratory tract, *Nature,* 211, 1254, 1969.

42. **Hounam, R. F., Balck, A., and Walsh, M.,** The deposition of aerosol particles in the nasopharyngeal region of the human respiratory tract, *J. Aerosol Sci.,* 2, 341, 1971.

43. **Lippmann, M.,** Deposition and clearance of inhaled particles in the human nose, *Ann. Otol. Rhinol. Laryngol.,* 79, 519, 1970.

44. **Heyder, J. and Rudolph, G.,** Deposition of aerosol particles in the human nose, in *Inhaled Particles IV,* Part I, Walton, W. H., Ed., Pergamon Press, Oxford, 1977, 107.
45. **Albert, R. E., Lippmann, M., Peterson, H. T., Jr., Berger, J., Sanborn, K., and Bohning, D.,** Bronchial deposition and clearance of aerosols, *Arch. Intern. Med.,* 131, 115, 1973.
46. **Morrow, P. E.,** Factors determining hygroscopic aerosol deposition in airways, *Physiol. Rev.,* 66, 330, 1986.
47. **Howell, W. E.,** The growth of cloud drops in uniformly cooled air, *J. Meteorol.,* 6, 134, 1949.
48. **Mason, B. J.,** *The Physics of Clouds,* Clarendon Pess, Oxford, 1957, 92.
49. **Winkler, P. and Junge, C.,** The growth of atmospheric aerosol particles as a function of relative humidity, *J. Rech. Atmos.,* 4, 617, 1972.
50. **Pruppacher, H. R. and Klett, J. D.,** *Microphysics of Clouds and Precipitation,* D. Reidel, Boston, 1978.
51. **Orr, C., Hurd, F. K., and Corbett, W. J.,** Aerosol size and relative humidity, *J. Colloid Sci.,* 13, 472, 1958.
52. **Orr, C., Hurd, F. K., Hendriz, W. P., and Junge, C.,** The behavior of condensation nuclei under changing humidities, *J. Meteorol.,* 14, 240, 1958.
53. **Derjagiun, B. V., Durghin, L. A., Rosenzweig, L. A., and Fedoseyer, V. A.,** Study of passivation of condensation growth of drops of water and salt solutions, *J. Colloid Interface Sci.,* 37, 484, 1971.
54. **Azarniouch, M. K., Bobkowicz, A. J., Cooke, N. E., and Farkas, E. J.,** Growth of sulfuric acid droplets exposed to water vapor, *Can. J. Chem. Eng.,* 51, 590, 1973.
55. **El Golli, S., Brichard, S., Turpin, P. Y., and Treiner, C.,** The evaporation of saline droplets, *J. Aerosol Sci.,* 5, 273, 1974.
56. **Nair, P. V. N. and Vohra, K. G.,** Growth of aqueous sulfuric acid droplets as a function of relative humidity, *J. Aerosol Sci.,* 6, 265, 1975.
57. **Tang, I. N. and Munkelwitz, H. R.,** Aerosol growth studies. III. Ammonium bisulfate aerosols in a moist atmosphere, *J. Aerosol Sci.,* 8, 321, 1977.
58. **Ferron, G. A., Haider, B., and Kreyling, W. G.,** A method for the approximation of the relative humidity in the upper human airways, *Bull. Math. Biol.,* 47, 565, 1985.
59. **Ferron, G. A.,** The size of soluble aerosol particles as a function of the humidity of the air. Application to the human respiratory tract, *J. Aerosol Sci.,* 8, 251, 1977.
60. **Ferron, G. A., Haider, B., and Kreyling, W. G.,** Aerosol particle growth in the human airways using a calculated humidity profile, *J. Aerosol Sci.,* 14, 196, 1983.
61. **Ferron, G. A., Hornik, S., Kreyling, W. G., and Haider, B.,** Comparison of experimental and calculated data for the total and regional deposition in the human lung, *J. Aerosol Sci.,* 16, 133, 1985.
62. **Blanchard, J. D. and Willeke, K.,** Total deposition of ultrafine sodium chloride particles in human lungs, *J. Appl. Physiol.,* 57, 1850, 1984.
63. **Fazio, F., Santolicandro, A., Solfanelli, S., Palla, A., Fornai, E., and Giuntini, C.,** Lung imaging following inhalation of technetum 99m-labelled microspheres: a comparison with the krypton-81m ventilation technique, in *Clinical and Experimental Applications of Krypton 81-m,* Lavender, J. P., Ed., British Institute of Radiology, London, 1978, 130.
64. **Kim, C. S., Brown, L. K., Lewars, G. G., and Sackner, M. A.,** Deposition of aerosol particles and flow resistance in mathematical and experimental airway models, *J. Appl. Physiol.,* 55, 154, 1983.
65. **Love, R. G. and Muir, D. C. F.,** Aerosol deposition and airway obstruction, *Am. Rev. Resp. Dis.,* 114, 891, 1976.
66. **Lourenco, R. V., Lodenkemper, R., and Carton, R. W.,** Patterns of distribution and clearance of aerosols in patients with bronchiectasis, *Am. Rev. Resp. Dis.,* 106, 857, 1972.
67. **Agner, J. E., Bateman, J. R. M., Pavia, D., and Clarke, S. W.,** Radionuclide demonstration of ventilatory abnormalities in mild asthma, *Clin. Sci.,* 66, 525, 1984.
68. **Weiss, T., Dorrow, P., and Felix, R.,** Continuous aerosol inhalation scintigraphy in the evaluation of early and advanced airways obstruction, *Eur. J. Nucl. Med.,* 9, 62, 1984.
69. **Lin, M. S. and Goodwin, D. A.,** Pulmonary distribution of an inhaled radioaerosol in obstructive pulmonary disease, *Radiology,* 118, 645, 1976.
70. **Garrard, C. S., Gerrity, T. R., Schreiner, J. F., and Yeates, D. B.,** Analysis of aerosol deposition in the healthy human lung, *Arch. Environ. Health,* 36, 184, 1981.
71. **Svartengren, M., Philipson, D., Linnman, L., and Camner, P.,** Airway resistance and deposition of particles in the lung, *Exp. Lung Res.,* 7, 257, 1984.
72. **Palmes, E., Altshuler, B., and Nelson, N.,** Deposition of aerosols in the human respiratory tract during breath holding, in *Inhaled Particles and Vapours II,* Davies, C. N., Ed., Pergamon Press, New York, 1967, 339.
73. **Palmes, E. D., Goldring, R. M., Wand, C. S., and Altschuler, B.,** Effect of chronic obstructive pulmonary disease on rate of deposition of aerosols in the lung during breath holding, in *Inhaled Particles and Vapous II,* Davies, C. N., Ed., Pergamon Press, New York, 1971, 123.
74. **Palmes, E. D., Wang, C. S., Goldring, R. M., and Altschuler, B.,** Effect of depth of inhalation on aerosol persistence during breath holding, *J. Appl. Physiol.,* 34, 356, 1973.
75. **Lapp, N. L., Hankinson, J. L., Amandus, H., and Palmes, E. D.,** Variability in the size of airspaces in normal human lungs as estimated by aerosols, *Thorax,* 30, 293, 1975.

76. **Hankinson, J. L., Palmes, E. D., and Lapp, N. L.,** Pulmonary air space size in coal miners, *Am. Rev. Resp. Dis.,* 119, 391, 1979.
77. **Gebhart, J., Heyder, J., and Stahlhofen, W.,** Use of aerosols to estimate pulmonary air-space dimensions, *J. Appl. Physiol.,* 51, 465, 1981.
78. **Bennett, W. D. and Smaldone, G. C.,** Use of aerosols to estimate mean airspace size in chronic obstructive pulmonary disease, *J. Appl. Physiol.,* 64, 1554, 1988.
79. **Rosenthal, F.,** A model for determining alveolar and small airway dimensions from aerosol recovery data, *J. Appl. Physiol.,* 58, 582, 1985.
80. **Heyder, J. and Davies, C. N.,** The breathing of half micron aerosols. III. Dispersion of particles in the respiratory tract, *Aerosol Sci.,* 2, 437, 1971.
81. **Heyder, J., Blanchard, J. D., and Brain, J. D.,** Examining convective gas mixing by aerosols, *Prog. Resp. Res.,* 21, 111, 1986.
82. **McCawley, M. and Lippmann, M.,** Development of an aerosol dispersion test to detect early changes in lung function, *Am. Ind. Hyg. Assoc. J.,* 49, 357, 1988.
83. **Heyder, J., Blanchard, J. D., Feldman, H. A., and Brain, J. D.,** Convective mixing in human respiratory tract: estimates with aerosol boli, *J. Appl. Physiol.,* 64, 1273, 1988.
84. **Lee, P. S., Gerrity, T. R., Hass, F. J., and Lourenco, R. V.,** A model for tracheobronchial clearance of inhaled particles in man and a comparison with data, *IEEE Trans. Biomed. Eng.,* BME-26, 624, 1979.
85. **Yeates, D. B., Aspin, N., Levinson, H., Jones, M. T., and Bryan, A. C.,** Mucociliary tracheal transport in man, *J. Appl. Physiol.,* 39, 487, 1975.
86. **Foster, W. M., Langenback, E., and Bergofsky, E. H.,** Measuement of tracheal and bronchial mucus velocities in man: relation to lung clearance, *J. Appl. Physiol.,* 48, 965, 1980.

Chapter 2

TOXICOLOGIC RESPONSES TO INHALED AEROSOLS AND THEIR INGREDIENTS

David J. Velasquez

TABLE OF CONTENTS

I. INTRODUCTION

In one day, a normal person breathes approximately 13,000 l of air. The inspired air can contain numerous airborne contaminants including a variety of dusts, gaseous pollutants, smokes, various types of aerosols, and microorganisms. In order to deal with this wide variety of potential insults, a number of lung defenses have evolved (Figure 1). These defenses include the mucociliary escalator, which is composed of a mucus lining layer which covers the surface of the trachea, bronchi, and bronchioles, including the terminal bronchioles, and which is moved by the ciliated epithelium. In the pulmonary region, alveolar macrophages are present. These are phagocytic cells which scavenge particulate material which penetrates to the alveolar region of the lung and which are capable of recruiting additional cells if the particulate load is large. They also play a role in effecting immune responses to a variety of types of inhaled material, although the exact mechanism by which a response is elicited is not well understood. These two primary defense systems are augmented by additional host defenses such as the mechanical cough response in the upper airways, and by the lymphatic drainage system in the pulmonary region. Relative solubilities of deposited particles are of considerable importance in determining which clearance pathways will be dominant. When studying the fate of administered therapeutic aerosols, it is important to understand the nature of the defense systems in the lung and the types of toxicologic responses which can result from imprudent or inappropriate aerosol formulation and administration.

II. GENERAL RESPIRATORY SYSTEM ANATOMY

The tracheobronchial tree provides a rapid and efficient means of transporting inspired air to the peripheral gas exchange regions (Figure 2). This rapidly branching structure is maintained by cartilage rings in the larger airways which give way to cartilage plates in the middle airways. The cartilaginous structure gradually disappears in the smaller bronchi, while airway smooth muscle and connective tissue become prominent in the medium and smaller airways. The epithelium of the tracheobronchial tree is comprised largely of ciliated and secretory cells, although a wide variety of supportive and specialty cell types are also present. Also dispersed throughout the tracheobronchial tree are several types of nerve cells which serve to monitor the local environment as well as control the response to various stimuli perceived. The entrance configuration to the tracheobronchial tree, the oro- or nasopharynx, is also important for its role in treating the inspired air by humidifying and warming it to body temperature. Additionally, it serves to act as a gross filter by collecting larger particles, and, in fact, is a major deposition site for inspired particles.

The rapidly branching nature of the tracheobronchial tree, the resulting increase in numbers of airways, and the gradual decrease in airway diameter serve to provide an efficient distribution system for inspired air (Figure 3). The initial inspiratory airflow is gradually slowed and distributed to the periphery of the lung. Efficient gas exchange occurs due to the small diffusion distance and the large surface area in the pulmonary region of approximately 80 m². The epithelium of the gas exchange region is characterized by flattened type I and cuboidal type II alveolar cells. The type I cell presents a diffusion thickness of less than 1 μm which allows inspired oxygen to cross easily for uptake in the pulmonary capillaries.

III. AEROSOL SYSTEMS

A. AEROSOL GENERATORS

Aerosols can be generated by a variety of mechanisms. Four general aerosol generation devices are discussed here. The jet atomizer (Figure 4A) operates using a compressed air source which can help to form as well as break up a thin film or jet of liquid. A baffle system is usually

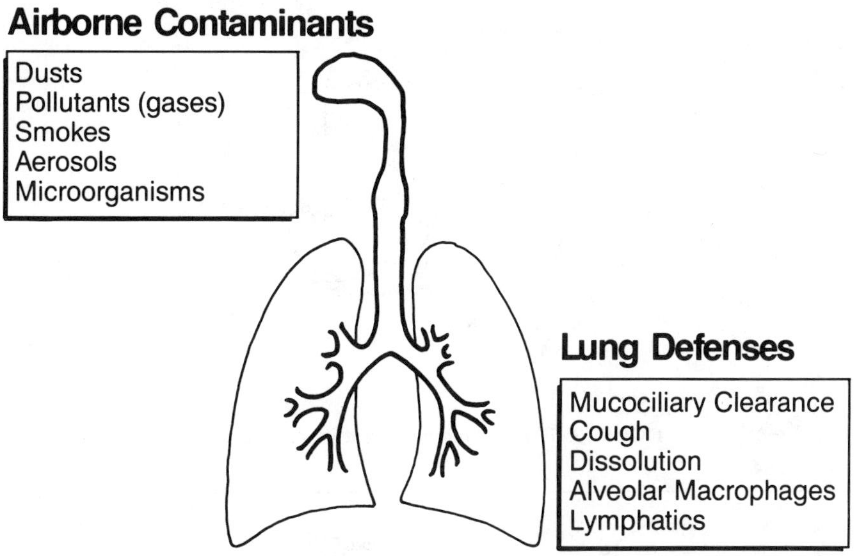

Airborne Contaminants

Dusts
Pollutants (gases)
Smokes
Aerosols
Microorganisms

Lung Defenses

Mucociliary Clearance
Cough
Dissolution
Alveolar Macrophages
Lymphatics

FIGURE 1. Airborne challenges and lung defenses.

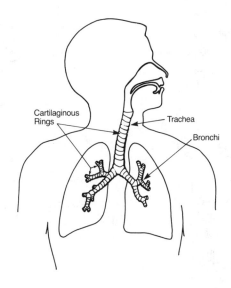

FIGURE 2. The human trachea and major bronchi.

present to further reduce the size of the aerosol droplets. The aerosol characteristics and output are controlled by the driving air pressure.

Another type of device is the ultrasonic generator (Figure 4B) which uses a high frequency, usually piezoelectric, crystal to impart energy into and through a liquid conducting medium and subsequently into the nebulizer solution. The high frequency oscillations cause miniature liquid fountains to form at the liquid surface and these fountains ultimately break up to form the aerosol droplets. A controlled flow of air is passed over the surface of the liquid to entrain the aerosol and carry it out of the nebulizer.

The metered dose inhaler (MDI) is a portable unit which operates using a low boiling point propellant in which the active ingredient is dissolved or dispersed (Figure 4C). A valve system

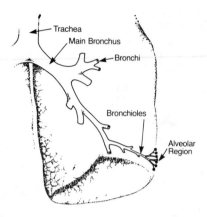

FIGURE 3. Bronchi, bronchioles, and alveolar region.

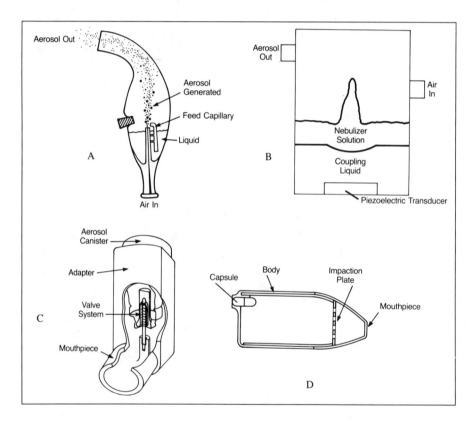

FIGURE 4. (A) Devilbiss atomizer, (B) ultrasonic generator, (C) metered dose inhaler, (D) rotahaler powder generator.

isolates a fixed volume of the formulation when actuation of the unit is begun. This volume is moved to an expansion chamber (at atmospheric pressure) as actuation proceeds, where the propellant flash vaporizes and creates an aerosol of the active agent. Depending on the chemical nature of the drug, it can be dispersed within the propellant as a suspension or may be dissolved in the propellant, usually with the aid of a cosolvent.

Powder inhalers are available in several different configurations (Figure 4D). In general, a predetermined dose of the dry therapeutic agent, sometimes mixed with a dry carrier material to ensure proper dispersion, is loaded into a gelatin capsule or similar type of container. This unit is opened or pierced within the inhaler when dosing is required, and the contents are entrained in an airstream generated by a mechanical device or by the patient's own efforts. Usually a baffle system is used to help break up aggregates.

B. GENERATOR CHARACTERISTICS

Some characteristics of the four types of generators mentioned can be described. The jet atomizer is a continuous-flow, relatively low concentration system. The aerosol output is "wet" and the formulation requires an aqueous carrier, the active ingredient, a preservative, and possibly a cosolvent. Either a compressed air source or a rubber bulb is required to provide airflow to the atomizer.

The ultrasonic generator is a continuous-flow, relatively high concentration system. The aerosol is "wet" and the formulation requires an aqueous carrier, the active ingredient, a preservative, and possibly a cosolvent. Electricity is required as the energy source. The aerosol concentration is controlled by the airflow introduced to the system so that a broad concentration range is possible.

The MDI is a single-pulse, relatively high concentration system. The aerosol is "dry" and the formulation requires a propellant, the active ingredient, a surfactant, a preservative, and possibly a cosolvent. The unit is self-contained and delivers the dose at a relatively high velocity due to rapid propellant expansion and evaporation.

Powder generators are usually single-dose, potentially high-concentration systems. The aerosol is dry and the formulation usually consists of an inert "extender" such as lactose and the active ingredient. The energy for aerosol generation is usually generated by the patient's breathing, but pressurized air can be used, either with a rubber bulb or a compressed air source. The efficiency of aerosolization can vary widely because particle entrainment and deagglomeration usually requires inspiratory efforts from the patient which may not be very efficient in these systems.

The above classes of generators generally deliver aerosols having different size characteristics. Several studies have been performed to measure the particle or droplet size produced by these generators (Table 1).[1-3] The droplet size of aerosols generated from a jet nebulizer generally ranges from 3 to 8 μm with geometric standard deviations (S.D.) ranging from 1.5 to 2.0. The ultrasonic generators deliver 6 to 9 μm droplets with geometric S.D. between 1.4 and 1.7. Metered dose inhalers deliver particles ranging in size from approximately 1 to 4 μm with geometric S.D. of 1.5 to 4.0, a wide variation. Powder generators are more difficult to characterize, especially if the aerosol characteristics of only the drug particles are desired. As noted earlier, lactose is usually present in the powder formulation to help deagglomerate the drug particles, and the lactose particles are usually at least 20 μm in diameter.

These generation systems produce a wide range of particle sizes and each type displays a fairly large variation in sizes, as indicated by the relatively large geometric S.D. It is important to be aware of the particle size characteristics of these systems because particle size is a primary determinant, not only of the fraction of aerosol deposited in a particular region, but also of the deposition site itself. It is also important to note that the method of measuring particle size has a direct influence on the size reported. For example, in the MDI, particle size initially changes very rapidly as the propellants vaporize, and therefore the size distribution is dynamic in nature. Depending on the time of sampling or the position of the sampler, a different size distribution may be seen. Similarly, sampling at the point of emission of a jet atomizer and ultrasonic generator will measure the initial droplet size. Sampling from an aerosol line at some distance removed from the point of generation results in measuring an aerosol that has aged somewhat (i.e., dried or possibly coagulated) and therefore will result in a different median diameter and size distribution. These differences are important considerations, especially when comparing particle size distributions reported for different studies.

The relationship between aerodynamic size and deposition site in the respiratory tract has

TABLE 1
Aerosol Size Measurements

Jet

Unit	Droplet Size Mass Median Diameter	Distribution Geometric Standard Deviation
Vaponefrin	5.6μ	1.8
Penisol	2.9	—*
Bennett No. 633	3.9	—*
Bennett Twin Jet No. 2814	6.8	1.8
Bennett Twin Neb No. 3012	7.7	1.8
DeVilbiss No. 640	6.3	1.9
DeVilbiss Experimental	4.9	2.0
Mist O$_2$ Gen Gette ET-IT	3.9	1.8
Mist O$_2$ Gen Gette ET-IP	3.5	—*
Mist O$_2$ Gen Gemini Twin Jet	8.9	2.1
Mist O$_2$ Personal	6.1	1.9
Puritan 126-051 (40 mm)—unheated	6.5	1.9
Puritan 126-051 (40 mm)—heated	5.7	—*
Mist-O$_2$-Gen MC-11C	3.5	1.9
Mist-O$_2$-Gen VT-11C	6.7	1.7
(Baffle set in normal position)		

MDI

Unit	Particle Size Mass Median Aerodynamic Diameter	Distribution Geometric Standard Deviation
Bronkometer	1.2μ	3.9
Mistometer	1.9	3.3
Medihaler—Duo	2.4	—*
Medihaler—Epi	2.6	—*
Respihaler—decadron	1.4	2.1
Respihaler—prodecadron	1.3	2.3

*Not log-normally distributed

Physical Characteristics of Aerosols

Trade Name	MMAD	GSD
Duo-Medihaler	3.6	1.7
Medihaler-Epi	3.1	1.7
Medihaler-Iso	2.8	1.8
Norisodrine Aerotrol	3.9	2.1
Alupent	3.5	1.7
Metaprel	3.5	1.5
Isuprel Mistometer	4.3	2.1
Bronkometer	3.5	1.7
Asthma-Meter	3.4	1.7

Ultrasonic

Nebulizer	Operating frequency (kHz)	Mass median diameter (μm)	Geometric standard deviation[c]
DeVilbiss[a]	1350	6.9	1.6
Mist-O$_2$-Gen[b]	1400	6.5	1.4
Mead Johnson	800	9.0	1.7

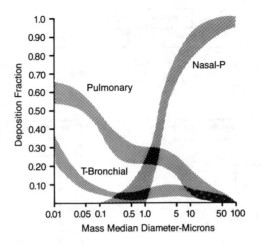

FIGURE 5. Regional aerosol deposition probabilities.[7]

been studied by many investigators.[4-6] A typical representation of regional deposition characteristics was published by the Task Group on Lung Dynamics.[7] Regional deposition as a function of particle size and the type of overlap are shown in Figure 5.

IV. TOXICOLOGIC CONSIDERATIONS

A. TOXIC RESPONSES

A toxic response is characterized by several components. First, a chemical or physical agent, the toxin, is required. In this context, it can be the aerosol or vapor, or some component thereof. The second requisite is a biologic system, in this case, the respiratory tract, an organ system of considerable complexity. Third, a mechanism for causing an interaction is needed. Deposition of the aerosol within the respiratory tract and subsequent dissolution are the predominant mechanisms. These are influenced by the particle size distribution, breathing patterns, geometry of the respiratory tract, and the physicochemical characteristics of the region of the respiratory tract where deposition occurs. Finally, a response to the agent is elicited. There can be different responses in different regions of the respiratory tract or different responses in the same region to different doses. It is apparent that a multitude of variables must be considered to determine whether a response elicited by an inhaled agent in the respiratory tract may be considered a toxic response or may ultimately lead to a toxic response.

B. FACTORS DETERMINING RESPONSES

Looking at the above elements in detail, some factors which may influence the toxicity of inhaled agents can be described. The physical characteristics, chemical composition, and solubility of the aerosol/drug components are important. Also of interest is the nature of the formulation vehicle and excipients which are required to maintain stability. In the biologic system, the age, sex, weight, and (especially) state of health are important considerations when evaluating the response to aerosol exposure. The method of administration, frequency, and duration of exposure are also important considerations when evaluating toxic responses. For example, if an aerosol is administered at the beginning of a deep inspiration, its deposition pattern will be considerably different than if it were administered midway through a shallow breathing maneuver. Frequency and duration of administration determine the total dose received. A metered dose inhaler delivers a short, relatively high dose while a jet atomizer delivers a lower concentration, but may be administered over a much longer time frame. The

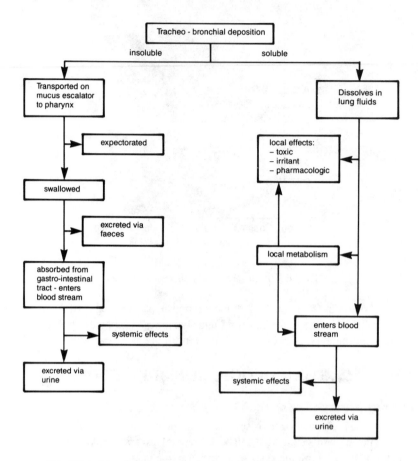

FIGURE 6. Fate of inhaled particles deposited in the tracheobronchial region.[8]

types of responses which may be seen depend on the deposition site and are examined in the following section.

C. PARTICLE FATE FOLLOWING DEPOSITION

Using a compartmentalized approach to separate the different functional regions of the tracheobronchial region (Figure 6),[8] it is possible to determine some possible consequences for either soluble or insoluble particles which are deposited. Insoluble particles will be removed via the mucociliary system and will be either swallowed or expectorated. If swallowed, they can either be excreted, or, if solubilized during passage through the gastrointestinal tract, may enter the bloodstream. Particle constituents may be excreted in the urine or deposit in one or more organs and possibly cause systemic effects. Soluble particles deposited in the tracheobronchial region can dissolve in lung fluids and exert local effects such as toxic, irritant, or pharmacologic responses. The solute may also become metabolized and cause similar responses. The solute can also enter the bloodstream and be delivered to various organs where it may exert an effect. Excretion will occur primarily through the urine. Physiologic responses to soluble particles can also be viewed as indications of efficacy for a drug which elicits beneficial effects.

The fate of particles deposited in the pulmonary region can be similarly described (Figure 7).[8] Insoluble particles will probably be engulfed by alveolar macrophages and transported to the mucociliary system. At that point they will be carried up the mucociliary escalator to the pharyngeal region where they may be expectorated or swallowed. If swallowed, they may be solubilized upon passage through the gastrointestinal tract with the parent material entering the bloodstream. Further systemic effects may be elicited with subsequent excretion via the urine.

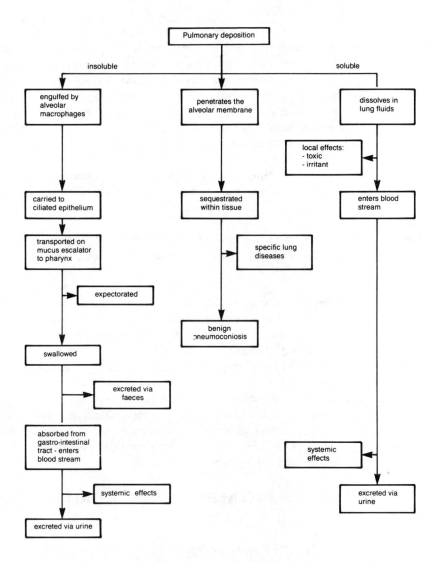

FIGURE 7. Fate of inhaled particles deposited in the pulmonary region.[8]

Nonsolubilized particles would be excreted in the feces. Insoluble particles in the alveolar region which are not phagocytized may become sequestered in the pulmonary tissue. If sequestered for a long period, some solubilization may occur and, depending on the chemical nature of the material, adverse tissue reactions may lead to to a fibrotic response. Alternatively, a relatively benign pneumoconiosis may result with no immediate adverse responses seen. Soluble particles which reach the pulmonary region will dissolve in the lung milieu and may exert local toxic, irritant, or pharmacologic effects. The material can also enter the bloodstream and exert systemic effects and ultimately be subject to excretion via the urine.

An additional clearance pathway for the alveolar region is the lymphatic drainage. Although the mechanism is not completely understood, it appears that some fraction of the alveolar macrophages and their contents can be cleared through the lymphatics and that particulate material as well may find its way into the lymphatic system.

D. DRUG INTERACTIONS

Adverse drug reactions are usually seen in only a small percentage of the population. There are several different types of reactions which can be called adverse. One type is an allergic reaction which is usually due to an immune response, and, as such, may be an immediate or delayed reaction. These hypersensitivity reactions have been further subclassified into at least four groupings, depending on the types of antibodies involved, reaction time, and reaction mechanism.[9] One type of hypersensitivity response is an anaphylactic reaction which is usually quite severe in its symptoms, affects the respiratory and cardiovascular systems, and may be life threatening. Another type of adverse reaction is hypersusceptibility to the drug. This reaction occurs primarily because of biologic variability among patients. Drugs are approved for use based on a statistically insignificant occurrence of adverse reactions during well-controlled studies, but a certain number of people in the general population may develop an undesirable response to the drug. Hypersusceptibility may also result due to the presence of disease which may make a person overly sensitive to a drug's negative effects. Tachyphylaxis, or tolerance, can be considered to be an adverse reaction because tolerance or resistance to a drug's effects negates the drug's utility.

Adverse effects may also occur when several drugs are administered concurrently and result in a modification of the nominal therapeutic effects of any single drug.[10] Several types of interactions can be identified as follows:

- Addition occurs when effects from two drugs taken simultaneously are similar to the additive effects which would be expected from the drugs taken separately.
- Synergism occurs when drugs of similar activity which are taken together show responses greater than would be expected based on additive effects.
- Potentiation occurs when drugs with different actions are taken together and show greater effects than when taken separately.
- Antagonism occurs when drugs which act to produce opposing effects are taken together and cause a subsequent reduction in overall efficacy. Although these interactions may not induce an adverse response, the uncharacteristic nature of some of them may alter the intended therapeutic effect. One final adverse reaction is a toxic response to the drug itself, and may be generally termed a side effect of the drug.

V. ADVERSE REACTIONS TO AEROSOLS IN THE RESPIRATORY TRACT

A recent reference work, *PDR's 1988 Index of Drug Interactions and Side Effects,*[11] lists drugs, known interactions, side effects, and associated products. *The Physicians' Desk Reference,*[12] itself, is a useful compendium of approved drugs which lists the drugs with a wide variety of information including manufacturer, chemical description, indications and contraindications for the drug, and adverse reactions which have been reported. Several classes of drugs are indicated for the treatment of pulmonary disorders. Those which can be administered in an aerosolized form are discussed.

A. DRUG-RELATED RESPONSES

In asthmatic patients, aerosolized β-2 agonists are frequently used to dilate the airways. Precautions listed include paradoxic bronchospasm, and adverse reactions reported include cardiovascular effects such as tachycardia and hypertension, central nervous system effects including tremor and headache, and throat irritation.

Aerosolized sympathomimetics have been reported to also cause paradoxic bronchospasm and tachycardia, blood pressure changes, tremor, and headache. Adverse reactions to aerosolized mast cell stabilizers include throat irritation, cough, and wheezing. Aerosolized steroids can also be administered, but should be taken with caution because of potential side effects.[13,14] They have been known to cause dysfunction of the hypophyseal-pituitary-adrenal axis and candidiasis in the oropharynx,[15] where deposition of the drug by impaction can be quite high. This complication can be treated and may be reduced with the use of aerosol spacers and by gargling.[16,17] Additional gastrointestinal and central nervous system effects have been noted as well as respiratory infections, hoarseness, and dermatologic effects. However, these side effects are usually seen only when steroids are administered in high concentrations.

A list of trade name commercial aerosolized products is shown in Table 2.[12] Also listed is the pharmacologic compound, its mode of action, and the ingredients in the aerosol formulation. The excipients present are numerous and varied and include the propellants themselves. The various classes of excipients and their effects in the lung are discussed below.

B. PROPELLANT EFFECTS

Propellants are a significant component of metered dose aerosol systems. The commonly used propellants are Freon 11 (trichlorofluoromethane), Freon 12 (dichlorodifluoromethane), and Freon 114 (dichlorotetrafluoroethane). These propellants have been studied for their toxic effects by several authors.[18-21] A summary of one set of studies is shown in Table 3.[18] Various propellants are classified as low or high pressure propellants of low, intermediate, or high toxicity. The most prevalent toxicological finding for the chlorofluorocarbon propellants is induction of or sensitization to cardiac arrhythmias in the mouse or dog when epinephrine is administered shortly after the propellant exposure.[22] The studies reported were generally run at relatively high concentrations (several percent or more, by volume, in air). Figure 8[23] shows the concentration in blood of Freon 11 and Freon 12 following aerosol administration of 2 puffs from an MDI. The Freon concentrations are seen to rise sharply and fall off rapidly. However, in order to reach concentrations which would cause sensitization to arrhythmia in dogs, more than 12 puffs would be required in a short time span.

C. EXCIPIENT STUDIES

Other excipients in aerosol formulations include antioxidants, preservatives, and stabilizers. Such compounds as oleic acid, sorbitan trioleate, and benzalkonium chloride are found in various formulations. When aerosolized, these materials have been reported to cause an irritant response;[24,25] however, it is difficult to adequately characterize their chemical toxicity at low concentrations. Nevertheless, studies of aerosol formulations administered with and without the active agent have shown a bronchoconstrictive response when the active agent is absent.[26,27] This type of response can lead to the paradoxical bronchoconstriction seen in some studies, especially in a hypersensitive population of patients.

Other studies have looked specifically at the actions of sodium sulfite and bisulfite.[32,33] In guinea pigs, sodium sulfite is much more potent than sulfur dioxide in inducing bronchoconstriction.[30] In sulfite-sensitive asthmatics, Koepke et al.[31] (Figure 9A) found a marked decrease in FEV_1 following inhalation of a 0.3% metabisulfite solution. This concentration is equivalent to that found in commercial preparations of isoetharine and other drug formulations used in nebulizer solutions. The FEV_1 value returned to baseline levels after administration of isoetharine. In other studies, Koepke et al.[32] and Witek and Schachter[33] measured SO_2 concentrations following administration of commercial aerosol formulations containing sodium metabisulfite and found values ranging from 2 to 6 ppm (Figure 9B).[33] Concentrations of 1 ppm SO_2 have been shown to induce bronchoconstriction in some asthmatics. The method of aerosol generation and formulation can affect the concentration of SO_2 present as shown in Table 4.[33] The range of concentrations seen suggests that responses in patients may also vary depending on the method of aerosol generation used.

D. LOCAL AIRWAY EFFECTS

Another aspect of aerosol formulation considerations is the local effect of deposited aerosol on ionic composition and pH in the respiratory tract.[34,35] Studies have shown that pH values <2.0

TABLE 2
Aerosol Products, Active Agents, Mode of Action, and Excipients

Aerobid	Flunisolide	Steroid	F11, F12, F114 sorbitan trioleate
{ Beclovent	Beclomethasone dipropionate	Steroid	F11, F12 Oleic acid
Vanceril			
Brethaire	Terbutaline sulfate	β_2-Adrenergic	F11, F12, F114 sorbitan trioleate
Decadron	Dexamethasone	Steroid	Chlorofluoro-hydrocarbons
Respihaler	Sodium phosphate		2% alcohol
{ Proventil	Albuterol	β_2-Adrenergic	F11, F12
Ventolin			Oleic acid
Tornalate	Bitolterol mesylate	β-Adrenergic	F12, F114 38% alcohol Ascorbic acid, saccharin, menthol
Alupent	Metaproterenol	β-Adrenergic	Chlorofluoro-hydrocarbons
	Sulfate		Sorbitan trioleate
		Solution	pH-adjusted aqueous solution, benzalkonium chloride, edetate disodium
Bronkosol	Isoetharine	β_2-Adrenergic	
		Solution	Acetone sodium bisulfite, glycerin, parabens, water, sodium chloride, sodium citrate
Bronkometer	Isoetharine Mesylate	β_2-Adrenergic	F12, F114 30% alcohol, 0.1% ascorbic acid, menthol, saccharin
Duo-Medihaler	Isoproterenol Hydrochloride	Sympathomimetic	F11, F12, F114 Cetylpyridinium chloride
	Phenylephrine bitartrate		sorbitan trioleate
{ Isuprel	Isoproterenol hydrochloride	β-Adrenergic	F12, F114 33% alcohol,
Mistometer			ascorbic acid
Norisodrine			
Aerotrol		*Solution*	0.5% chlorobutanol, 0.3% sodium metabisulfite, citric acid, glycerin, water, sodium chloride (saccharin sodium, sodium citrate)

TABLE 2 (Continued)
Aerosol Products, Active Agents, Mode of Action, and Excipients

Medihaler-Epi	Epinephrine bitartrate	Sympathomimetic	F11, F12, F114 Cetylpyridinium chloride, sorbitan trioleate
Medihaler-Iso	Isoproterenol sulfate	Sympathomimetic	F11, F12, F114 Sorbitan trioleate
Intal	Cromolyn sodium	Mast cell stabilizer	F12, F114 Sorbitan trioleate

or >8.0 can stimulate the rapidly responding airway receptors in the epithelium and induce cough.[28,36] A buffered solution at low or high pH is a more efficient bronchoconstrictor than an unbuffered solution.[37] By comparison, studies by Schanker and Less[38] have suggested that the airway pH in dogs is 6.6. Concerns regarding the effects of extremes in pH on physiologic responses should be weighed against the need to adjust the pH of the aerosol formulation in order to solubilize or stabilize the active ingredient. Adjustments in the formulation may be in order if an unusually high or low pH is required to stabilize the drug.

A further concern regarding localized effects from administered aerosols are the possible changes in tonicity of the liquid lining layer caused by local deposition.[39] Studies have shown that distilled water, hypotonic saline (0.3% and 7.5 mosm), and hypertonic saline (3.6 and 4.0%) can induce bronchoconstriction.[40,41] Similar effects were seen when distilled water, 0.3 and 3.6% saline caused 20 to 40% decreases in FEV_1.[42,43] The mechanisms which induce the bronchoconstriction may be different.[44-46] Some of the postulated effects of changing the local tonicity are provocation of lung irritant receptors, stimulation of mast cells to release histamine (hypotonic and hypertonic solutions), and stimulation of basophils to release histamine (hypertonic solutions).[47,48] An additional complicating factor is the possibility that the local osmolarity may change in different regions of the respiratory system. Boucher et al.[49] has reported measurements of tracheal osmolarity in dogs at 330 mosm and a value of 304 mosm in 0.5 cm bronchi. Studies in asthmatic patients have shown similar bronchoconstrictive responses. Allegra and Bianco[50] (Figure 10) showed the effects of a distilled water aerosol on asthmatics and normals and the effect of a saline aerosol on asthmatics. The distilled water aerosol caused a pronounced increase in airway resistance in asthmatics and had no effect in normals while the asthmatics did not respond to the saline aerosol. In this study, pulmonary function measurements indicated that airway resistance was more strongly affected, with a lesser but still significant decrease in FEV_1 seen compared to baseline values.

E. OTHER PHYSIOLOGIC RESPONSES

Another physiologic response of interest following aerosol therapy is lung clearance. Bronchodilators usually stimulate mucociliary clearance after administration, probably by increasing ciliary beat frequency, opening the airways (thereby increasing internal surface area), and stimulating secretion, all of which are regarded as beneficial effects. However, effects on alveolar clearance have not been well characterized. An interesting comparison of a nonaerosolized respiratory drug is shown in Figures 11A and B.[51,52] Oral aminophylline caused an increase in mucociliary clearance. However, a comparison of the ability of alveolar macrophages to kill intrapulmonary bacteria following aminophylline administration indicated that the phagocytic ability of the alveolar macrophages had been compromised. These studies illustrate the importance of determining not only the effects on mucociliary clearance but also how pulmonary clearance might be altered based on aerosolized respiratory drug actions.

A topic which deserves mention and requires detailed investigation is the immunologic potential of inhaled aerosols in the normal population. With the proliferation of therapeutic

TABLE 3
Summary of Pattern of Effects on Circulatory and Respiratory Systems of Inhalation of Propellants

Fluorocarbon No.; Chemical Name (Frequency of Use in Aerosols)	Cardiac Arrhythmia			Tachycardia		Hypotension		Bronchoconstriction		
	Induce	Sensitive								
	Mouse	Mouse	Dog	Dog	Monkey	Dog	Monkey	Rat	Dog	Monkey
Low-pressure propellants of high toxicity										
FC 11; Trichloro-fluoromethane (93)	++	++	++	++	++	+	++	++	0	0
FC 21; Dichloromono-fluoromethane (0)	++	++	++	++	+	+	+	0	+	0
FC 113; Trichloro-trifluoroethane (0)	++	++	++	++		+			+	0
Trichloroethane (1)	+	+	++	+	+	0	+		0	
Methylene chloride (8)	+	+	++							
Low-pressure propellants of intermediate toxicity										
FC 114; Dichloro-tetrafluoroethane (36)	0	+	+	+	0	+	0	+	+	0
FC 142b; Monochloro-difluoroethane (2)	0	0	+	+		+			+	
Isobutane (37)	0	+	+	0	0	0	0	++	+	+
FC C-318; octafluorocyclo-butane (0)	0	+	+	0	0	0	0	+	+	
High-pressure propellants of intermediate toxicity										
FC 12; Dichlorodi-fluoromethane (153)	0	0	+	+	0	0	0	0	+	0
FC 22; Monochlorodi-fluoromethane (0)	0	+	+							
Propane (6)	0	++	+							
Vinyl chloride (1)	++	++	+							
High-pressure propellants of low toxicity										
FC 115; Chloropenta-fluoroethane (0)	0	+	+	+		+		++	+	
FC 152a; Difluoro-ethane (5)	0	0	+	0	0	0	0	0	0	0

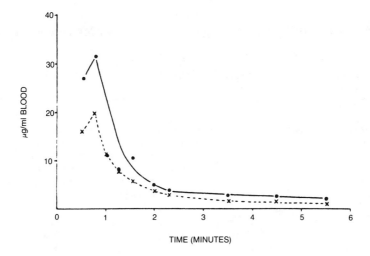

FIGURE 8. Freon 11 (solid circles) and Freon 12 (x-x) blood concentrations following 2 puffs of a Ventolin inhaler separated by 30 s and with a 10- s breath-hold.[23]

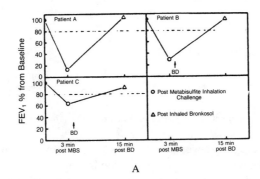

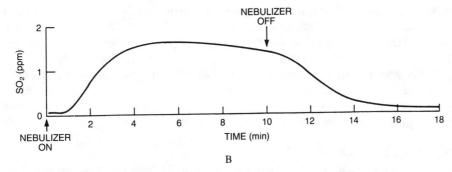

FIGURE 9. (A) Changes in FEV_1 following metabisulfite inhalation.[31] (B) SO_2 concentrations from an MDI containing bisulfite.[33]

TABLE 4

Sulfur Dioxide (ppm) Generated Using Different Delivery Methods and Drug Lots

Different drugs (via compressed air at 10 psi: same lot of each drug)

Isoetharine (n = 5)	Isoproterenol (n = 5)	Metaproterenol (n = 5)	Sterile water (n = 5)
2.66 ± 0.32	1.94 ± 0.22	0	0

Different delivery methods (lot W00211 of isoetharine)

	Air tank 10 psi (n = 5)	Bulb nebulizer (2 puffs) (n = 5)	Bulb nebulizer (10 puffs) (n = 10)
	2.66 ± 0.32	0.26 ± 0.09	0.64 ± 0.18

(Lot W00712 of isoetharine)

	Pulmo-aide (2 puffs) (n = 5)	Bulb nebulizer (10 puffs) (n = 5)	Bulb nebulizer (10 puffs) (n = 10)
	2.7 ± 0.50	0.30 ± 0.04	0.74 ± 0.15

Different drug lots (compressed air [10 si])

Metaproterenol (n = 5) #713007	Metaproterenol (n = 5) #693914
0	0

Isoetharine (bulb nebulizer [10 puffs]) (n = 5) #W00712	Isoetharine (n = 5) #W00211
0.74 ± 0.15	0.64 ± 0.18

Note: Values represent the average of peak concentrations (mean ± S.D.).

drugs resulting from the rapidly developing field of biotechnology, the possibility of immune responses in this population following administration by any route must be kept in mind.

Netter[53] has illustrated a variety of mechanisms which can lead to bronchoconstriction in asthmatics. These mechanisms include immunologic responses, β-adrenergic blockade, biochemical deficiency, and neural or neurotransmitter defects, and illustrate the variety of responses which may be seen in a particular susceptible population. When these mechanisms are examined along with the numerous types of agents and excipients in a typical aerosol formulation, it leads to an appreciation of the various types of responses which can result. For other disease states, the results are equally complex. Such an exercise points up the difficulty in identifying specific causative agents if an adverse response is seen in an individual, particularly if a disease state is already present.

F. DEATHS FROM ASTHMA

Deaths due to asthma rose worldwide beginning about 20 years ago and then declined (Figure 12).[54] This trend has been analyzed by many and several conclusions have been drawn.[55-59] The increased number of deaths was correlated with an increased number of MDI prescriptions. One possible cause of the increase seen in the U.K. might also have been the approval of more potent formulation of isoproterenol, which was five times stronger than the existing formulation. A change in the coding system for reporting deaths also artificially increased the number of reported deaths. The asthmatic population itself may also have increased. Better reporting procedures have probably developed over time so that a more efficient reporting system is in place. However, the most widely believed cause of the increased death rate was poor patient management by the physician, although poor patient compliance in spite of good management

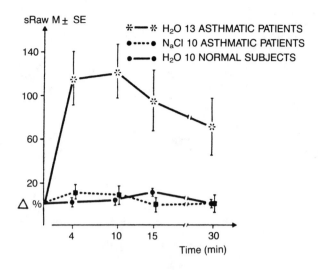

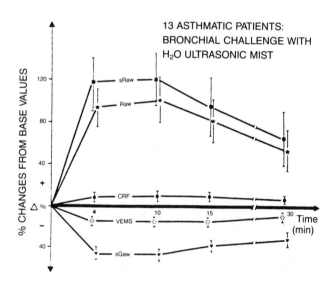

FIGURE 10. (Upper) Changes in airway resistance after ultrasonic distilled water in asthmatics and normals and ultrasonic saline in asthmatics. (Lower) Airway changes (resistance, FRC, FEV_1, and conductance) after ultrasonic distilled water in asthmatics.[50]

would have the same effect. Reliance on the MDI as an optimal form of therapy, without conscientiously following up on the patient's condition and considering alternative or supplemental therapies if symptoms worsen, may lead to a relatively poor treatment regimen. If the asthma gradually progresses into a more severe form, the existing MDI therapy for a patient may not be appropriate, and without further evaluation by the physician, more frequent usage of the MDI (which gradually becomes less effective) may result. Such overusage of inappropriate medication has been cited as the possible cause of death in many cases, although it is usually difficult to obtain good data to support such claims. It is now recommended that the asthmatic patient consult his physician whenever symptoms worsen or the MDI therapy is no longer effective so that a re-evaluation of the appropriate therapy can be made. An Asthma Mortality Task Force summary addressing this issue in depth has been published.[60]

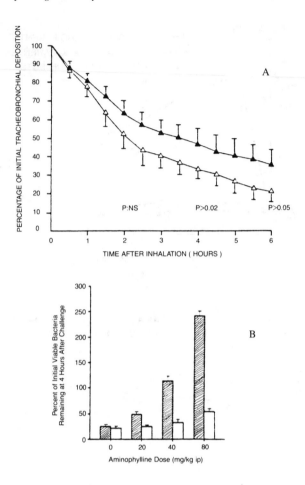

FIGURE 11.   (A) Mean tracheobronchial clearance curves for 12 patients with obstructive lung disease following therapy with oral aminophylline (open triangle) and placebo (closed triangle).[51] (B) Comparison of intrapulmonary killing of *S. aureus* (open column) and *P. mirabilis* (hatched column) during treatment with various doses of aminophylline (mean +/- standard error of 12 to 16 determinations).[52]

VI. REQUIREMENTS FOR DRUG APPROVAL

The Food and Drug Administration (FDA) has the responsibility to insure that the medications available to the public are safe and effective. These judgments are based on submissions of large data packages which contain the results of a variety of mandated tests as well as substance information. For a company to obtain approval for a new chemical entity (NCE), several requirements must be met. Initially (the pre-IND phase), research and development will lead to a promising candidate. This compound will be synthesized, analytical techniques developed for its characterization and detection, and limited bioavailability and metabolic studies will be run. Adherence to GLP's is also needed during this stage. The next step is to obtain an investigational new drug (IND) classification from the FDA for the candidate drug. For this to occur, a data package must be submitted. Animal safety and efficacy studies must be performed which evaluate the pharmacology, metabolism, pharmacokinetics, and toxicity of the drug. Toxicity studies include acute, subacute, and mutagenicity studies. Chronic toxicity studies as well as teratology and carcinogenicity evaluations are usually completed later and

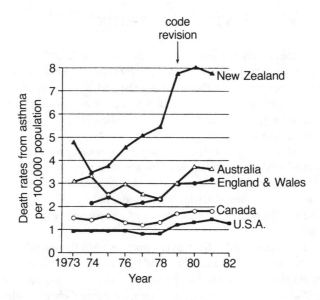

FIGURE 12. Mortality rates from asthma.[54]

included as part of the submission package to the FDA. The manufacturing and control processes for the drug must be documented. Synthesis in bulk is necessary, and formulation, manufacturing, and stability data are needed. Quality control data are also required, including reference standard data and specifications. Normally, the company would have acquired patent protection by this time.

The next step is to obtain clinical information on human safety and efficacy. In phase 1 of the IND, clinical pharmacology is determined. The drug doses are established using normal, healthy volunteers who are closely monitored in studies usually lasting less than 1 year. The drug's pharmacokinetics, metabolism, and bioavailability of the drug in man are characterized. Phase 2 involves clinical trials using populations for which the drug is intended. These studies should take place in established medical centers and should be well-controlled, well-designed studies performed by established investigators. Drug dosages are fine-tuned using this patient population. Following these studies, it may be advisable to meet with the FDA to review the data and examine protocols and the experimental design of the studies which are being proposed for the next stage, phase 3 clinical trials. In this phase, definitive efficacy and safety studies are performed. The affected patient population is used in multicenter studies to evaluate the utility of the drug. These studies are well-controlled and require that the drug formulation be well understood and stable. The data from these studies must yield good statistics, show a sound experimental design, and should include positive control results. When all studies are completed, the entire data package is submitted as a new drug application (NDA) to FDA for its review and subsequent approval or rejection of the NCE candidate.

In order to proceed effectively with an NDA, it is important to follow procedures which the FDA has established. For the new drug, emphasis should be on its bioavailability, the relative pharmacokinetics following different routes of administration, its systemic toxicity, histopathological findings, and data with appropriate statistics and proper controls. For a new administration route, there are no absolute guidelines in place. Comparison of efficacy with existing administration routes for existing entities is important. Specific guidelines can be established or modified if a good case can be made using sound scientific arguments. Again, use of statistics with appropriate controls is mandatory. Communicating with the FDA at any phase of the development process is encouraged, but especially regarding study design and data collection.[61,62]

VII. CONCLUSION

Toxicologic responses to inhaled aerosols are the result of undesirable interactions between the aerosols and the respiratory tract. The respiratory tract is a complex biological system which is composed of myriad cell types and therefore can respond in a variety of ways to the agents present in an aerosol formulation. Specific excipients in a formulation can be altered, following administration, to a more reactive form in the lung milieu. The pH and/or osmolarity of a formulation may also evoke a biological response.

The FDA is charged with responsibly evaluating therapeutic agents for efficacy and safety. Their evaluations are based on examination of information regarding the characteristics and behavior of a drug in its formulated state as well as examining its therapeutic effects following administration in a series of clinical trials. When approved by the FDA, the drug becomes available for public use. In general, the incidence of toxicologic responses to pharmaceutic aerosols is quite low.

The ideal aerosol system should deliver an accurate, optimal therapeutic drug dose and will be formulated in such a way that any excipients will be benign in the lung environment. The pH and osmolarity should closely match that of the airway lining layer. However, even for an ideal aerosol, a pragmatic observation made by Paracelsus, a medieval chemist who established the role of chemistry in medicine, should be kept in mind: "All substances are poisons; there is none which is not a poison. The right dose differentiates a poison and a remedy."

REFERENCES

1. **Hiller, C., Mazumder, M., Wilson, D., and Bone, R.,** Aerodynamic size distribution of metered-dose bronchodilator aerosols, *Am. Rev. Respir. Dis.,* 118, 311, 1978.
2. **Mercer, T. T., Goddard, R. F., and Flores, R. L.,** Output characteristics of several commercial nebulizers, *Ann. Allergy,* 23, 314, 1965.
3. **Mercer, T. T.,** *Aerosol Technology in Hazard Evaluation,* Academic Press, New York, 1973, 347.
4. **Davies, C. N.,** Deposition and retention of dust in the human respiratory tract, *Ann. Occup. Hyg.,* 7, 169, 1964.
5. **Lippmann, M. and Albert, R. E.,** The effect of particle size on the regional deposition of inhaled aerosols in the human respiratory tract, *Am. Ind. Hyg. Assoc. J.,* 30, 257, 1969.
6. **Morrow, P. E.,** Experimental studies of inhaled materials. A basis for respiratory models, *Arch. Int. Med.,* 126, 466, 1970.
7. Task Group on Lung Dynamics, Deposition and retention models for internal dosimetry of the human respiratory tract, *Health Phys.,* 12, 173, 1966.
8. **Clark, D. G.,** The toxicological evaluation of aerosols, in *Proc. Eur. Soc. Study of Drug Toxicol. XV. Experimental Model Systems in Toxicology and their Significance in Man,* Duncan, W. A. M., Ed., Excerpta Medica, Amsterdam, 1974, 252.
9. **Lehnert, B. E. and Schachter, E. N.,** *The Pharmacology of Respiratory Care,* C. V. Mosby, St. Louis, 1980, 69.
10. **Ariens, E. J.,** Adverse drug interactions. Interaction of drugs on the pharmacodynamic level, in *Proc. Eur. Soc. Study Drug Toxicol. XIII. Toxicological Problems of Drug Combinations,* Baker, S. B. de C. and Neuhaus, G. A., Eds., Excerpta Medica, Amsterdam, 1972, 137.
11. *PDR'S 1988 Index of Drug Interactions and Side-Effects,* Medical Economics Company, Inc., Oradell, NJ, 1988.
12. *Physicians' Desk Reference,* Medical Economics Company, Inc., Oradell, NJ, 1988.
13. **Clark, T. J. H.,** Safety of inhaled corticosteroids, *Eur. J. Resp. Dis.,* 63(Suppl.), 235, 1981.
14. **Dunlap, N. E. and Fulmer, J. D.,** Corticosteroid therapy in asthma, *Clin. Chest Med.,* 5, 669, 1984.
15. **Birdseye, S.,** Letter, *Med. J. Aust.,* 147, 469, 1987.
16. **Toogood, J. H., Jennings, B., Greenway, R. W., and Chuang, L.,** Candidiasis and dysphonia complicating beclomethasone treatment of asthma, *J. Allergy Clin. Immunol.,* 65, 145, 1980.
17. **Toogood, J. H., Baskerville, J., Jennings, B., Lefcoe, N. M., and Johansson, S.,** Use of spacers to facilitate inhaled corticosteroid treatment of asthma, *Am. Rev. Resp. Dis.,* 129, 723, 1984.

18. **Aviado, D. M. and Belej, M. A.,** Toxicity of aerosols, *J. Clin. Pharm.,* 15, 86, 1975.

19. **Aviado, D. M. and Smith, D. G.,** Toxicity of aerosol propellants in the respiratory and circulatory systems. VIII. Respiration and circulation in primates, *Toxicology,* 3, 241, 1975.

20. **Aviado, D. M. and Dremal, J.,** Five fluorocarbons for administration of aerosol bronchodilators, *J. Clin. Pharm.,* 15, 116, 1975.

21. **Belej, M. A. and Aviado, D. M.,** Cardiopulmonary toxicity of propellants for aerosols, *J. Clin. Pharmacol.,* 15, 105, 1975.

22. **Clark, D. G. and Tinston, T. J.,** The influence of fluorocarbon propellants on the arrhythmogenic potential of adrenaline and isoprenaline, in *Proceedings of the European Society for the Study of Drug Toxicology XIII: Toxicological Problems of Drug Combinations,* Baker, S. B. de C. and Neuhaus, G. A., Eds., Excerpta Medica, Amsterdam, 1972, 212.

23. **Dollery, C. T., Williams, F. M., Draffan, G. H., Wise, G., Sahyoun, H., Paterson, J. W., and Walker, S. R.,** Arterial blood levels of fluorocarbons in asthmatic patients following use of pressurized aerosols, *Clin. Pharmacol. Ther.,* 15, 59, 1974.

24. **Beasley, R., Rafferty, P., and Holgate, S.,** Letter — benzalkonium chloride and bronchoconstriction, *Lancet,* 2(8517), 1227, 1986.

25. **Shim, C. S. and Williams, M. H.,** Cough and wheezing from beclomethasone dipropionate aerosol are absent after triamcinolone acetonide, *Ann. Intern. Med.,* 106, 700, 1987.

26. **Bryant, D. H. and Pepys, J.,** Bronchial reactions to aerosol inhalant vehicle, *Br. Med. J.,* 1, 1319, 1976.

27. **Yarbrough, J., Mansfield, L. E., and Ting, S.,** Metered dose inhaler induced bronchospasm in asthmatic patients, *Ann. Allergy,* 55, 25, 1985.

28. **Fine, J. M., Gordon, T., and Sheppard, D.,** The roles of pH and ionic species in sulfur dioxide- and sulfite-induced bronchoconstriction, *Am. Rev. Resp. Dis.,* 136, 1122, 1987.

29. **Sher, T. H. and Schwartz, H. J.,** Bisulfite sensitivity manifesting as an allergic reaction to aerosol therapy, *Ann. Allergy,* 54, 224, 1985.

30. **Chen, L. C., Lam, H. F., Ainsworth, D., Guty, J., and Amdur, M. O.,** Functional changes in the lungs of guinea pigs exposed to sodium sulfite aerosols, *Toxicol. Appl. Pharmacol.,* 89, 1, 1987.

31. **Koepke, J. W., Staudenmayer, H., and Selner, J. C.,** Inhaled metabisulfite sensitivity, *Ann. Allergy,* 54, 213, 1985.

32. **Koepke, J. W., Selner, J. C., and Dunhill, A. L.,** Presence of sulfur dioxide in commonly used bronchodilator solutions, *J. Allergy Clin. Immunol.,* 72, 504, 1983.

33. **Witek, T. J. and Schachter, E. N.,** Detection of sulfur dioxide in bronchodilator aerosols, *Chest,* 86, 592, 1984.

34. **Godden, D. J., Borland, C. Lowry, R., and Higgenbottam, T. W.,** Chemical specificity of coughing in man, *Clin. Sci.,* 70, 301, 1986.

35. **Higgenbottam, T.,** Cough induced by changes of ionic composition of airway surface liquid, *Clin. Resp. Physiol.,* 20, 553, 1984.

36. **Higgenbottam, T.,** Anticholinergics and cough, *Postgrad. Med. J.,* 63(Suppl. 1b), 75, 1987.

37. **Fine, J. M., Gordon, T.,** Thompson, J. E., and Sheppard, D., The role of titratable acidity in acid aerosol-induced bronchoconstriction, *Am. Rev. Resp. Dis.,* 135, 826, 1987.

38. **Schanker, L. S. and Less, M. J.,** Lung pH and pulmonary absorption of nonvolatile drugs in the rat, *Drug Metab. Dispos.,* 5, 174, 1977.

39. **Finney, M. J. B., Anderson, S. D., and Black, J. L.,** The effect of non-isotonic solutions on human isolated airway smooth muscle, *Resp. Physiol.,* 69, 277, 1987.

40. **Belcher, N. G., Rees, P. J., Clark, T. I. H., and Lee, T. H.,** A comparison of the refractory periods induced by hypertonic airway challenge and exercise in bronchial asthma, *Am. Rev. Resp. Dis.,* 135, 822, 1987.

41. **Mattoli, S., Foresi, A., Corbo, G. M., Valente, S., Patalano, F., and Ciappi, G.,** Increase in bronchial responsiveness to methacholine and late asthmatic response after the inhalation of ultrasonically nebulized distilled water, *Chest,* 90, 726, 1986.

42. **Bascom, R. and Bleecker, E. R.,** Bronchoconstriction induced by distilled water, *Am. Rev. Resp. Dis.,* 134, 248, 1986.

43. **Schoeffel, R. E., Anderson, S. D., and Altounyan, R. E.,** Bronchial hyperreactivity in response to inhalation of ultrasonically nebulized solutions of distilled water and saline, *Br. Med. J.,* 283, 1285, 1981.

44. **Boushey, H. A.,** Bronchial challenge by physical agents, *Clin. Rev. Allergy,* 3, 411, 1985.

45. **Higgenbottam, T., Borland, C., Barber, B., and Chamberlain, A.,** Pulmonary epithelial permeability after inhaled distilled water "fog", *Chest,* 87(Suppl.), 156S, 1985.

46. **Smith, C. M., Anderson, S. D., and Black, J. L.,** Methacholine responsiveness increases after ultrasonically nebulized water but not after ultrasonically nebulized hypertonic saline in patients with asthma, *J. Allergy Clin. Immunol.,* 79, 85, 1987.

47. **Eggleston, P. A., Kagey-Sobotka, A., Schleimer, R. P., and Lichtenstein, L. M.,** Interaction between hyperosmolar and IgE-mediated histamine release from basophils and mast cells, *Am. Rev. Resp. Dis.,* 130, 86, 1984.

48. **Findlay, S. R. and Lichtenstein, L. M.,** Basophil "releasability" in patients with asthma, *Am. Rev. Resp. Dis.,* 122, 53, 1980.
49. **Boucher, R. C., Stutts, M. J., Bromberg, P. A., and Gatzy, J. T.,** Regional differences in airway surface liquid composition, *J. Appl. Physiol.,* 50, 613, 1981.
50. **Allegra, L. and Bianco, S.,** Non-specific broncho-reactivity obtained with an ultrasonic aerosol of distilled water, *Eur. J. Resp. Dis.,* 61(Suppl. 106), 41, 1980.
51. **Sutton, P. P., Pavia, D., Bateman, J. R. M., and Clarke, S. W.,** The effect of oral aminophylline on lung mucociliary clearance in man, *Chest,* 80(Suppl.), 889, 1981.
52. **Nelson, S., Summer, W. R., and Jakab, G. J.,** Aminophylline-induced suppression of pulmonary antibacterial defenses, *Am. Rev. Resp. Dis.,* 131, 923, 1985.
53. **Netter, F. H.,** *Respiratory System,* Vol. 7, Sect. IV, Plate 15, CIBA Collection of Medical Illustrations, CIBA Pharmaceutical, Summit, NJ, 1979.
54. **Sly, R. M.,** Increases in deaths from asthma, *Ann. Allergy,* 53, 20, 1984.
55. British Thoracic Society, Death from asthma in two regions of England, *Br. Med. J.,* 285, 1251, 1982.
56. **Esdaile, J. M., Feinstein, A. R., and Horwitz, R. I.,** A reappraisal of the United Kingdom epidemic of fatal asthma. Can general mortality data implicate a therapeutic agent?, *Arch. Intern. Med.,* 147, 543, 1987.
57. **Jackson, R. T., Beaglehole, R., Rea, H. H., and Sutherland, D. C.,** Mortality from asthma: a new epidemic in New Zealand, *Br. Med. J.,* 285, 771, 1982.
58. **Keating, G., Mitchell, E. A., Jackson, R., Beaglehole, R., and Rea, H.,** Trends in sales of drugs for asthma in New Zealand, Australia, and the United Kingdom, 1975-81, *Br. Med. J.,* 289(6441), 348, 1984.
59. **Speizer, F. E., Doll, R., and Heaf, P.,** Observations on recent increases in mortality from asthma, *Br. Med. J.,* 1, 335, 1968.
60. Proc. Asthma Mortality Task Force, Sheffer, A. L., Buist, A. S., Eds., *J. Allergy Clin. Immunol.,* 80(Spec. issue), 1987.
61. **Doyle, M.,** personal communication, 1988.
62. **McRight, A.,** personal communication, 1988.

Chapter 3

DRUG APPLICATION TO THE RESPIRATORY TRACT: METABOLIC AND PHARMACOKINETIC CONSIDERATIONS

Peter A. Crooks and Lyaquatali A. Damani

TABLE OF CONTENTS

I. INTRODUCTION

The respiratory system is subdivided, for descriptive purposes only, into the "upper respiratory tract" consisting of the nose, nasopharynx, and larynx and the "lower respiratory tract" comprising the trachea, bronchi, and the lungs. Formulations may be designed for delivering drugs to one or both of these sites, either for local action or for systemic effects. It is clearly important to have an idea of the likely contribution of different parts of the respiratory tract to metabolism of such drugs during their contact and/or absorption from areas of application, since this may ultimately influence drug effect. Unfortunately, most of the data in the literature at present are confined to the pulmonary system, i.e., the lower respiratory tract. The general picture emerging is that the lungs play an important role in the biotransformation of certain classes of drugs, irrespective of whether exposure to lung tissue is via the alveolus (i.e., inhaled drugs) or via the pulmonary vasculature (i.e., drugs in the systemic circulation). The upper respiratory tract appears to be less important insofar as metabolism during absorption is concerned. However, this view is based on limited experimentation, and more detailed studies are required to elucidate the metabolizing capabilities of cells in the nasal mucosa. In view of the disproportionate information in the literature, this review is based largely on "pulmonary metabolism" — this is not a personal bias but a constraint placed on the authors by the limited data available.

By way of introduction, prior to reading this review on metabolism in the respiratory tract, an understanding of certain aspects of respiratory system physiology and pathology is essential, and the reader is encouraged to read appropriate texts on those subjects. In addition to this introduction, this review is divided into nine other parts: an overview of drug metabolism for the benefit of those not familiar with basic concepts in this scientific discipline (Section II); a discussion of extrahepatic metabolism, to define the scope of the problem insofar as the respiratory tract is concerned (Section III); a description of the drug metabolizing capabilities of the respiratory tract, particularly the nature of the enzyme activities detected and their location in specific cell types, if known (Section IV and V); Section VI deals with drug accumulation and/or clearance in the lungs when drug application is at a point distant to the respiratory system, and where exposure is therefore via the respiratory vasculature; the next two sections will address absorption (Section VII), metabolism, and pharmacokinetics of drugs administered directly to the respiratory tract (Section VIII); a section on the metabolism and absorption of peptides administered to respiratory tissues is also included (Section IX); a concluding section follows (Section X).

II. DRUG METABOLISM — AN OVERVIEW

A. DEFINITIONS

Drugs and other foreign compounds are often collectively called "xenobiotics", and the term "drug or xenobiotic metabolism" is almost invariably used in its strictest meaning of biotransformation, that is, structural alterations to xenobiotics mediated by endogenous enzyme systems. In its broadest meaning, drug metabolism is taken to include the processes of absorption, distribution, biotransformation, and elimination, and it suits the purpose of the present reviewers to use this wider definition to include other aspects (e.g., pharmacokinetics). Biochemical alterations of lipophilic drugs to polar metabolites are essential in order to facilitate their elimination from the body, and a group of enzymes collectively called the drug metabolizing enzymes, appear to act primarily in preparing drugs for rapid excretion. Drug biotransformations occur predominantly in the liver, but extrahepatic sites such as the skin, lungs, gastrointestinal tract, etc., are also important in many cases (see Section III).

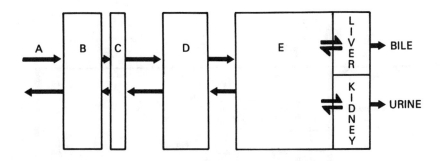

FIGURE 1. Diagrammatic representation of drug absorption from "external" surfaces, e.g., the respiratory membrane (see text in Section III.A).

B. DRUG METABOLISM PATHWAYS

Drug metabolism is a biphasic process with most drugs undergoing an initial phase I or functionalization reaction followed by a phase II or conjugation reaction. The former may be an oxidation, reduction or hydrolytic reaction, usually resulting in the introduction or unmasking of a reactive functional group (e.g., -OH, $-NH_2$, -COOH). Phase II pathways involve reaction of the phase I metabolites with endogenous molecules (e.g., glucuronic acid, sulfate), to generate highly polar, water-soluble conjugates which can readily be eliminated from the body. Enzyme systems mediating drug biotransformations are located at various subcellular sites, e.g., the cytosol, mitochondria, and smooth endoplasmic reticulum. Enzymes on the endoplasmic reticulum are called mixed function oxidases or monooxygenases, and have deservedly received considerable attention from investigators in the last 2 decades in view of their importance in detoxication, and in some instances of toxication reactions via reactive intermediate formation. The scientific literature devoted to drug metabolism has increased in recent years and readers who feel the need for additional enlightenment are referred to *Introduction to Drug Metabolism* by Gibson and Skett[1] and to the earlier classic, *Drug Metabolism: Chemical and Biochemical Aspects* by Testa and Jenner.[2]

The major emphasis throughout the rest of this chapter is on pulmonary metabolism, the capacity of the lungs to carry out drug biotransformations. This knowledge is useful for two reasons: (1) an understanding of metabolic and pharmacokinetic factors is useful in the design of drugs for targeting to the respiratory tract and (2) drug or chemical toxicity to the lung can often be explained by selective metabolic activation within specific cell types.

III. EXTRAHEPATIC DRUG METABOLISM

A. METABOLISM AT SITES OF DRUG APPLICATION

The sites of extrahepatic drug metabolism are often the portals of entry or excretion of the body: the lungs, kidney, skin, and gastrointestinal mucosa.[3] Cells in such sites have been demonstrated to possess almost all the drug metabolizing enzymes that are present in hepatic cells, albeit in much lower concentrations. The rate and total capacity of extrahepatic drug metabolism is generally considered to be much lower than in the liver, but nonetheless biotransformation at such sites may have an important influence on the ultimate fate and effect of the drug.

When drugs are administered by the more common routes, such as the dermal, gastrointestinal or respiratory routes, they inevitably come into contact with various epithelial cell types during absorption from these sites. A simple diagrammatical representation of drug absorption from such external surfaces is depicted in Figure 1. A is the site of drug application, which may, for example, be the respiratory membrane; B represents the anatomic barrier, comprised of one

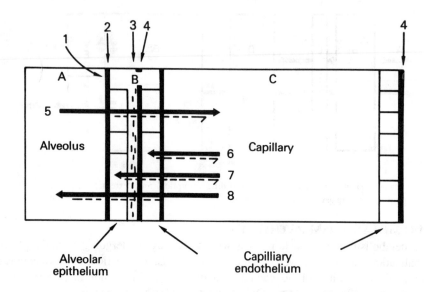

FIGURE 2.   Diagrammatic representation of the ultrastructure of the respiratory membrane (see text in Sections III.C and III.D for key to 1 to 8). Arrows indicate passage of drugs (horizontal dotted line) through the respiratory membrane after alveolar or capillary exposure, or of metabolites (vertical dotted line) generated in the epithelial or endothelial layers.

or several layers of various epithelial cell types; C is the vasculature associated with this membrane; D is the systemic circulation; and E represents the body tissues and organs. Drug passage across the anatomic barrier may occur by one of several mechanisms (passive diffusion, facilitated transport, active transport, etc.) into the circulatory system followed by transport to various tissues and organs. The reverse may occur in some instances, e.g., elimination of volatile gaseous anesthetics into expired air. In general, drugs that enter the systemic circulation undergo metabolism in the liver, and the metabolites are excreted via urine or bile. However, drugs are confronted with a variety of drug metabolizing enzymes at extrahepatic sites. Although the enzymes in most such tissues are generally present at a much lower concentration than in the liver, their contribution to overall drug metabolism in many cases is significant. This may be due to a variety of factors, e.g., organ size or area, rate of blood flow, period of contact with metabolizing cells, etc.

B. FIRST-PASS METABOLISM

Many drugs undergo what is referred to as first-pass metabolism on transit through unit B-C (Figure 1). The term "first-pass metabolism" was originally used to describe hepatic first-pass metabolism for drugs administered orally, rectally, or by peritoneal injection. It is now recognized that a gastrointestinal or pulmonary first-pass effect may also preclude a significant fraction of the administered drug from reaching peripheral circulation. If the drug effect is required at the site of application, then this metabolism, and presumably pharmacological inactivation, is an advantage in that it limits total drug exposure to localized sites (see Section VIII for further discussion and examples). The central theme of this review is the description of the events that occur at unit B-C in Figure 1 insofar as the respiratory tract is concerned. Whereas full details of metabolism at different sites of the respiratory tract are lacking, a considerable amount of information has accumulated for the lungs.

C. ULTRASTRUCTURE OF THE RESPIRATORY MEMBRANE

The unique features of the lung which bring it into such close contact with the environment are illustrated in Figure 2, which is a diagrammatic representation of the ultrastructure of the respiratory membrane. (*Note:* Figure 2 is essentially a more detailed version of unit B-C in Figure 1.) The respiratory membrane consists of two main layers. (a) The first is the alveolar epithelium which is comprised of at least three different cell types, alveolar type I, II and III or brush cells, in addition to the migratory alveolar macrophages. The epithelial layer has a thin fluid film (2, Figure 2), which itself is covered with a monomolecular layer of surfactant (1). (b) The capillary endothelium with its capillary basement membrane (4), separated from the epithelium by an interstitial space (3) is the second layer. What makes the respiratory membrane unique is the fact that despite the large number of layers (see Figure 2), the overall thickness is less than 1 μm, and in some areas it is as low as 0.1 μm. Since the average diameter of the pulmonary capillaries is only about 7 μm, the red blood cells (average diameter 8 μm) must actually squeeze through the capillaries. Such an arrangement, therefore, brings the membrane of the red blood cell into close contact with the respiratory membrane, allowing diffusion of oxygen in one direction and carbon dioxide in the other.

D. ALVEOLAR AND VASCULAR EXPOSURE OF THE LUNGS TO DRUGS

The architecture represented in Figure 2, in addition to allowing gaseous exchange, also allows the entry of potential toxicants via the alveolus (5, Figure 2), because of the direct contact between the environmental air and the functional elements of the lungs. The kind of hazardous materials which can find their way into the lungs include (1) gases and vapor, (2) particulate matter, e.g., inorganic dusts or organic materials, and (3) xenobiotics, including drugs that are intentionally targeted to this area (see Tables 1 and 2).

Exposure to lung tissue can also occur via the vasculature. It is important to realize that venous drainage from virtually the entire body perfuses through the alveolar-capillary unit. Xenobiotics that have found their way into the circulation at sites distant to the lungs are therefore brought into very close contact with lung tissues because of the unique facilities that have evolved for gaseous exchange. Unionized lipophilic drugs can be transferred from the circulation to cells of the capillary endothelium (6, Figure 2), or to cells of the alveolar epithelium (7), or may even by transferred through these layers to the alveolar air (8), and therefore eliminated in the expired air (see Figure 2). Certain endogenous and exogenous compounds (e.g., basic amines) are also selectively taken up in pulmonary tissues by mechanisms other than simple passive diffusion (see Section VI).

The lung also serves as an organ of excretion for certain classes of drugs (e.g., volatile anesthetics). As such, the lung may be exposed to a higher concentration of the compound for a longer time period. It is, therefore, not surprising that the lung has developed a biochemical defense mechanism to protect itself against such chemical insults. One form of this defense is drug biotransformation. Lungs, therefore, do not play a passive role in drug handling. They can and do influence the biological activities of inhaled and circulating drugs and other xenobiotics as subsequent sections of this review demonstrate.

E. DRUGS TARGETED TO THE RESPIRATORY TRACT

A survey of the data summarized in Tables 1 and 2 reveals that by far the majority of the drugs targeted to the respiratory tract are applied for their local action, e.g., nasal decongestion, bronchodilation, etc. The lining of the upper respiratory tract (i.e., nasal mucosa) and the airways may also be used for absorption of a compound for its systemic effect (see Section VIII). This is an area that has attracted a considerable amount of attention, and numerous studies have demonstrated that drugs can be administered systemically by application to the respiratory tract, either to the nasal mucosa or to the lungs. However, apart from the use of anesthetic gases and the occasional use of antidiabetic hormonal preparations via this route, no other drugs are at present administered systemically via the respiratory tract. Even with the limited number of drugs applied to the respiratory tract (see Tables 1 and 2), the role of the target organ in the metabolism of such compounds is not known in all cases. Indeed, comparative pharmacokinetic

TABLE 1
Drugs Applied to the Respiratory Tract for Their Local Action

Drug type	Generic name	Proprietary name(s)
A. Bronchodilators (inhalational preparations)		
1. β_2-adrenoceptor stimulants		
(selective)	Salbutamol	Ventolin
	Terbutaline sulfate	Bricanyl
	Rimiterol hydrobromide	Pulmadil
	Fenoterol hydrobromide	Berotec
	Pirbuterol	Exirel
	Reproterol hydrochloride	Bronchodil
(nonselective)	Epinephrine	Medihaler-Epi
	Isoproterenol	Medihaler-Iso
	Orciprenaline	Alupent
2. Anticholinergic bronchodilators		
	Ipratropium bromide	Atrovent
	Atropine methonitrate	Eumydrin
B. Corticosteroids (inhalational preparations)		
	Beclomethasone dipropionate	Becotide
	Beclomethasone dipropionate (nasal)	Beconase
	Betamethasone valerate	Bextasol
	Budesonide	Pulmicort
	Budesonide (nasal aerosol)	Rhinocort
	Flunisolide (nasal spray)	Syntaris
C. Prophylactic antiasthmatics (inhalational preparations)		
	Sodium cromoglycate	Intal
	Sodium cromoglycate (nasal insufflation, drops, and spray)	Rynacrom
D. Topical nasal decongestants and antihistamines (nasal drops and sprays)		
	Ephedrine hydrochloride	—
	Oxymetazoline hydrochloride	Afrazine
	Phenylephrine hydrochloride	Neophryn
	Xylometazoline hydrochloride	Otrivine
E. Inhalation mucolytics (nebulized solutions)		
	Acetylcysteine	Airbron
	Tyloxapol	Alevaire
F. Vapors and inhalations		
	Benzoin tincture	—
	Menthol and benzoin inhalation	—
	Menthol and eucalyptus inhalation	—
G. Anti-infective nasal preparations		
	Various compound preparations (drops, creams, inhalations)	Naseptin, Betnesol-N Dexa-Rhinaspray, Locabiotal

data after oral, intravenous, intrabronchial, and inhalational administration is available for only a few of the compounds listed in Table 1 (see Section VIII for further discussion). The data in Tables 1 and 2 have been compiled from information in the British National Formulary (July 1986), and do not therefore include nebulized antibiotics, e.g., mixtures of carbenicillin and

TABLE 2
Drugs Applied to the Respiratory Tract for Absorption and Systemic Effects

Drug type	Generic name	Proprietary name(s)
A. Inhalation anesthetics (gases)		
	Halothane	Fluothane
	Enflurane	Alyrane, Ethrane
	Isoflurane	Aerrane, Forane
	Trichloroethylene	Trilene
	Cyclopropane	—
	Diethylether	—
	Nitrous oxide	—
B. Antidiabetic hormonal preparations (insufflations, nasal sprays and solutions)		
	Posterior pituitary lobe	Di-Sipidin
	Desmopressin	DDAVP
	Lypressin	Syntopressin
C. Insulin and other polypeptides		
	Experimental stage — no products on market as yet (see text)	
D. Steroids and other drugs subject to significant first-pass metabolism		
	Experimental stage — no products on market as yet (see text)	

gentamicin, prophylatic agents such as ketotifen, clemastine, prostaglandins, local anesthetics, surfactants, and vaccines against influenza and tuberculosis.[4]

IV. DRUG-METABOLIZING ENZYMES IN RESPIRATORY TISSUES

Pulmonary drug- and xenobiotic-metabolizing enzymes function primarily to protect the lung against chemical insult, thus reducing the residence time of the xenobiotic in the pulmonary tissue, by forming polar products generally possessing lower pharmacological or toxological activity that can be rapidly cleared. It is remarkable that prior to 1970, very little was known about the drug-metabolizing capabilities of the lung.[5] Subsequent studies[6,7] have shown that, as is the case with hepatic drug-metabolizing enzymes, the lung enzymes generally have characteristically broad substrate specificity, which is due to their existence in several isozymic forms; lung enzymes also have relatively high K_m values, compared to the K_m of pulmonary enzymes involved in intermediary metabolism. Thus, lung-metabolizing enzymes usually function below saturating concentrations of substrate under normal circumstances.

Metabolism of a xenobiotic in the lung will usually lead to the formation of more than one metabolite, and the metabolic profile will be dependent on a number of factors, such as: relative ease of access of the xenobiotic to the active site of a particular enzyme, availability of co-factors involved in the enzyme mechanism, physicochemical properties of the enzyme (i.e., V_{max}, K_m), and possible competition at the active site with other exogenous and possible endogenous substrates and with inhibitors, inducers, or activators of the enzyme activity. Other factors influencing the nature of xenobiotic metabolites formed in the lung are age, health, and cell type. The latter is of some importance with respect to drug delivery, and is discussed in Section V. In addition, metabolic profile may vary with dose.

Almost all the major xenobiotic metabolizing enzymes have been detected in both the lung and the nasal cavity in several animal species. Table 3 gives characteristics such as subcellular location, co-factor requirements, substrate type, and known inducers and inhibitors of xenobiotic-metabolizing enzymes in the lung. Of these, cytochrome P-450 and flavin-containing monooxygenases, epoxide hydrolases, esterases, dehydrogenases, and the phase II enzymes introduce, uncover, or transfer water-soluble groups to the xenobiotic substrate, thus aiding their excretion via the kidney.

V. LOCALIZATION OF DRUG-METABOLIZING ENZYMES IN THE RESPIRATORY TRACT

A. UPPER RESPIRATORY TRACT

The division between the upper and lower airways may be taken as the junction of the larynx and trachea. The nasal vestibule or entrance is lined by skin (with sebaceous glands and strong hairs), whereas elsewhere the nasal epithelium is comprised of columnar ciliated and nonciliated, basal, and goblet cells. The olfactory epithelium is located in the upper part of the nasal cavity and appears to possess drug-metabolizing enzymes. There is a transition from columnar ciliated to stratified squamous epithelium in the nasopharynx and larynx. The above description serves to emphasize the complex nature of the linings of the upper airways and the heterogeneity of the cell types. Only recently have detailed studies been carried out on the metabolizing capabilities of the nose, nasopharynx, and larynx. This work has shown that cytochrome P-450 is present in the nasal area. Interestingly, for some subtrates the tissues in the nasal cavity have greater metabolic activities on a per gram tissue basis than the lung or even the liver. The cytochrome P-450 activity present within the nasal cavity appears to be nonuniformly distributed.

The olfactory epithelium is far more easy to study than the respiratory epithelium because of the more localized and organ-like structure of the former. The olfactory epithelium of several species contains cytochrome P-450 and is capable of metabolizing drugs.[8] Interestingly, although the levels of cytochrome P-450 are lower than in liver, the specific activities, when expressed as product formed per unit time per nanomole P-450, are much higher in the olfactory epithelium.[9] The physiological significance of this insofar as olfaction is concerned is unknown, but the total drug-metabolizing capacity is unlikely to be significant in view of the very small size of the olfactory region in man. Nevertheless, with regard to the use of the nasal cavity as a portal of entry for systemic drugs, this may be an important factor to consider. In this respect, it is important to note that the olfactory mucosa usually possesses higher activities of cytochrome P-450 than the respiratory mucosa, and this difference in activity is also observed for other drug-metabolizing enzymes.[10] Flavin-containing monooxygenase activity is high in the nasal ethmoturbinates of rabbit respiratory tract in the area of the olfactory mucosa, having amounts exceeding those found in the liver;[11] epoxide hydrolase activity has also been reported in the nasal cavity.[12] The olfactory mucosa has been shown to contain a higher carboxylesterase activity than in nasal mucosa, the former activity being mainly located in the sustentacular cells and the acinar cells of Bowman's glands.[13,14]

Two isozymes of aldehyde hydrogenase (aldehyde dehydrogenase I and II) and formaldehyde dehydrogenase have been detected in the nasal cavity.[15] The specific activities of aldehyde dehydrogenase II and formaldehyde dehydrogenase in homogenates of olfactory epithelia were higher than in respiratory epithelial homogenates.

The phase II enzymes, which include glucuronyl transferases, glutathione transferases and sulfate transferases have been detected in rat nasal tissue, however, their activities may be dependent upon the activated co-factor in these tissues.[12,16] Recent immunohistochemical techniques in combination with enzyme histochemistry have shown that Bowman's gland contains the greatest amounts of cytochromes P-450 BNF-B and MC-B, whereas cytochrome

TABLE 3
Characteristics of Xenobiotic-Metabolizing Enzymes in the Lung[7]

Enzyme system	Subcellular location	Co-factor and other requirements	Type of substrate	Inducers	Inhibitors
Phase I					
Cytochrome P-450	Endoplasmic reticulum	$NADPH+O_2$	Numerous	Rat: 3-MC, TCDD, PCBs, Rabbit: unresponsive	α-Naphthoflavone
Amine oxidase (flavin-containing monoxygenase)	Endoplasmic reticulum	$NADPH+O_2$	Secondary and tertiary amines, sulfur compounds	—	Piperonyl butoxide
Reductase	Endoplasmic reticulum	NADPH/NADH	Cytochrome P-450, azodyes, paraquat	—	—
Epoxide hydrolase	Endoplasmic reticulum	Water	Epoxides	Rabbit: phenobarbitone, 3-MC Unresponsive	1,2-Epoxy-3,3,3 trichloropropane
Esterase	Inclusion bodies, vacuoles	Water	Esters, amides thioesters	—	—
Phase 2					
Glucuronyl transferase	Endoplasmic reticulum	UDP-glucuronic acid	Phenols, thiols, amines carboxylic acids	Rat: 3-MC, TCDD Rabbit: unresponsive	—
Sulfotransferase	Cytosol	PAPS	Phenols	—	—
N-Acetyltransferase	Cytosol	Acetyl CoA	Amines	—	—
Methyltransferase	Cytosol	S-Adenosyl methionine	Catechols, phenols, thiols	—	—
Glutathione S-transferase	Cytosol	Glutathione	Electrophiles	Rat: phenobarbitone Rabbit: unresponsive	—
Monoamine oxidase	Mitochondria	O_2	Monoamines	—	Propargylamines, cyclopropylamines, hydrazines
Alcohol dehydrogenase	Cytosol	NAD	Primary, secondary and poly alcohols	—	Pyrazoles imidazoles

TABLE 3 (continued)
Characteristics of Xenobiotic-Metabolizing Enzymes in the Lung[7]

Enzyme system	Subcellular location	Co-factor and other requirements	Type of substrate	Inducers	Inhibitors
Aldehyde dehydrogenase	Cytosol, mitochondria, endoplasmic reticulum	NAD or flavine	Most aldehydes	Phenobarbitone, TCDD-induced cytosolic isozyme	Disulfiram, cyanamide
Aldehyde reductase	Cytosol	NADPH	Most aldehydes + some ketones	—	Barbiturates, flavonoids
Ketone reductase	Cytosol	NADPH	Ketones + some aldehydes	—	—
Xanthine oxidase	Cytosol	FAD, H_2O	Purines + other heterocyclics	—	Cyanide
Aldehyde oxidase	Cytosol	FAD, H_2O	Similar to xanthine oxidase	—	Cyanide, nonionic detergents, estradiol progesterone
Superoxide dismutase	Cytosol, mitochondria	—	$O_2^{\cdot-}$	Redox-active compounds, increased PO_2	—
Prostaglandin synthetase	Endoplasmic reticulum	Arachidonic acid O_2	Co-oxidation of aromatic amines etc.	—	Indomethacin, aspirin
Glutathione peroxidase	Cytosol, mitochondria	Glutathione	H_2O_2, organic hydroperoxides	—	—

| Catalase | Peroxisomes | — | H$_2$O$_2$ | — |
| Rhodanese | Mitochondria | Thiosulfate or sulfite | Cyanide, inorganic sulfides | — |

Abbreviations: 3-MC, 3-methylcholanthrene; PCB, polychlorinated biphenyl; TCDD, 2,3,7,8-tetrachlorodibenzo-*p*-dioxin.

P-450 PB-B is concentrated to the greatest extent within respiratory ephithelial cells, and cytochrome P-450 PCN-E is distributed quite uniformly throughout the nasal mucosa.[17] The authors comment that the olfactory region exhibits significantly greater monooxygenase activity than does the respiratory region and appears to represent the major site for the oxidative metabolism of xenobiotics in the untreated rat nasal cavity. In the same study, identical amounts of glutathione-S-transferase E were found in the olfactory and respiratory epithelia, however, the olfactory region contained the greatest amounts of NADPH-cytochrome P-450 reductase and glutathione-S-transferase B, and the respiratory region contained the highest levels of epoxide hydrolase and glutathione-S-transferase C.

Some reports have described studies which suggest a low drug-metabolizing ability of the nasal mucosa. These data come mostly from *in vivo* studies comparing plasma levels of drugs after oral, nasal, and intravenous adminstration. Drugs such as propranolol, which suffer an extensive gastrointestinal and hepatic first-pass metabolism after oral administration, are rapidly absorbed unmetabolized after intranasal administration.[18] The AUCs after equivalent intravenous and nasal doses of propranolol are identical, indicating the efficiency and rapidity of absorption from the nasal mucosa. Several other studies of this nature give circumstantial evidence of the lower capacity of the nasal mucosa for biotransformation. In view of the fact that a large proportion of inhaled particulate matter is trapped in the nasal cavity by inertial impaction, it would be surprising if the epithelial cell layer has not evolved a biochemical defense in the form of metabolizing enzymes.

Future studies will need to focus on the complete characterization of the enzyme activities at different sites in the upper airways and their localization within specific cell types in man. This is important for two reasons; first, this information may provide an explanation of the higher rates of nasal tumors from certain classes of chemicals,[19] and second, these data will allow an estimation of the total capacity of this organ for drug clearance. The latter will, of course, be of prime importance if the nasal mucosa is to be used as a target for systemic drug delivery (see Section VIII.A).

B. LOWER RESPIRATORY TRACT

The lower respiratory tract may be divided into the tracheobronchiolar, bronchiolar, and alveolar regions. In general terms, the airways are lined by pseudostratified columnar ciliated epithelium, beneath which are mucus glands, connective tissue, cartilage, smooth muscle, and nerves. The trancheobronchiolar region consists of pseudostratified epithelium and comprises at least ten cell types in man,[20] these being basal, ciliated, mucus, serous, Clara, "special type", intermediate, brush cells, Kultschitsky, and migratory lymphocyte cells. Cytochrome P-450 activities are distributed throughout the tracheobronchial region, although they are apparently not highly concentrated in a few cells, as is the case for the lower portion of the lung.[21] Interestingly, in the rabbit, flavin-containing monooxygenase activity appears to be absent in the larynx and trachea, whereas in the carina, the conducting airways, and the pulmonary and small airway portion of the lungs, activities of this enzyme are comparable or exceed those found in the liver.[22] Esterase activity can be detected in the trachea of the Syrian hamster, however, the activity is lower than that observed in the maxillo and ethmo regions of the nasal cavity. Aldehyde dehydrogenase activity is relatively low in the tracheal epithelial cells compared to lung levels.[15] From immunohistochemical studies[17,23] it has been shown that cytochromes P-450 PB-B and PCN-E, NADPH-cytochrome P-450 reductase, epoxide hydrolase, and glutathione-S-transferases B, C, and E have relatively high activities in tracheal epithelial cells, thus demonstrating that the tracheal epithelium represents another site within the respiratory tract at which xenobiotics can be oxidatively metabolized, epoxides can be hydrated, and electrophiles can be enzymatically conjugated with reduced glutathione.

The bronchiolar region is characterized by the presence of a columnar epithelium comprising mainly two types of cells: the ciliated and the Clara cells. The latter are among the more metabolically active cells in the lungs and have a high concentration of cytochrome P-450, although monooxygenase activity is present in other epithelial cell types.[24,25] This region of the conducting airways also has significant flavin-containing monooxygenase activity and the distal bronchioles have high levels of aldehyde dehydrogenase located in the Clara cells.

The alveolar region or the respiratory unit consists of three cell types, type I pneumonocytes (thin-flattened cells), type II pneumonocytes (cuboidal cells), and brush alveolar or type III cells. In addition this region has the migratory alveolar macrophages. Type I and II cells have been demonstrated to possess monooxygenase activity, and this is a partial explanation of the site-specific toxicity of certain chemicals.[26]

The above data emphasize the complex nature of the lower respiratory tract. In fact, over *40 different cell types* are encountered depending on the animal species. In addition, the endothelial and smooth muscle cells of the pulmonary vasculature may also contribute to drug biotransformation.[27] Almost all the drug-metabolizing enzymic activities detected in the liver have now been detected in the lung, albeit at much lower levels.[28-31] The lung can therefore carry out monooxygenations mediated by cytochrome P-450 and by the flavin-containing monooxygenase system, and it can reduce, hydrolyze, and conjugate most substrates.[32] Interestingly, not all the isozymes of P-450 seen in the liver are observed in the lung[33] and this may account for the qualitative differences in metabolism between these two organs. Immunohistochemical and histochemical studies generally confirm that the bronchus, bronchiole, and alveolar wall are the major sites for xenobiotic metabolism within the lung.[17] Results have shown that untreated rat lungs contain very low levels of cytochrome P-450 BNF-B and absence of cytochrome P-450 MC-B. However, Clara cells appear to contain the greatest concentrations of cytochrome P-450 PB-B, NADPH-cytochrome P-450 reductase, and epoxide hydrolase.

The induction of drug-metabolizing enzymes in the lower respiratory tract does not always follow the same pattern as in the liver. This again allows for further qualitative and quantitative differences, and accounts in some cases for site-specific lung toxications. Bioactivation of the lung toxin, 4-ipomeanol, is mediated specifically via cytochrome P-450 PB-B in the rat. The toxicity of 4-ipomeanol is directed predominantly to Clara cells, a major site of cytochrome P-450 PB-B activity.[17] The herbicide, paraquat, is selectively accumulated in type II alveolar cells by an energy-dependent process.[34] Studies with such pulmonary toxins are, in part, responsible for the increased information on cellular localization of drug-metabolizing enzymes. The lower respiratory tract, as can be deduced from the above information, is metabolically an active organ, and in some cases the relative participation of the lung in clearance may be greater than predicted solely on the basis of whole-organ metabolic potentials.[35]

The lung's capacity to metabolize xenobiotics is highly variable from one species to another.[32] A limited amount of data on enzymatic activities in human respiratory tissues and cells is available,[36] but the majority of studies, on which the above overview is based, utilize animal tissues, and therefore caution is required when extrapolating to man.

VI. DRUG ACCUMULATION IN THE RESPIRATORY TRACT

A. DRUG AND ENDOGENOUS SUBSTANCE CLEARANCE IN THE LUNGS

The respiratory tract plays a vital role in the maintenance of oxygen supply to the body and the elimination from it of carbon dioxide. Whereas this role is rightly emphasized by physiologists, the immunologic and homeostatic roles are often not given prominence. Many endogenous substances, for example, circulating vasoactive peptides, vasoactive amines, and prostaglandins, can be removed from the blood by the lungs. This selective removal of such bioactive materials results in the regulation of their systemic concentration and constitutes the lung's homeostatic function. A large number of drugs and other xenobiotics also undergo such systemic clearance by the lungs, very often because of their structural similarity to the endogenous materials.[27,31] Exposure to the respiratory tissues in these cases is via the pulmonary vasculature, i.e., drugs are administered at targets other than the alveolus, but are cleared from systemic circulation during their passage through the lungs. Compounds that accumulate in the lungs are represented in almost every therapeutic class, e.g., narcotic analgesics (morphine), antihistamines (diphenhydramine), tranquilizers (imipramine), antimalarials (quinacrine), anesthetics (thiopentone), anorectics (chlorphentermine), antiarrhythmics (procainamide) and β-adrenergic blockers (propranolol). Notable exceptions are drugs used in the treatment of diseases of the lungs and the airways, where selective uptake from circulation might be an advantage (see next section).

B. CONSEQUENCES OF DRUG ACCUMULATION IN THE LUNG

Localization of drugs in the lungs in some cases may be an advantage in that the lung acts as a depot which maintains therapeutic blood levels for several days. In other cases, accumulation in the lung results in selective toxicity to this organ.[36] For example, the persistence of certain amine drugs (e.g., chlorphentermine) in the lungs appears important in drug-induced phospholipidosis.[37] The selective uptake and toxicity of 4-ipomeanol and paraquat have already been discussed in Section V.

This chapter is a consideration of the role of the lung metabolism when drugs are administered by aerosols. The reader may then rightly wonder why the authors have apparently digressed into this section where exposure is via the blood. One reason is that drugs used in the treatment of respiratory disorders are not always administered via the alveolus; whereas the site of action of such drugs is not known with certainty, *inhaled drugs appear to have a faster onset of action than drugs administered systemically*. Drugs administered via other routes therefore rely on transport via the systemic circulation to the lungs, and diffusion into the smooth muscle, endothelial or epithelial cells, or to other presumed topical sites of action. Clearly, any selective uptake in the pulmonary tissues would localize drug action and allow the administration of lower doses, thereby protecting the rest of the body from high concentration of the drug. An understanding of the mechanisms of uptake for vasoactive amines such as 5-hydroxytryptamine and for drugs such as chlorphentermine could, therefore, be of importance in designing systemic drugs for the treatment of respiratory diseases. This is unlikely to be easy since the common characteristic essential for lung uptake (i.e., the presence of basic amino functionalities) is very often not present in drugs used in the treatment of lung diseases (see Tables 1 and 2). A second reason why a knowledge of lung uptake processes is essential is because of the real chance of drug-endogenous substrate and drug-drug interactions of clinical importance when drugs are targeted to this organ. Effects of such drugs on the homeostatic functions of the lung, and on displacement of other drugs concurrently administered and also liable to be accumulated should be thoroughly investigated.

VII. ABSORPTION OF DRUGS FROM RESPIRATORY SURFACES

A. DEPOSITION OF AEROSOLIZED DRUGS

Drug absorption may occur from the nasal mucosal surface, the oropharynx, the conducting airways, and the respiratory or gas exchange surfaces. Absorption in the lung periphery appears to be particularly rapid, in part due to the very thin boundary, and in part due to the high degree of vascularity in the respiratory units. Deposition of aerosolized liquid and solid particulate matter has been discussed elsewhere in this book. As has been pointed out, particles greater than 5 μm are mostly deposited in the upper respiratory tract by inertial impaction, but particles smaller than 5 μm may reach the alveolar region and deposit by sedimentation or by Brownian movement. Since the absorption and metabolizing characteristics of different segments of the respiratory tract vary considerably, differential deposition will lead to differences in pharmacokinetics and possibly pharmacodynamics of an aerosolized drug. The rapid onset of action of inhaled drugs would imply a topical site of action, although absorption from various sites and redistribution to the lungs via systemic circulation may contribute partially to the pharmacological action. In this respect it is worth noting that drugs absorbed from the large airways would be redistributed to the lungs without any hepatic clearance. This is because the bronchiolar region is drained by the bronchial veins, and drugs absorbed in this region are transported back to the lungs without passage through the liver. The smaller airways and the alveolar regions are drained by the pulmonary veins, and drugs absorbed in the periphery are therefore subject to hepatic first-pass metabolism before being circulated back to the lungs. In general, the respiratory tract lining may be considered to be a typical lipoid-pore membrane. However, the actual structure and absorption characteristics are vastly different in the upper and lower respiratory tracts.

B. ABSORPTION OF DRUGS FROM THE UPPER RESPIRATORY TRACT

In addition to drugs targeted to the nasal cavity for local or systemic action, a large proportion of particulate drug inhaled by nose or mouth is deposited in the naso- and oropharynx, respectively; some of this drug may be absorbed, but a significant amount is swallowed. Quantitative data on the absorption of inhaled drugs from the oral, pharyngeal, and bronchial mucosa are limited, due to the obvious practical difficulties in differentiating between absorption from nasal, tracheobronchiolar, bronchiolar, and alveolar regions. A wide range of locally applied compounds have, over the years, been shown to cross the nasal mucosa in human and animal studies, among which are polypeptides (e.g., insulin, luteinizing hormone-releasing hormone), steroid hormones (e.g., progesterone), and other drugs (e.g., propranolol). The systemic side effects observed occasionally after nasal administration of decongestants and antihistamines (e.g., phenylephrine and antazoline, respectively) would suggest that a significant amount of locally applied dose is either absorbed or swallowed. Similarly, the success of antidiabetic pituitary gland preparations (see Table 2), when used as insufflations, nasal solutions, and sprays, would imply systemic absorption from this site. Attempts have been made over the last 2 decades to deliver doses of insulin by the nasal route.[38,39] Hirai et al.[38] demonstrated in dogs that insulin was absorbed reliably from this site and that acidic solutions and the presence of surfactants enhanced this process. Limited clinical data are now also available from Salzman et al.[40] This group reports the successful use of aqueous nasal applications of insulin in patients over a period of 6 months as an adjunct to subcutaneous therapy. This approach to drug delivery is now being extended to other polypeptides (e.g., LH-RH, interferons, and influenza vaccines).

The most widely used drugs for the treatment of nasal disorders are α-adrenoceptor agonists (e.g., phenylephrine, a vasoconstrictor), cholinoceptor antagonists (e.g., ipratropium bromide), antiallergenics (e.g., disodium cromoglycate), and corticosteroids (e.g., beclomethasone dipropionate). Quantitative data on the absorption of these topically applied drugs into the systemic circulation is not available. However, the work of Hussain et al.[41-44] on the intranasal instillation of propranolol and progesterone and related steroids in man and rat, respectively, demonstrates that conventional drugs may be readily absorbed from the nasal cavity. Whereas orally administered propranolol and progesterone undergo extensive metabolism in the gastrointestinal wall, remarkably, the bioavailability of intranasally administered solutions or gels is identical to that obtained with intravenous administration (see Table 4). The lower drug-metabolizing capacity of the nasal mucosa (see Section V.A) is only a partial explanation for the difference between oral and nasal routes. There appears to be a fundamental difference in absorptive characteristics from these two sites, since compounds not absorbed from the gastrointestinal tract are often readily absorbed from the nasal mucosa. If the problems of local irritancy can be overcome by appropriate formulation design, aerosolized nasal application of drugs may be used more routinely in the future to circumvent the alteration of drugs in the gastrointestinal tract or to overcome the inconvenience of parenteral drug administration.

TABLE 4

Mean Area Under Serum Level-Time Curve for Propranolol (Human Data) and Progesterone (Rat Data) Administered by Three Routes[18,41]

	Propranolol	Progesterone
Route	Mean $AUC_{0-\infty}$ ±SE (dose in mg) $(ng \times hr)$ ml^{-1}	Mean $AUC_{0-\infty}$ ±SE (dose in μg) $(ng \times min)$ ml^{-1}
Intravenous	175.4 ± 20.4 (10 mg)	1612.2 ± 80.8 (50 μg)
Nasal	190.3 ± 17.6 (10 mg)	1659.0 ± 109.2 (50 μg)
Oral[a]	349.5 ± 35.2 (80 mg)	19.0 ± 4.6 (50 μg)

[a] Intraduodenal administration of progesterone to rats.

C. ABSORPTION OF DRUGS FROM THE LOWER RESPIRATORY TRACT

Most of the fundamental research on absorption through the lungs has, of necessity, been carried out in animals. Experiments are usually performed using perfused lung preparations or are carried out in the intact animal. In the former case the bronchial circulation is disrupted and therefore estimates of absorption reflect passage across the alveolar membranes. In the intact animal, estimates of absorption reflect the combined permeability of the tracheobronchiolar, bronchiolar, and alveolar epithelia. In general, lipid-soluble drugs are more readily absorbed than hydrophilic compounds, most drugs being transported by passive diffusion across the lipoid-pore membrane. In contrast, the nonlipid-soluble compounds are absorbed by diffusion through aqueous membrane pores. The uptake of such hydrophilic drugs is usually by a nonsaturable diffusion process, the absorption rates being inversely related to their molecular weights (see Table 5, and references cited therein). Although intratracheal injection of drug solutions at the point of bifurcation of the trachea allows administration of accurate doses for experimental work, aerosolized drugs are in general much better absorbed, presumably because of greater deposition in the alveolar regions. Appropriate models have now been developed for the study of absorption of aerosolized drugs from the rat lung.[45] The absorption characteristics of the respiratory membranes appear to differ from those of the gastrointestinal mucosa, and many compounds not absorbed after oral administration are readily absorbed after aerosolized delivery. For example, disodium cromoglycate is very poorly absorbed from the gastrointestinal tract, but is well absorbed after deposition in the lungs.[46]

There are numerous methodological problems in estimating absorption of inhaled drugs in humans, not the least being the fact that normal doses are in the microgram range and require highly sensitive assay methods. Such studies invariably use ^{3}H- or ^{14}C-labeled drugs; after aerosolization, the amount of drug in the apparatus, in mouthwashings, and in plasma and urine is estimated. Davies and co-workers[47] have carried out elegant studies with isoproterenol. These investigators measure the drug and its metabolites in plasma and urine after oral and inhalational administration, and estimate from these measurements the amount of drug deposited in the oropharynx, the proportion subsequently swallowed, and by difference the amount deposited in the periphery (and presumably absorbed via the lungs). More recent studies by the same group[48] have obtained more direct estimates of deposition and absorption from the human lung by using activated charcoal. The oral administration of activated charcoal to subjects immediately after inhalation of terbutaline prevents gastrointestinal absorption of the swallowed drug. The drug appearing in the plasma then reflects the absorption of the drug deposition in the lower parts of the respiratory tract. With disodium cromoglycate, which is not significantly absorbed from the gastrointestinal tract, estimation of absorption from the lungs is less troublesome. Peak plasma levels of this prophylactic antiasthmatic are achieved within 15 min after inhalation of radiolabeled drug, indicating rapid absorption from the airways.[49]

TABLE 5
**Absorption of Drugs Through Adult Rat Lungs After Intratracheal
Administration[45,78-80]**

Compound	Mol wt	Absorption rate (min. for 50% absorption)
Lipid soluble drugs		
Salicylic acid	138	1.0
Barbitone	206	1.4
Sulfafurazole	267	3.4
Procainamide	236	5.7
Nonlipid soluble drugs		
Urea	60	4.7
p-Aminohippuric acid	194	41
Sucrose	342	87
Enulin	5,000	220
Dextran	75,000	688

VIII. METABOLISM AND PHARMACOKINETICS OF DRUGS APPLIED TO THE RESPIRATORY TRACT

A. DRUGS APPLIED FOR ABSORPTION AND SYSTEMIC ACTION

The most widely used drugs in this context are the anesthetic gases, e.g., cyclopropane, enflurane, etc. (see Table 2). The total amount of drug absorbed via the lungs during surgical anesthesia is large (~10 to 30 g), but most of this is exhaled unchanged over a period of time after the discontinuance of anesthesia. Blood levels achieved are in tens or even hundreds of milligrams per liter. For example, blood levels of halothane range from 80 to 260 mg/l, but drop to the low milligram (1 to 20 mg) range rapidly during the postanesthetic period.[50] Over 80% of the dose of halothane has been estimated to be eliminated unchanged. Halothane metabolites in urine, e.g., trifluoroacetic acid, account for a smaller proportion (20%) of the dose, and reductive metabolism to reactive metabolites in the liver has been linked to the hepatotoxicity of this agent. Halothane is the most extensively metabolized of the volatile anesthetic agents; only 0.5% and 2.4% of cyclopropane and enflurane, respectively, are reported to undergo metabolism. The role of pulmonary tissues in the metabolism of the anesthetic gases is unknown, but the high dose and rate at which the lung is exposed to these agents would possibly lead to saturation of this organ's capacity for biotransformation.

The pharmacokinetics of propranolol in humans after oral, nasal, and intravenous administration (Figure 3A) have recently been investigated in an attempt to exploit the nasal cavity as a portal of entry for drugs which suffer an extensive gastrointestinal first-pass metabolism.[41] For nasal application, 10 mg of propranolol hydrochloride in 0.5 ml of 2% methylcellulose gel was placed in the nasal cavity while the subjects were in a sitting position. Remarkably, the bioavailability of 10 mg propranolol was identical after intravenous and nasal application, whereas bioavailability for an 80-mg oral dose was calculated at 25%. Propranolol is extensively metabolized in the gastrointestinal tract and liver by several routes (see Figure 3B), but apparently escapes this first-pass effect in the nasal mucosa. Similar pharmacokinetic and metabolic data are available for progesterone (see Figure 4), 17-β-estradiol, and 17-α-ethynyl estradiol in the rat (see Table 4),[42-44] but in general, data on the respiratory tract metabolism of drugs applied for systemic effects is lacking.

B. DRUGS APPLIED FOR TOPICAL ACTION

The data generated with isoproterenol and other inhalational bronchodilators (Figure 5) clearly illustrates the importance of metabolism and pharmacokinetics in deposition and

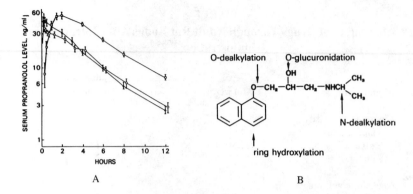

FIGURE 3. (A) Time course of the average serum propranolol levels in 6 male subjects following nasal administration of 10 mg/subject (△), intravenous administration of 10 mg/subject (○), and oral administration of 80 mg/subject (☐). (B) Structure of propranolol and routes of its biotransformation. (Reproduced by permission, American Physiological Association.)

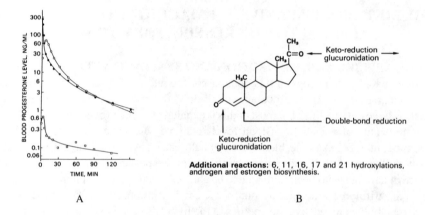

FIGURE 4. (A) Mean blood levels of unchanged progesterone in rats following the intravenous (●), nasal (○), and oral (☐) administration of 50 μg/rat progesterone.[18] (B) Structure of progesterone and its biotransformation pathways. (Reproduced by permission, American Physiological Association.)

absorption studies. Isoproterenol is metabolized in man along two main pathways[47] (see Scheme 1). Orally administered isoproterenol is mainly converted to isoproterenol *O*-sulfate in the gastrointestinal tract, whereas isoproterenol deposited in the airways is *O*-methylated to afford *O*-methyl isoproterenol sulfate as a urinary metabolite. Unlike epinephrine, isoproterenol is resistant to metabolism by monoamine oxidases. Comparative pharmacokinetic and urinary metabolic studies after intravenous, intrabronchial, oral, and inhalational administration of ^{3}H-isoproterenol revealed that the inhaled dose behaves like the orally administered drug (see Table 6). A large amount of *O*-methylated isoproterenol, in the free and sulfated forms, was detected in urine after administration via the intravenous and intrabronchial routes, whereas the major urinary metabolite after the oral and inhalation route was the *O*-sulfate. These data allowed the following conclusions: (1) *O*-methylation mainly occurs in the airways and lungs, but *O*-sulfation occurs in the gastrointestinal wall and liver, and (2) a large proportion (>90%) of inhaled drug is deposited in the oropharynx and is eventually swallowed. These indirect methods were the first to demonstrate the inefficiency of this mode of drug delivery. Isoproterenol has a biphasic elimination profile after intravenous administration. The initial half-life is only a few

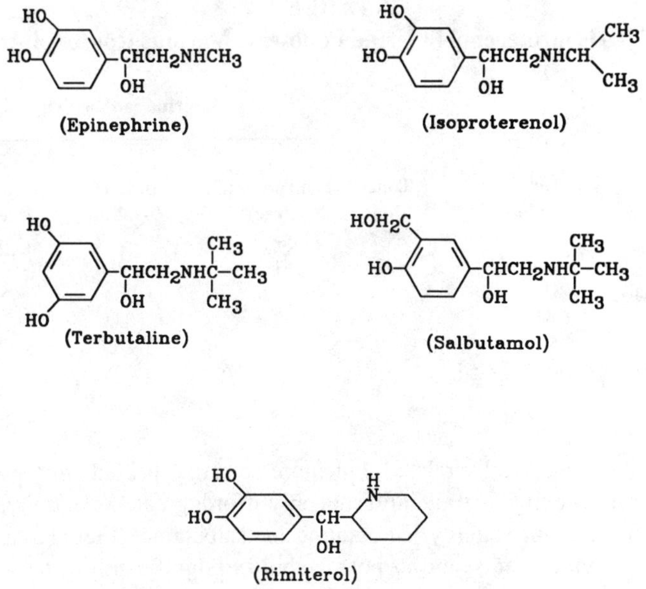

79

FIGURE 5. Structures of some clinically used inhaled bronchodilator drugs.

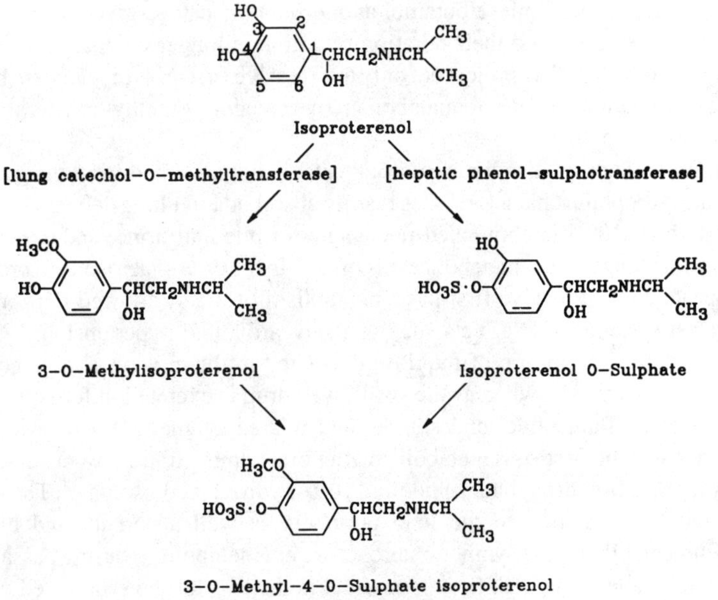

SCHEME 1. Metabolism of isoproterenol in man. (Adopted from Davies, Reference 47.)

minutes, whereas the terminal half-life is several hours. After inhalation, the duration of action is for about 2 h; with both modes of administration the entire dose is eliminated in urine within 24 h.[51]

TABLE 6

Metabolites of ^{3}H-Isoproterenol in Urine Following Various Routes of Administration[47]

			% urine radioactivity as		
Route	Dose (μg/kg)	Time (hr)	Isoproterenol (free)	Isoproterenol O-sulfate	3-O-Methyl-isoproterenol (free & conjugated)
Intravenous	0.44	22	51.6	0	45.8
Intrabronchial	0.03	50	8.8	6.3	65.9
Oral	44	48	9.2	84.2	4.0
Inhalation (pressurized aerosol)	5.7	48	3.5	86.1	7.3

The fate of some chemically related, but more selective β-2-adrenoceptor stimulants is somewhat different. The chemical alteration not only affords greater selectivity, but also confers a small degree of metabolic stability. Terbutaline and salbutamol (Figure 5) are not substrates for catechol-*O*-methyltransferase and are not metabolized significantly by the lungs. Unlike isoproterenol, salbutamol does not appear to be sulfated in the gastrointestinal mucosa, but is subject to first-pass metabolism in the liver; half the dose is excreted in urine as the sulfate conjugate, the rest is eliminated unchanged. The half-life of salbutamol is dependent on the route of administration, the longest $t_{1/2}$ being after inhalation. Terbutaline is metabolized in the liver and possibly the gut to afford mostly the sulfate conjugate, but some free drug and glucuronide are also excreted in urine. Both salbutamol and terbutaline can be given orally in reasonable doses (c.f., isoproterenol), and their duration of action is longer compared to isoproterenol. Rimiterol, on the other hand, is subject not only to extensive first-pass metabolism by sulfate and glucuronide conjugation, but also to metabolism by catechol-*O*-methyltransferases, and therefore has a very short half-life.[51]

The antiasthmatic drug, disodium cromoglycate, is not absorbed from the gastrointestinal tract due to its hydrophilic character, but is readily absorbed after lung delivery. The fraction of the dose absorbed (10%) is eliminated unchanged in bile and urine, and experiments have demonstrated that lungs do not metabolize this drug.[52] In the case of aerosolized bronchodilators such as isoproterenol, extensive first-pass metabolism of the swallowed portion of the dose protects against systemic side effects such as tachycardia and hypertension. With disodium cromoglycate, the small portion of the dose deposited in the airways and alveolar region is responsible for prophylaxis, whereas the swallowed drug is excreted in feces.

Beclomethasone, flunisolide, budesonide, and related synthetic glucocorticosteroids undergo extensive hepatic first-pass metabolism after oral administration. Budesonide is metabolized mostly to the 6-β-hydroxybudesonide and 16-α-hydroxyprednisolone.[53] The portion of the drug delivered by inhalation to the lung periphery is well absorbed, and high systemic availability indicates that these synthetic steroids are not metabolized during passage across the respiratory membranes. The high first-pass effect in the liver of the swallowed portion of the dose probably protects against systemic side effects. The pharmacokinetics of ^{3}H-budesonide have been studied; after the administration of 500 μg of ^{3}H-labeled drug by a pressurized aerosol, peak-plasma levels were achieved within 10 min, after which the plasma concentration of the unchanged drug declined exponentially with time.[54]

C. PRO-DRUGS AND TISSUE TARGETING

The lung targeting of drugs via the pro-drug approach has the potential for improving selectivity, prolonging the therapeutic effect, and conferring or enhancing pulmonary activity. Effective pro-drug design affords compounds that have high affinity for lung tissue, and for which the lungs exhibit a high rate of metabolic conversion to the active component relative to

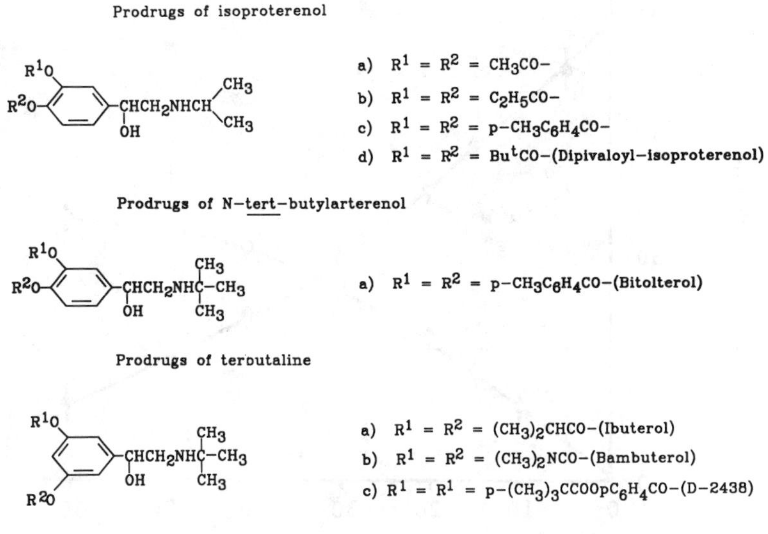

Prodrugs of isoproterenol

a) $R^1 = R^2 = CH_3CO-$

b) $R^1 = R^2 = C_2H_5CO-$

c) $R^1 = R^2 = p-CH_3C_6H_4CO-$

d) $R^1 = R^2 = Bu^tCO-$ (Dipivaloyl-isoproterenol)

Prodrugs of N-tert-butylarterenol

a) $R^1 = R^2 = p-CH_3C_6H_4CO-$ (Bitolterol)

Prodrugs of terbutaline

a) $R^1 = R^2 = (CH_3)_2CHCO-$ (Ibuterol)

b) $R^1 = R^2 = (CH_3)_2NCO-$ (Bambuterol)

c) $R^1 = R^1 = p-(CH_3)_3CCOOpC_6H_4CO-$ (D-2438)

FIGURE 6. Structures of some prodrugs of isoproterenol, *N*-tert-butylarterenol, and terbutaline.

other tissues; this provides a means for improving selectivity of drug action in the lung relative to effects in other organs and tissues. Pulmonary pro-drugs should, therefore, be selectively taken up by the lung, undergo metabolic conversion specifically in the lung, and the resulting parent drug should be effectively 'trapped' in the lung tissue, after which should always follow a carrier washout period.

The pulmonary pro-drugs, dipivaloylisoproterenol and bitolterol (Figure 6), have both been shown to exhibit decreased cardiac side effects, and both compounds possess increased antiasthmatic properties compared to the administration of the parent drug. Both bambuterol and ibuterol (Figure 6), pro-drugs of terbutaline, exhibit a prolonged therapeutic effect when compared to terbutaline itself. These observations have been attributed to the resistance of these diesters to extensive first-pass metabolism by sulfation, improved absorption of the more lipophilic diester derivative, and metabolic conversion of these drugs specifically by lung esterases to the active component. Lung tissue targeting by molecular modification is discussed in detail in Chapter 4.

IX. METABOLISM AND ABSORPTION OF PEPTIDES ADMINISTERED TO RESPIRATORY TRACT TISSUE

Peptide drugs have the potential to become the most promising group of medicinal agents in modern times. However, their susceptibility to rapid enzymic degradation in the gastrointestinal tract by peptidases has made it necessary to administer such drug entities parenterally.

Although several drug types are absorbed rapidly and quantitatively following nasal administration (see Section VIII.B), peptides have generally exhibited low nasal bioavailabilities, and there is a lack of good data on bioavailability of peptides administered to other parts of the respiratory tract. Studies with insulin,[38] the antidiuretic agent 1-desamino-8-D-arginine-vasopressin (DDAVP),[55,56] and the luteinizing hormone-releasing hormone (LHRH) analog, nafarelin acetate,[57] show clearly that considerably greater nasal than parenteral doses are required to produce similar pharmacological effects. Even low molecular weight peptides appear to exhibit poor nasal bioavailability. The tripeptide, L-pyro-2-aminoadipyl-L-histidyl-L-thiazolidine-4-carboxyamide (MK-771), an analog of thyrotropine-releasing hormone, has only 13% nasal bioavailability in rats compared to that of the intravenous dose.[58] Studies with

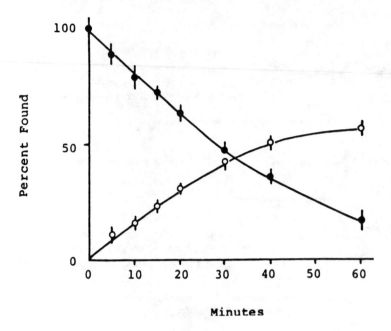

FIGURE 7. The disappearance of Leu-enkephalin (●), and the appearance of Gly-GlyPheLeu (o) in the nasal perfusate of the rat. The symbols represent the mean and standard error from 4 animal experiments. (Reproduced by permission of Academic Press.)

dipeptides indicate that such compounds undergo extensive enzymic hydrolysis by peptidases in the nasal cavity, and that this may be the prime cause of the low nasal bioavailability exhibited by these drug types.[59,60]

The pentapeptides Leu- and Met-enkephalin, have been studied in some detail with respect to respiratory tract bioavailability. Hussain et al.[60,61] have examined the nasal metabolism and absorption of Leu-enkephalin in rats using an *in situ* perfusion technique and have found that this peptide rapidly disappeared from the nasal perfusate with concomitant formation of GlyGlyPheLeu (see Figure 7) and its subsequent metabolic products. Kinetic analysis clearly showed that the overall disappearance of Leu-enkephalin from the nasal perfusate was due to enzymic hydrolysis, and that the absorption, if any, was less than 10%. Interestingly, hydrolysis of Leu-enkephalin in nasally perfused buffer was considerably reduced by the addition of a large excess of di- or tripeptide containing either a tyrosine or phenylalanine unit (see Figure 8), suggesting that co-administration of a pharmacologically inactive peptide which competes as a substrate for the nasal peptidases may be a useful approach to improving the bioavailability of nasally administered peptides.

Structural modification of small peptides and its effect on peptide absorption from the nasal cavity has been studied by Huang et al.[60] Unlike terminal *N*-acylation, esterification of the free carboxylic acid moiety of simple peptides increases lipophilicity and absorption considerably, however, such derivatives are rapidly hydrolyzed by peptidases in the nasal cavity. Huang et al.[60] have studied the nasal absorption of simple L-tyrosine analogs and conclude that the polarity and/or lipophilicity of amino acid derivatives do not have significant effects on the extent of their nasal absorptions, but that the net charge on the molecule does. Thus, positively charged molecules pass through the membrane more easily than the negatively charged, and carboxylic ester derivatives effectively mask the negative charge of the carboxylate moiety. It has been suggested that a combination of a peptide pro-drug (such as an ester) and a peptidase inhibitor may provide a useful approach to the enhancement of peptide absorption from the nasal cavity.[60] Esterification of the terminal carboxylate function of dipeptides and related compounds, and

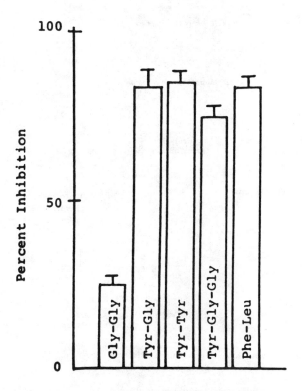

FIGURE 8. The influence of competing peptidase substrates on the hydrolysis of Leu-enkephalin in Ringer's buffer precirculated through the nasal cavity of the rat; values are the mean and standard error from 4 experiments. (Reproduced by permission of Academic Press.)

even some tripeptides, can result in an unwanted intramolecular aminolysis reaction, which affords a diketopiperazine product.[63-67] Such degradation products have been detected in studies with methyl esters of dipeptides such as GlyGly, GlyAla, AlaGly, and GlySar, with the methyl ester isoLeuGly and GlyisoLeu, AspPhe (Aspartame), and with the ethyl ester of the angiotensin-converting enzyme (ACE) -inhibitor dipeptide, RS-10085. In the case of Aspartame, diketopiperazine formation is illustrated in Scheme 2. This type of intramolecular reaction can occur in aqueous solution in the pH range 5.0 to 8.5 at 25°C and is self-catalyzed. At values of pH around neutrality, the rate of cyclization (k_2) has been shown to be faster than the rate of hydrolysis of the ester (k_1).[68] The six-membered diketopiperazine product results from nucleophilic attack of the N-terminal amine function at the activated (i.e., esterified) carboxylic acid function. The transformation is accompanied by extensive racemization at the asymmetric centers in the diketopiperazine product. Thus, subsequent hydrolysis back to the parent dipeptide (route a) may result in considerable reduction in biological activity due to loss of chiral integrity. In addition, hydrolysis of the diketopiperazine may result in the formation of a new dipeptide (route b), structurally unrelated to the parent dipeptide (see Scheme 2). It is conceivable that deactivating intramolecular reactions of this type could occur in larger carboxyl-derivatized peptides with the involvement of internal trifunctional amino acid residues containing nucleophilic functionalities (e.g., lysine and arginine).

An alternative approach to enhancing the nasal absorption of peptides is via the coadministration of surfactant molecules. Hussain[58] has shown that the effect of 1% sodium glycocholate on the rate and extent of absorption of the thyrotropine releasing hormone tripeptide analog, MK-771, from the nasal cavity of rats results in an enhancement of nasal bioavailability (calculated from the areas under the nasal and intravenous blood level curves)

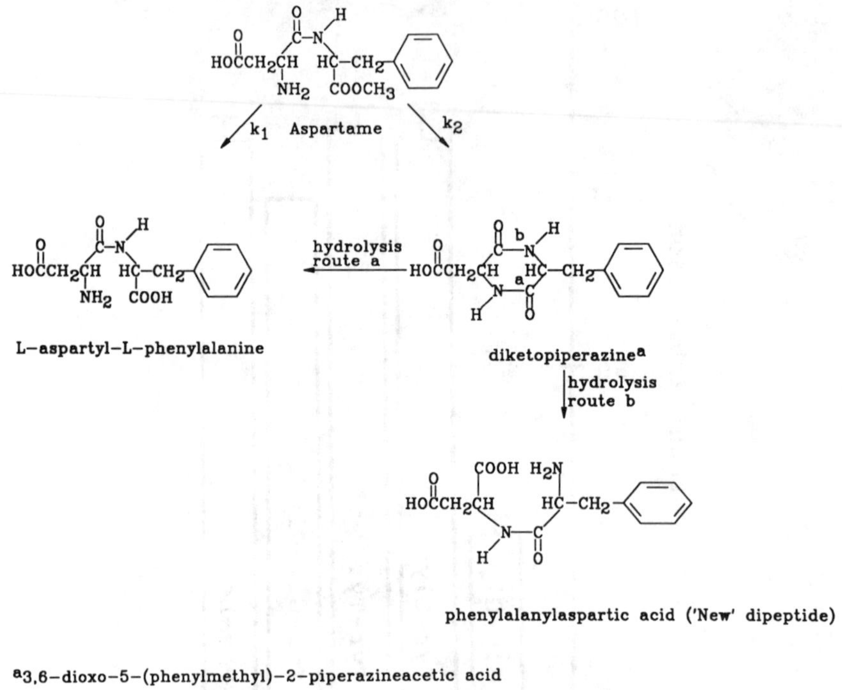

SCHEME 2.   Intramolecular aminolysis of L-aspartyl-L-phenylalanine methyl ester (Aspartame) and subsequent hydrolysis of the resulting diketopiperazine derivative.

of up to 78% of that of the intravenous dose. Similar results were obtained by Su et al.[69] with the enkephalin analog TyrD-AlaGlyL-PheD-Leu-OH (DADLE). Recent studies have indicated that surfactants such as sodium glycocholate may exert their effect by damaging the nasal membrane and producing large fissures through which the peptide molecules are able to penetrate.

The lung is recognized as having an important role in the metabolism of a variety of neurohumoral substances,[70-72] and contains several enzymes known to degrade peptides, including ACE, amino-peptidase, and enkephalinase.[73,74] Studies by Gillespie et al.[75] have shown that both Leu- and Met-enkephalin are rapidly metabolized in a curvilinear, time-dependent manner during transit through the isolated perfused rat lung (see Figures 9 and 10). The inhibitor, captopril, abolished the enzymic degradation of both enkephalins to TyrGlyGly, and attenuated somewhat the formation of tyrosine, whereas bestatin, an aminopeptidase inhibitor, effectively blocked the formation of tyrosine and augmented the production of TyrGlyGly (see Figure 11). The enkephalinase inhibitor, thiorphan, failed to influence the degradation of either of the enkephalins, although this may be due to inaccessibility of the substrates for this enzyme.[76] Thus, in the perfused rat lung, aminopeptidase may play the most significant role in degrading exogenous Leu- and Met-enkephalins, and ACE and aminopeptidase may be functionally linked. This study also indicated that although the lung rapidly metabolizes exogenous enkephalins, it does not appear to avidly sequester either the parent compounds or their metabolites, although treatment of isolated perfused rat lung with a combination of captopril and bestatin does augment the pressor effect of Leu-enkephalin.[77]

X. CONCLUSIONS

This review has outlined some of the metabolic and pharmacokinetic factors that need to be

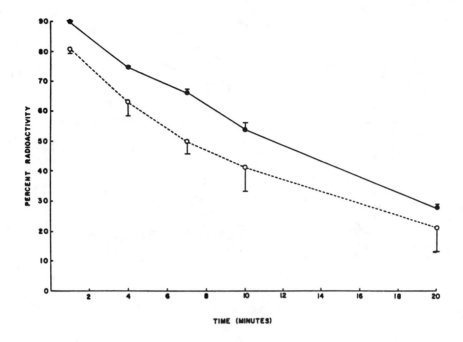

FIGURE 9. The disappearance of [³H]-enkephalins from isolated rat lung perfusate; [³H]-Leu-enkephalin (●), [³H]-Met-enkephalin, (o). Each datum point represents the mean and standard error from 3 experiments. (Reproduced by permission, American Society of Pharmacology and Experimental Therapeutics.)

considered when designing drugs for inhalational use. In view of the vastly different structures and the presence of heterogeneous cell types in different segments of the respiratory tract, the absorptive and metabolizing capabilities of these areas are likely to be different. Metabolism, and therefore bioavailability, of different formulations of even the same drug may vary if deposition patterns are not identical. A knowledge of the xenobiotic-metabolizing enzymes in the respiratory tract could be useful in the design of inhalation drugs, either for local action or for absorption and systemic action. The ability of the lungs to take up certain types of chemicals from the circulation could also be utilized in the design of pro-drugs which undergo selective metabolism in the lung to release the active agent. The interpretation of metabolic and pharmacokinetic data after inhalation exposure is not easy; the early (minutes) plasma levels are probably due to the inhaled drug, whereas the latter plasma levels (hours) are probably due to that portion of the drug that was deposited in the oropharynx and subsequently swallowed. In only a few cases is it possible to define clearly the role of the pulmonary tissues in metabolism of aerosolized drugs. Peptide delivery via the respiratory tract presents an interesting alternative to the parenteral route. However, the high metabolic instability and low bioavailability of these drug types when applied to the respiratory tract are major obstacles that must be overcome.

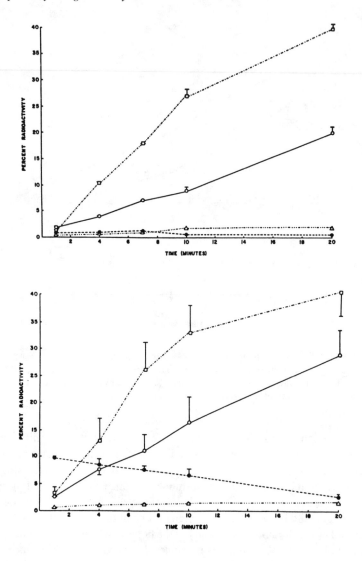

FIGURE 10.   Formation of metabolites after administration of (top) [³H]-Leu-enkephalin and (bottom) [³H]-Met-enkephalin to rat lung perfusate; tyrosine (o), TyrGly (Δ), TyrGlyGly (□), TyrGlyGlyPhe (●). Each datum point represents the mean and standard error from 3 experiments. (Reproduced by permission, American Society of Pharmacology and Experimental Therapeutics.)

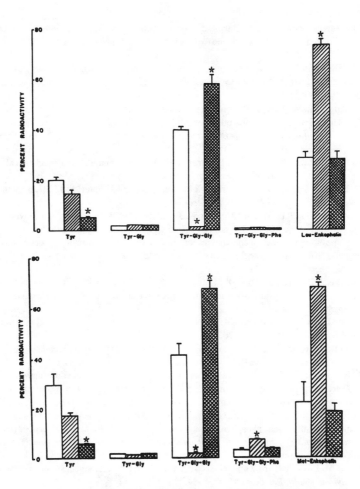

FIGURE 11.   Effect of peptidase inhibitors on (top) [³H]-Leu-enkephalin metabolism, and (bottom) [³H]-Met-enkephalin metabolism in isolated perfused rat lungs; control (□), captopril (18.4 mM) (▨), bestatin (116 mM) (▩). Data are expressed as mean and standard error from 3 experiments; *differs significantly from control at p, 0.05.[75] (Reproduced by permission, American Society of Pharmacology and Experimental Therapeutics.)

REFERENCES

1. **Gibson, G. G. and Skett, P.,** *Introduction to Drug Metabolism,* Chapman & Hall, London, 1986.
2. **Testa, B. and Jenner, P.,** *Drug Metabolism: Chemical and Biochemical Aspects,* Marcel Dekker, New York, 1976.
3. **Vainio, H. and Hietanen, E.,** Role of extrahepatic metabolism in drug disposition and toxicity, in *Concepts in Drug Metabolism,* Part A, Jenner, P. and Testa, B., Eds., Marcel Dekker, New York, 1980, 251.
4. **Lourenco, R. V. and Cotromanes, E.,** Clinical aerosols. I. Characterization of aerosols and their diagnostic uses, *Arch. Intern. Med.,* 142, 2163, 1982.
5. **Tierney, D. F.,** Lung metabolism and biochemistry, in *Annu. Rev. Physiol.,* 36, 209, 1974.
6. **Gram, T. E.,** The metabolism of xenobiotics by mammalian lung, in *Extrahepatic Metabolism of Drugs and Other Foreign Compounds,* Gram, T.E., Ed., MTP Press, Lancaster, England, 1980, 159.
7. **Benford, D. J. and Bridges, J. W.,** Xenobiotic metabolism in lung, *Prog. Drug Metab.,* 9, 53, 1986.
8. **Dahl, A. R., Hadley, W. M., Benson, J. M., Hahn, F. F., and McCleallan, R. O.,** Cytochrome P-450 dependent monooxygenase in olfactory epithelium of dogs: possible role in tumorigenicity, *Science,* 216, 57, 1982.
9. **Reed, C. J., Lock, E. A., and De Matteis, F.,** NADPH: cytochrome P-450 reductase in olfactory epithelium. Relevance to cytochrome P-450 dependent reactions, *Biochem. J.,* 240, 585, 1986.

10. **Voigt, J. M., Guengerich, F. P., and Baron, J.,** Localization of xenobiotic metabolizing enzymes in nasal tissues of untreated and 3-methylcholanthrene (MC) and aroclor 1254(A) pretreated rats, *Toxicologist,* 5, 162, 1985.

11. **Sabourin, P. J. and Dahl, A. R.,** Distribution of the FAD-containing monooxygenase in respiratory tract tissues, Annual Report LMF-114, Medinsky, M.A and Muggenburg, B.A., Eds., National Technical Information Service, Springfield, VA, 1985, 156.

12. **Baron, J., Voigt, J. M., Whitter, T. B., Bawabata, T., Knapp, S. A., Guengerich, F. P. and Jakoby, W. B.,** Identification of intratissue sites for xenobiotic activation and detoxification, in *Biological Reactive Intermediates III. Molecular and Cellular Mechanisms of Action in Animal Models and Human Disease,* Snyder, R., Ed., Plenum Press, New York, 1988 in press.

13. **Bogdanffy, M. S., Randall, H. W., and Morgan, K. T.,** Histochemical and biochemical detection of carboxyesterase activity in the rat nasal passages, *Toxicologist,* 6, 145, 1985.

14. **Dahl, A. R., Bond, J. A., Petridou-Fischer, J., Sabourin, P. J., and Whaley, S. J.,** Effects of the respiratory tract on inhaled materials, *Toxicol. Appl. Pharmacol.,* 33, 484, 1988.

15. **Bogdanffy, M. S., Randall, H. W., and Morgan, K. T.,** Histochemical localization of aldehyde dehyrogenase in the respiratory tract of the Fischer-344 rat, *Toxicol. Appl. Pharmacol.,* 82, 560, 1985.

16. **Bond, J. A.,** Some biotransformation enzymes responsible for polycyclic aromatic hydrocarbon metabolism in rat nasal turbinates; enzyme activities of in vitro modifiers and intraperitoneal and inhalation exposure of rats to inducing agents, *Cancer Res.,* 43, 4804, 1983.

17. **Baron, J., Burke, J. P., Guengerich, F. P., Jakoby, W. B., and Voigt, J. M.,** Sites for xenobiotic activation and detoxication within the respiratory tract: implications for chemically induced toxicity, *Toxicol. Appl. Pharmacol.,* 93, 493, 1988.

18. **Hussain, A. A., Hirai, S., and Bawarshi, R.,** Nasal absorption of natural contraceptive steroids in rats—progesterone absorption, *J. Pharm. Sci.,* 70, 466, 1981.

19. **Jenner, J. and Dodd, G. H.,** Xenobiotic metabolism in the nasal epithelia, *Drug Metab. Drug Interact.,* 1988 in press.

20. **Jeffery, P. K.,** Structure and function of mucus-secreting cells of cat and goose airway epithelium, in *Respiratory Tract Mucus,* Ciba Found. Symp. No. 54, Elsevier/North-Holland, Amsterdam, 1978, 5.

21. **Autrup, H.,** Carcinogen metabolism in human tissues and cells, *Drug Metab. Rev.,* 13, 603, 1982.

22. **Sabourin, P. J., Tynes, R., Smyser, B., Dahl, A., and Hodgson, E.,** The FAD-containing monooxygenase: oxidation of nitrogen-, sulfur-, and phosphorus-containing compounds, in *Biological Reactive Intermediates III. Molecular and Cellular Mechanism of Action in Animal Models and Human Disease,* Snyder, R., Ed., Plenum Press, New York, 1988 in press.

23. **Trump, B. F., McDowell, E. M., and Harris, C. C.,** Chemical carcinogenesis in the tracheobronchial epithelium, *Environ. Health Perspect.,* 55, 77, 1984.

24. **Devereux, T. R. and Fouts, J. R.,** Isolation of pulmonary cells and use in studies on xenobiotic metabolism, *Methods Enzymol.,* 77, 147, 1981.

25. **Domin, B. A., Devereux, T. R., Fouts, J. R., and Philpot, R. M.,** Pulmonary cytochrome P-450: isozyme profiles and induction by 2,3,7,8-tetrachlorodibenzo-p-dioxin (TCDD) in Clara and type II cells and macrophages isolated from rabbit lung, *Fed. Proc.,* 45, 321, 1985.

26. **Boyd, M. R.,** Biochemical mechanisms in pulmonary toxicity of furan derivatives, *Rev. Biochem. Toxicol.,* 2, 71, 1980.

27. **Bend, J. R., Serabjit-Singh, C. J., and Philpot, R. M.,** The pulmonary uptake, accumulation and metabolism of xenobiotics, *Annu. Rev. Pharmacol. Toxicol.,* 25, 97, 1985.

28. **Oppelt, W. W., Zange, M., Ross, W. E., and Remmer, H.,** Comparison of microsomal drug hydroxylation in lung and liver of various species, *Res. Commun. Chem. Pathol. Pharmacol.,* 1, 43, 1970.

29. **Litterst, C. L., Mimnaugh, E. G., Reagan, R. L., and Gram, T. E.,** Comparison of *in vitro* drug metabolism by lung, liver and kidney of several common laboratory species, *Drug Metab. Disposition,* 3, 259, 1975.

30. **Gram, T. E.,** Comparative aspects of mixed function oxidation by lung and liver of rabbits, *Drug Metab. Rev.,* 2, 1, 1973.

31. **Brown, E. A. B.,** The localization, metabolism, and effects of drugs and toxicants in the lung, *Drug Metab. Rev.,* 3, 33, 1974.

32. **Hook, G. E. and Bend, J. R.,** Pulmonary metabolism of xenobiotics, *Life Sci.,* 18, 279, 1975.

33. **Philpot, R. M. and Wolf, C. R.,** The properties and deposition of the enzymes of pulmonary cytochromes P-450-dependent monooxygenase systems, *Rev. Biochem. Toxicol.,* 3, 51, 1981.

34. **Forman, H. J., Aldrich, T. K., Posner, M. A., and Fisher, A. B.,** Differential paraquat uptake and redox kinetics of rat granular pneumocytes and alveolar macrophages, *J. Pharmacol. Exp. Ther.,* 221, 428, 1982.

35. **Gillette, J. R.,** Sequential organ first-pass effects: simple methods for constructing compartmental pharmacokinetic models from physiological models of disposition by several organs, *J. Pharm. Sci.,* 71, 673, 1982.

36. **Witschi, H. and Cote, M. G.,** Biochemical pathology of lung damage produced by chemicals, *Fed. Proc.,* 35, 89, 1976.

37. **Heath, D., Smith, P., and Hasleton, P. S.,** Effects of chlorphentermine on the rat lung, *Thorax,* 28, 551, 1973.
38. **Hirai, S., Yashiki, T., and Mima, H.,** Effect of surfactants on the nasal absorption of insulin in rats, *Int. J. Pharm.,* 9, 165, 1981.
39. **Morimoto, K., Morisaka, K., and Kamada, A.,** Enhancement of nasal absorption of insulin and calcitonin using polyacrylic acid gel, *J. Pharm. Pharmacol.,* 37, 134, 1985.
40. **Salzman, R., Manson, J. E. M., Griffing, G. T., Kimmerle, R., Ruderman, N., McCall, A., Stoltz, E. I., Mullin, C., Small, D., Armstrong, J., and Melby, J. C.,** Intranasal aerosolized insulin. Mixed meal studies and long-term use in type I diabetes, *N. Engl. J. Med.,* 312, 1078, 1985.
41. **Hussain, A. A., Foster, S., Hirai, S., Kashihawa, T., Batenhorst, R., and Jones, M.,** Nasal absorption of propranolol in humans, *J. Pharm. Sci.,* 69, 1240.
42. **Hussain, A. A., Bawarshi-Nassar, R., and Huang, C. H.,** Physicochemical considerations in intranasal drug administration, in *Transnasal Systemic Medications,* Chien, Y.W., Ed., Elsevier, Amsterdam, 1985, 121.
43. **Bawarshi-Nassar, R. N., Hussain, A. A., and Crooks, P. A.,** Nasal absorption and metabolism of progesterone and 17β-estradiol in the rat, *Drug Metabol. Disposition,* in press, 1989.
44. **Bawarshi-Nassar, R. N., Hussain, A. A., and Crooks, P. A.,** Nasal absorption of 17β-ethinyl estradiol in the rat, *J. Pharm. Pharmacol.,* submitted, 1988.
45. **Brown, R. A., Jr. and Schanker, L. S.,** Absorption of aerosolized drugs in the rat lung, *Drug Metab. Disposition,* 11, 355, 1983.
46. **Curry, S. H., Taylor, A. J., Evans, S., Godfrey, S., and Ziedifard, E.,** Disposition of disodium cromoglycate administered in three particle sizes, *Br. J. Clin. Pharmacol.,* 2, 267, 1975.
47. **Davies, D. S.,** Pharmacokinetics of inhaled drugs, in *Evaluation of Bronchodilator Drugs,* Burley, D.M., Clarke, S.W., Cuthbert, M.F., Paterson, J.W., and Shelley, J.H., Eds., Trust for Education and Research in Therapeutics, London, 1975, 151.
48. **Davies, D. S.,** The fate of inhaled terbutaline, *Eur. J. Resp. Dis.,* 65 (Suppl. 134), 141, 1984.
49. **Pauwels, R.,** Pharmacokinetics of inhaled drugs, in *Aerosols in Medicine, Principles, Diagnosis and Therapy,* Moren, F., Newhouse, M.T., and Dolovich, M.B., Eds., Elsevier/North-Holland, Amsterdam, 1985, 219.
50. **Baselt, R. C.,** *Disposition of Toxic Drugs and Chemicals in Man,* Vol. 1, Biomedical Publications, Canton, CT, 1978, 48.
51. **Reynolds, E. F.,** Ed., *Martindale: The Extra Pharmacopoeia,* 28th Ed., Pharmaceutical Press, London, 1982.
52. **Walker, S. R., Evans, M. E., Richards, A. J., and Paterson, J. W.,** The fate of [^{14}C]-disodium cromoglycate in man, *J. Pharm. Pharmacol.,* 24, 525, 1972.
53. **Chaplin, M. D., Rooks, W., Swenson, E. W., Cooper, W. C., Nerenberg, C., and Chu, N. I.,** Flunisolide metabolism and dynamics of a metabolite, *Clin. Pharmacol. Ther.,* 27, 402, 1980.
54. **Ryrfeldt, A., Andersson, P., Edsbacker, S., Tonnesson, M., Davis, D., and Pauwels, R.,** Pharmacokinetics and metabolism of budesonide, a selective glucocorticoid, *Eur. J. Resp. Dis.,* 63 (Suppl. 122), 86, 1982.
55. **Vavra, I., Machova, A., Holecek, V., Cort, J. H., Zaoral, M., and Sorm, F.,** Effect of a synthetic analogue of vasopressin in animals and in patients with diabetes insipidus, *Lancet,* 1, 948, 1968.
56. **Mudler, J., Anderson, K. E., Arner, B., Aronson, S., Bachmann, R., and Hokfelt, B.,** Pharmacology of DDVP and its Clinical Trial in Cranial Diabetes Insipidus, Int. Congr. Ser. No. 256, Excerpta Medica, Amsterdam, 1972, 49.
57. **Fink, G., Gennser, G., Liedolm, R., Thorell, J., and Mulder, J.,** Comparison of plasma levels of luteinizing hormone-releasing hormone in men after intravenous or intranasal administration, *J. Endocrinol,* 63, 351, 1974.
58. **Hussain, A.,** personal communication.
59. **Huang, C. H.,** Enhancement of the Delivery of Peptides by the Administration of Their Pro-Drugs via the Nasal Route, Ph.D. Dissertation, University of Kentucky, Lexington, 1983.
60. **Huang, C. H., Kimura, R., Bawarshi, R., and Hussain, A.,** Mechanisms of nasal absorption of drugs. II. Absorption of L-tyrosine and the effect of structural modification on its absorption, *J. Pharm. Sci.,* 74, 1298, 1985.
61. **Hussain, A., Faraj, J., Aramaki, Y., and Truelove, J. E.,** Hydrolysis of leucine enkephalin in the nasal cavity of the rat — a possible factor in the low bioavailability of nasally administered peptides, *Biochem. Biophys. Res. Commun.,* 133, 923, 1985.
62. **Faraj, J. A.,** A Study of the Mechanisms of Nasal Absorption of Peptides in Rats, Ph.D. Dissertation, University of Kentucky, Lexington, 1986.
63. **Purdie, J. E. and Benoiton, N. L.,** Piperazinedione formation from esters of dipeptides containing glycine, alanine, and sarcosine: the kinetics in aqueous solution, *J. Chem. Soc. Perkin Trans. II,* 1845, 1973.
64. **Steinberg, S. M. and Bada, J. L.,** Peptide Decomposition in the neutral pH region via the formation of diketopiperazines, *J. Org. Chem.,* 48, 2295, 1983.
65. **Gu, L. and Strickley, R. G.,** Diketopiprazine formation, hydrolysis, and epimerization of the new dipeptide angiotensin-converting enzyme inhibitor RS-10084, *Pharm. Res.,* 4, 392, 1987.
66. **Dannan, H., Khawam, M. N., Bogardus, J. B., Hussain, A. A., and Crooks, P. A.,** S-Acylation of cysteine by O-acetylsalicylic anhydride: a possible mechanism for aspirin hypersensitivity?, *J. Pharm. Sci.,* 75, 1081, 1986.

67. **Steinberg, S. and Bada, J. L.,** Diketopiperazine formation during investigations of amino acid racemization in dipeptides, *Science,* 213, 544, 1981.

68. **Bouvette, R. E.,** Studies on the *In Vitro* and *In Vivo* Hydrolysis and Intramolecular Aminolysis of L-Aspartyl-L-Phenylalanine Methyl Ester, Ph.D. Dissertation, University of Kentucky, Lexington, 1986.

69. **Su, K. S. E., Campanale, K. M., Mendelsohn, L. G., Kerchner, G. A., and Gries, C. L.,** Nasal delivery of polypeptides. I. Nasal absorption of enkephalins in rats, *J. Pharm. Sci.,* 74, 394, 1985.

70. **Ben-Harari, R. R. and Youdim, M. B. H.,** The lung as an endocrine organ, *Biochem. Pharmacol.,* 32, 189, 1983.

71. **Hechtman, H. B. and Shapiro, D.,** Lung metabolism and systemic organ function, *Circ. Shock,* 9, 457, 1982.

72. **Pang, J. A. and Geddes, D. M.,** The biochemical properties of the pulmonary circulation, *Lung,* 159, 231, 1981.

73. **Ryan, J. W.,** Assay of peptidases and protease enzymes *in vivo, Biochem. Pharmacol.,* 32, 2127, 1981.

74. **Schwartz, J. C., Malfroy, B., and DeLa Baume, S.,** Biological inactivation of enkephalins and the role of enkephalin-dipeptidyl-carboxy-peptidase (enkephalinase) as neuropeptidase, *Life Sci.,* 29, 1715, 1981.

75. **Gillespie, M. N., Krechniak, J. W., Crooks, P. A., Altiere, R. J., and Olson,   J. W.,** Pulmonary metabolism of exogenous enkephalins in isolated perfused rat lungs, *J. Pharmacol. Exp. Ther.,* 232, 675, 1985.

76. **Llorens, C. and Schwartz, J. C.,** Enkephalinase activity in rat peripheral organs, *Eur. J. Pharmacol.,* 69, 113, 1981.

77. **Crooks, P. A., Bowdy, B. D., Reinsel, C. N., Iwamoto, E. T., and Gillespie,   M. N.,** Structure activity evidence against opiate receptor involvement in leu-enkephalin-induced pulmonary vasoconstriction, *Biochem. Pharmacol,* 33, 4095, 1984.

78. **Enna, S. J. and Schanker, L. S.,** Absorption of saccharides and urea from the rat lung, *Am. J. Physiol.,* 222, 409, 1972.

79. **Hemberger, J. A. and Schanker, L. S.,** Pulmonary absorption of drugs in the neonatal rat, *Am. J. Physiol.,* 234(2), C191, 1978.

80. **Schanker, L. S. and Hemberger, J. A.,** Relation between molecular weight and pulmonary absorption rate of lipid-insoluble compounds in neonatal and adult rats, *Biochem. Pharmacol,* 32, 2599, 1983.

Chapter 4

PRO-DRUGS FOR PULMONARY DRUG TARGETING

H. B. Kostenbauder and S. Sloneker

TABLE OF CONTENTS

I. INTRODUCTION

The number and variety of marketed pulmonary pro-drugs is quite small; therefore, much of what is presented here is presented as "potential" application. The following is a presentation of some background and theoretical considerations, however, some of the successful applications are discussed in detail.

II. POTENTIAL BENEFITS FROM LUNG TARGETING OF DRUGS VIA PRO-DRUGS

Some obvious potential benefits from lung targeting of drugs via pro-drugs would include improved selectivity of action in lung relative to effects on other organs, prolongation of therapeutic effect, and conferral of, or enhancement of, pulmonary activity.

A. IMPROVED SELECTIVITY OF ACTION IN LUNG RELATIVE TO EFFECTS ON OTHER ORGANS

Such selectivity might be achieved through systemic administration of pro-drugs which have high affinity for lung and/or for which lung exhibits a higher rate of metabolic conversion to active drug than do other tissues. Especially high selectivity might be obtained when pro-drugs such as those described above are administered locally by inhalation. Examples of pro-drugs exhibiting selectivity of action in lung are presented below.

1. Dipivaloyl Isoproterenol

Esterification of the catechol functions of isoproterenol to produce dipivaloyl ester yields a pro-drug (Figure 1) which itself is without pharmacologic activity, but which upon hydrolysis to isoproterenol *in vivo* yields several advantages relative to the parent drug.[1] When administered by aerosol to guinea pigs, the dipivaloyl ester of isoproterenol decreased cardiac side effects relative to isoproterenol, and increased antiasthmatic properties based on protection against histamine-induced bronchospasm.[1] Apparently this is because of preferential uptake of the lipophilic pro-drug by lung relative to heart, and to greater esterase activity of lung relative to heart tissue.

2. Bitolterol

Bitolterol (Figure 2), the di-*p*-toluoyl ester of *N-t*-butylarterenol, is widely recognized as the classic example of a pro-drug illustrating improved selectivity of action in lung relative to other organs. This drug is discussed in detail later in the chapter.

B. PROLONGATION OF THERAPEUTIC EFFECT

Bitolterol also falls into this category. The pro-drug bitolterol exhibits a substantially prolonged bronchodilator effect, relative to its parent drug *N-t*-butylarterenol, possibly by concentrating in lung and undergoing slow hydrolysis there.[2]

However, it is not essential that a pro-drug concentrate in lung and be hydrolyzed there in order to obtain a prolonged therapeutic effect. Bambuterol[3] (Figure 3) is a dimethylcarbamate of terbutaline. The dimethylcarbamate provides a quite stable linkage and protects the phenolic functions against metabolic conjugation; the dimethyl carbamate also increased lipophilicity and therefore reduces renal clearance relative to the parent terbutaline. The pro-drug thus has an increased residence time in the body and a sustained bronchodilator effect is achieved through the slow hydrolysis of the dimethylcarbamate linkage (this hydrolysis is primarily extrapulmonary) resulting in a substantial systemic release of terbutaline. This drug and other terbutaline pro-drugs are discussed in greater detail later in the chapter.

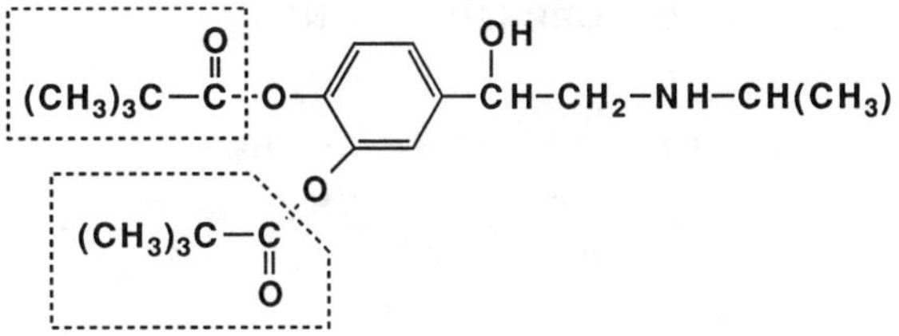

FIGURE 1. Dipivaloyl isoproterenol. The dotted lines enclose the pro-drug portion of the molecule.

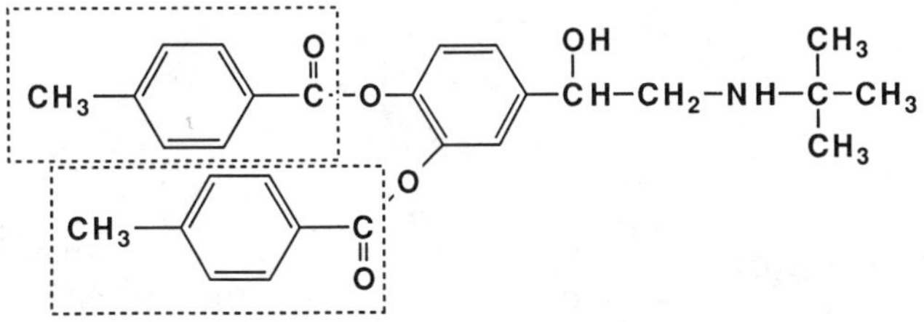

FIGURE 2. Bitolterol, the di-*p*-toluolyl ester of *N*-*t*-butylarterenol.

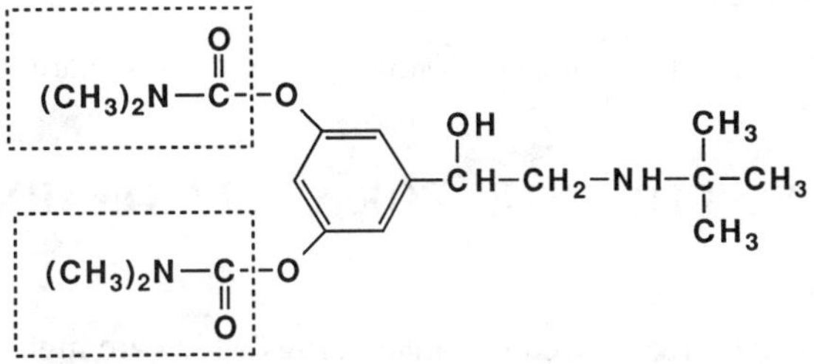

FIGURE 3. Bambuterol, the dimethylcarbamate of terbutaline.

C. CONFERRAL OF PULMONARY ACTIVITY OR ENHANCEMENT OF PULMONARY ACTIVITY

This would primarily involve modification that would deliver drugs to regions of the lung to which they normally had poor access. We are, in a later section, able to illustrate a theoretical pro-drug application involving drug metabolism, but for a therapeutic example it is necessary to resort to speculation.

Let us say, for example, that an agent which was an effective 5-lipoxygenase inhibitor in *in vitro* tests failed as an antiasthmatic drug when tested *in vivo* because the compound showed relatively poor lung uptake. Many such compounds possess -OH or -COOH functions which might be derivatized, as discussed below, to specifically enhance lung uptake of the agent and thus its antiasthmatic activity. It seems rather surprising that this approach does not seem to have been very actively explored.

In effect, this is the same principle indicated in earlier examples, except that in this case the goal is to achieve an effect in lung that is not achieved when the parent drug itself is administered.

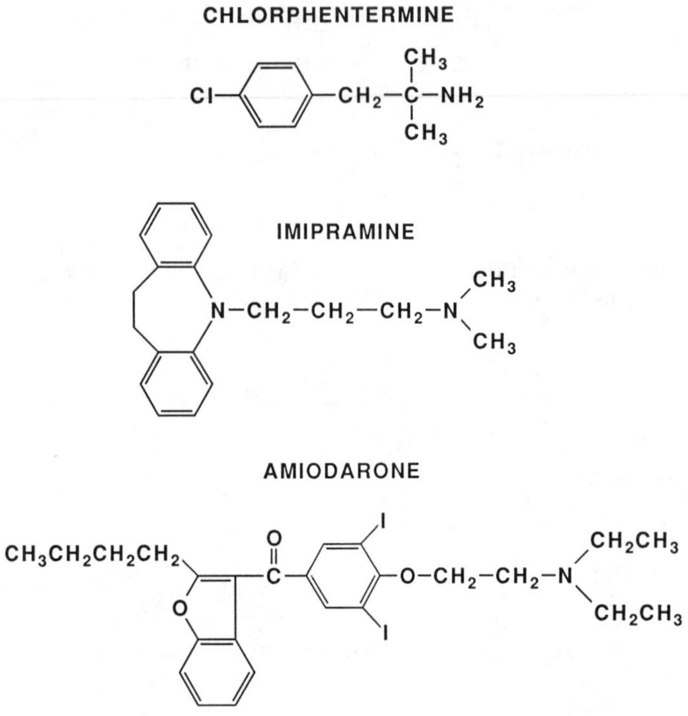

CHLORPHENTERMINE

IMIPRAMINE

AMIODARONE

FIGURE 4. Three drugs which form noneffluxable (very slowly effluxable) lung pools *in vivo.*

III. DESIRABLE ATTRIBUTES FOR A PULMONARY PRO-DRUG

A. LUNG UPTAKE

It has been rather widely recognized that many drugs which are highly lipophilic and are strongly basic amines (protonated at physiologic pH) show, upon systemic administration, a lung/plasma ratio quite a bit higher than the tissue/plasma ratio exhibited by other body organs. In isolated perfused lung studies, some of these drugs have been shown to efflux from lung in a way which can be represented as efflux from several kinetically distinct pools in lung tissue. For some drugs, efflux from one of the pools may be so slow as to be unobservable under the relatively short observation periods (a few hours) during which isolated perfused lung systems remain viable. Such drugs have been said to exhibit noneffluxable, or, more correctly, very slowly effluxable lung pools.

If, indeed, such very slowly effluxable pools exist *in vivo,* it would be expected that there would be an increase in lung/plasma ratios on repeated drug administration as well as persistence of drug in the lung long after it disappeared from other regions of the body. Experimental evidence exists to show that a few agents do exhibit these characteristics. Imipramine shows such persistence *in vivo* in rabbit lungs,[4] though not in the rat.[5] Chlorphentermine[6] and amiodarone[7] are other drugs for which such accumulation and persistence can be demonstrated *in vivo.* Structures for these compounds are shown in Figure 4.

At one point we reasoned that it might be possible to use a modification of the molecule of a proven noneffluxable pool (NEP) drug to direct pro-drugs to this lung uptake site to achieve a long residence of pro-drug in the lung.[8] We therefore took chlorphentermine, a classic example of drug exhibiting a noneffluxable pool and showing *in vivo* lung accumulation, and modified it by attaching a -COOH with which we could esterify a reputed pulmonary drug, as shown in

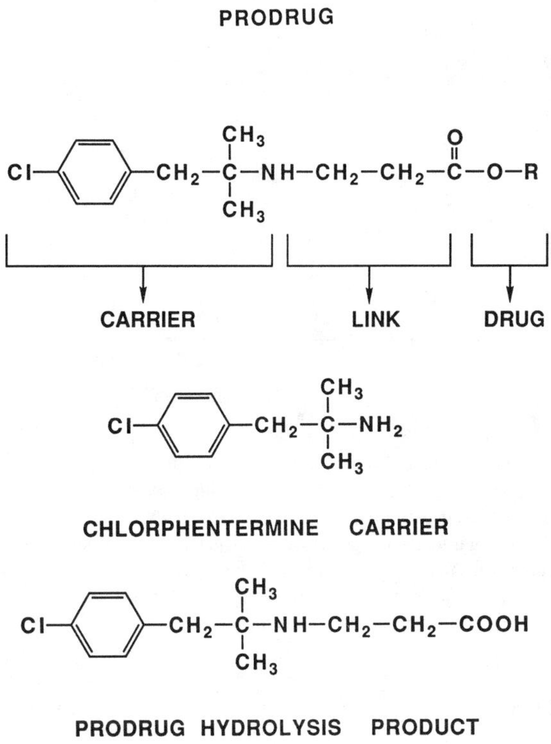

PRODRUG

FIGURE 5. Attempted use of a modified chlorphentermine carrier to
"anchor" a pro-drug in the lung NEP.

Figure 5. The hope was that the modified chlorphentermine would anchor the pro-drug in the noneffluxable pool site, and then, when the ester link hydrolyzed and released the free drug moiety, the negatively charged chlorphentermine carboxylate would rapidly wash out of the lung. It was found that the pro-drug did indeed compete with chlorphentermine for lung tissue binding, and that the ester link was hydrolyzed in lung. Figure 6 illustrates a study carried out to further test the hypothesis. Chlorphentermine was administered to a recirculating isolated perfused lung preparation and a steady-state was established between lung tissue and perfusion medium. (Chlorphentermine is not metabolized in lung.) At this point the pro-drug was administered and it displaced chlorphentermine as indicated by increased chlorphentermine concentration in the perfusion medium. When pro-drug infusion was terminated, the decline in chlorphentermine concentration in perfusion medium suggested that the pro-drug was being hydrolyzed and the carrier washed out of the lung, allowing chlorphentermine to return to its binding sites. *In vivo* activity of this pro-drug could not be evaluated, however, since the pro-drug itself was found to have a severe hypotensive effect, making it extremely toxic.

The above experience necessitated a closer look at just what were the structural features essential in a molecule to access the so-called NEP or slowly effluxable pool (SEP). We wished to determine what were the essential molecular features for this uptake. The first drug selected for study was verapamil (Figure 7), which is positively charged at physiologic pH, is highly lipophilic, and is not metabolized in lung.

Recirculating isolated perfused lung data (Figure 8) show extensive lung uptake of verapamil to produce a lung/perfusate ratio of 270/1 for artificial perfusion medium containing 3% bovine serum albumin. (The lung/plasma ratio *in vivo* is only about 67/1 because verapamil binds to α-1-acid glycoprotein present in rat plasma.)

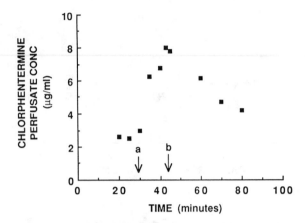

FIGURE 6. Demonstration that addition of the pro-drug shown in Figure 5 is capable of competing with chlorphentermine for lung binding sites in recirculating isolated perfused rabbit lung. Initiation of pro-drug infusion at point A causes displacement of chlorphentermine into perfusion medium from lung uptake sites; upon cessation of infusion at point B, chlorphentermine again is taken up by lung as the pro-drug is metabolized and vacates uptake sites.

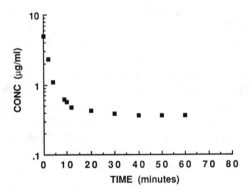

FIGURE 7. Verapamil, a drug with structural features required for lung uptake.

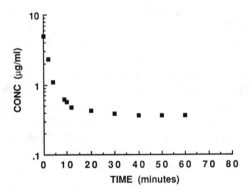

FIGURE 8. Uptake of verapamil by rat lung in a recirculating isolated perfused lung preparation.

Washout kinetics for verapamil in a nonrecirculating isolated perfused rat lung exhibit a biexponential plot (Figure 9) which provides evidence for two distinct effluxing pools that account for 54% of the drug taken up, and no efflux of the other 46% during the typical 1 to 2 h experimental period.

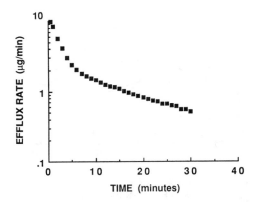

FIGURE 9. Rate of efflux of verapamil from a nonrecirculating isolated perfused rat lung preparation.

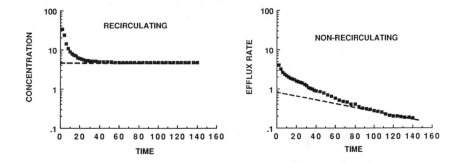

FIGURE 10. Simulation showing recirculating and nonrecirculating data for the same uptake and efflux parameters. Nonrecirculating data obtained up to 60 min show only 2 efflux components. However, by simultaneously analyzing nonrecirculating data up to just 60 min along with the recirculating data, one can accurately obtain the "unseen" third efflux component beyond 60 min (illustrated by the broken line).

A flow model was developed which adequately described kinetics of verapamil uptake and efflux for both recirculating and nonrecirculating studies.[9] By simultaneous fitting, using data from both the recirculating and nonrecirculating studies, it is possible to obtain more information and model parameters than from either study alone. The rationale is analogous to the fact that for a first-order reversible process, the rate constant for approach to equilibrium is the sum of the rate constants for the forward and reverse processes. Thus, when observation time is limited, use of equilibrium data along with efflux data make it possible to "see" efflux components not otherwise discernible over that period of observation. Simulated data are presented in Figure 10, to illustrate the point. In this example, efflux data obtained up to 1 h show just two efflux components. When efflux data up to just the 1 h point are, however, combined with nonrecirculating data for rate of approach to steady-state, model parameters are obtained which allow the efflux data beyond the 1 h point to be generated. Thus, the simultaneous fitting provided evidence for an additional efflux component which could not have been identified through the use of 1 h efflux data alone.

Application of this methodology to verapamil isolated perfused lung studies indicated that at a flow rate of 8 ml/min, efflux was experimentally observed from two lung pools with efflux $t\gamma_2$ of 1.4 and 14.6 min, respectively, and these pools accounted for 54% of the drug taken up by lung. Of the verapamil taken up by lung, 45% was in a so-called noneffluxable or slowly effluxable pool for which the predicted efflux half-life would be 17.2 h.

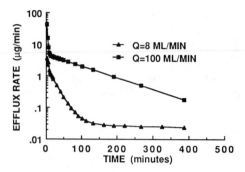

PREDICTED ER VS. TIME OBTAINED FROM BEST-FIT
ESTIMATES IN CUMULATIVE MODEL

FIGURE 11. Analysis of verapamil isolated perfused rat lung
data obtained at flow of 8 ml/min shows three efflux pools
with the third being an SEP with efflux half-life of 17.2 h. At
a simulated flow of 100 ml/min the SEP vanishes, and 100%
of the drug in the lung effluxes rapidly from pools 1 and 2.

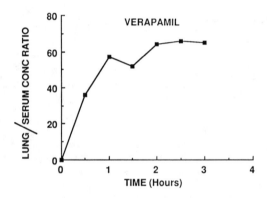

FIGURE 12. *In vivo* data for rats showing rapid attainment
of lung/serum steady-state for verapamil after i.v. bolus at
time zero. (n = 4)

However, isolated perfused rat lung preparations generally can run at only a fraction of *in vivo*
blood flow. Isolated perfused rat lungs will rapidly develop edema if flows are increased beyond
about 20 ml/min. *In vivo* blood flow in a rat, however, may more typically be in the range of 50
to 100 ml/min. Incremental increases in flow up to 20 ml/min showed a decrease in the NEP size,
and the flow model projection for a flow rate of 100 ml/min, illustrated in Figure 11, shows
evidence of only two efflux components and rapid washout of 100% of the drug. The prediction,
therefore, is that despite the 46% NEP observed at the 8 ml/min flow rate in the isolated perfused
lung studies, there would be no noneffluxable pool *in vivo* where flow rates would be 100 ml/
min or higher.

In vivo data for lung/serum ratios obtained from Sprague-Dawley rats at various times after
i.v. administration of verapamil indicate that, as shown in Figure 12, a constant lung/serum ratio
is attained within 2 h. There is no indication of a continued increase in lung/serum ratio that
would be expected if there were a noneffluxable pool *in vivo*. Thus, in agreement with model
prediction from isolated perfused lung (IPL) studies, there is no *in vivo* noneffluxable pool for
verapamil in rat lung.

It seems highly probable that most of the literature reports of amine drugs sequestering in lung and exhibiting NEPs or SEPs are artifacts arising from the necessary restriction on flow rates in isolated perfused lung preparations. While dozens of strongly basic lipophilic amines have been found to exhibit high lung uptake, very few have been found to truly sequester in lung and exhibit slowly effluxable pools *in vivo*.

These findings turned our efforts from seeking pro-drugs which would establish NEPs in lung to simply achieving high concentration of pro-drug in lung. Very simple amines such as octylamine show high affinity for lung tissue. Fowler et al.[10] found that in rabbits 70% of an i.v dose of octylamine was taken up by lung within 1 min. In studies in mice, Fowler et al.[11] also found that for a series of aliphatic amines, lung uptake increased with increasing chain length and uptake correlated with octanol/water partitioning. These workers also noted superior lung uptake for amine containing chains relative to other functions. Although octylamine itself is rapidly metabolized in lung, that does not detract from the observation that chemically simple, strongly basic, lipophilic amines will tend to concentrate in lung. Because complex molecules may result in new pharmacologic activities, it seem appropriate to keep structures as simple as possible and aim to achieve a high lung/plasma steady-state ratio, rather than be concerned about a mythical NEP. Any pro-drug having the characteristics of high lipophilicity and a strongly basic amine function might be expected to exhibit the desired lung uptake.

B. LUNG METABOLIC CAPABILITY TO CONVERT PRO-DRUG TO ACTIVE DRUG MOIETY

Lung tissue exhibits relatively high, though species dependent, nonspecific esterase activity. Thus drugs possessing hydroxyl or carboxyl functions may be readily derivatized to yield potential pro-drug linkages such as carboxylate or carbonate esters. Rates of *in vivo* cleavage can be altered by selection of aliphatic or aromatic coupling agents and by stereochemical factors. Lung tissue contains a variety of additional enzyme activities, but the above functions appear to represent the best opportunities.

C. RETENTION OF PARENT DRUG IN LUNG TISSUE AFTER RELEASE FROM PRO-DRUG

It might be anticipated that pro-drug approaches might serve little or no purpose if the pro-drug releases the drug at an action site at which the drug is not retained. Unlike the case of the blood-brain barrier, there is no basis for an expectation that small, relatively polar drug molecules would be strongly retained in lung when released intracellularly upon hydrolysis of the carrier pro-drug. Indeed, there is evidence that at least a substantial fraction of the released drug rapidly effluxes to the systemic circulation. Whether enhanced pharmacological response, which clearly occurs, might be attributed simply to a fleetingly higher local drug concentration or to entrapment of minute, but important, quantities of drug has not been established.

While no specific data can be cited from pro-drug pharmacologic studies correlating effect with drug concentration at an effector site, a striking example relative to pulmonary drug metabolism can be described.[12] Isosorbide dinitrate (ISDN) is a drug which is metabolized in lung homogenate by a typical A → B → C process: dinitrate to 2- or 5-mononitrate to isosorbide. Formation of the mononitrates occurs rapidly; then there is slow conversion to the completely denitrated isosorbide. However, if ISDN is administered to an isolated perfused rabbit lung, completely denitrated isosorbide appears ten times as fast as if one of the mononitrate intermediates was added to the lung.[12] In the isolated perfused lung, it appears that ISDN releases the mononitrates near metabolic sites that are not so accessible to the mononitrates themselves. This is of no clinical relevance, since ISDN is not a pulmonary drug, but it may be looked upon as a classic example of how a pro-drug might alter parent drug metabolism.

There are a number of other examples of enhanced lung metabolism following administration of a pro-drug. For example, isoproterenol is usually slowly metabolized by lung to 3-*O*-

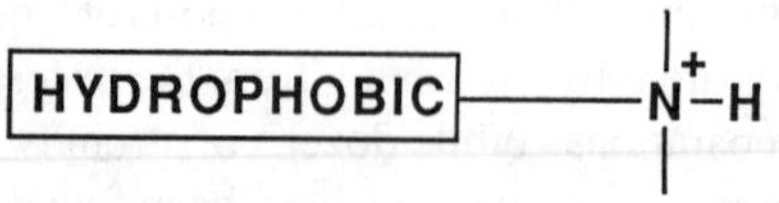

FIGURE 13. Characteristics for avid lung uptake: a substantial hydrophobic moiety and a strongly basic nitrogen.

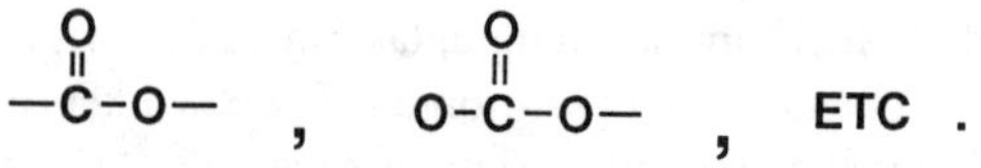

FIGURE 14.   Potential linking functions for lung pro-drugs.

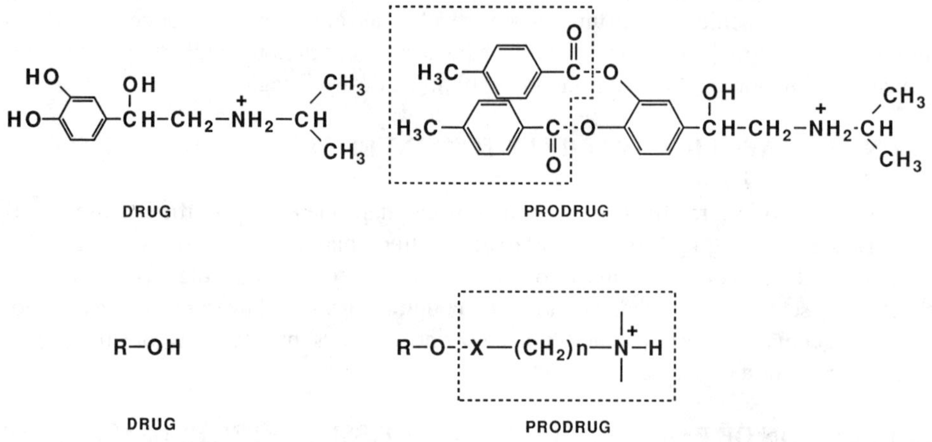

FIGURE 15.   Two approaches to lung-targeted pro-drugs. In the example in the upper half of the slide, the drug molecule provides the strongly basic nitrogen and the pro-drug moiety confers lipophilicity; in the example in the lower half of the slide the pro-drug contributes the basic nitrogen.

methylisoproterenol. When isoproterenol is administered to an isolated perfused rabbit lung as a di-*p*-toluoyl ester pro-drug, however, there is a huge increase in the rate of lung production of the 3-*O*-methyl metabolite.[13] If pro-drugs can deliver agents to sites where they are more efficiently metabolized, it is reasonable to expect that pro-drugs may also be capable of more efficient delivery to sites of pharmacologic action. This may be the case even in the absence of formidable barriers such as the blood-brain barrier.

IV. DESIGN OF PRO-DRUGS

From knowledge of optimal structural characteristics leading to preferential uptake by lung (Figure 13) and knowledge of lung metabolism of potential drug-carrier linking functions (Figure 14), it is possible to design pro-drugs to target a drug to the lung. There are a number of successful examples of the type illustrated in the top half of Figure 15 (bitolterol, for example). Examples of the type illustrated in the lower half of Figure 15 are at this time hypothetical, but would seen to have considerable potential.

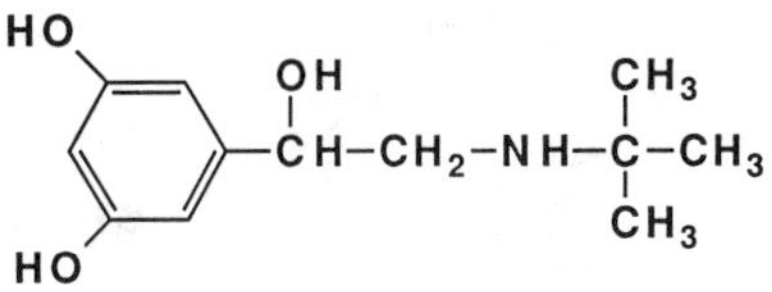

FIGURE 16. The bronchodilator drug, terbutaline.

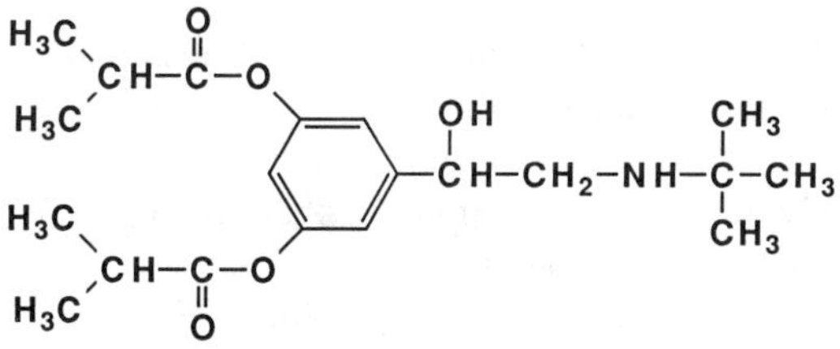

FIGURE 17. The terbutaline pro-drug, ibuterol.

V. PULMONARY PRO-DRUG EXAMPLES

A. TERBUTALINE PRO-DRUGS
1. Parent Drug

The bronchodilator terbutaline (Figure 16) is a relatively polar molecule with little affinity for lung tissue. Administered i.v., terbutaline exhibits an elimination half-life of about 4 h. The drug is rapidly absorbed following inhalation, with peak plasma concentrations occurring within 30 min. Following oral administration, the drug is slowly and incompletely absorbed, with peak plasma concentrations occurring at 1 to 4 h. Bioavailability is quite variable and of the order of 7 to 26%.[14] The drug undergoes substantial gut wall and liver first-pass metabolism, largely to sulfate conjugate. Pharmacologic effects have been correlated with plasma terbutaline concentrations.[15-17] The effect compartment apparently is relatively close to the central compartment, showing parallelism, with just a slight lag when comparing effects to plasma concentration.[17]

2. Ibuterol

The pro-drug ibuterol is the di-isobutyryl ester of the resorcinol functions of terbutaline (Figure 17). Ibuterol is rapidly hydrolyzed to terbutaline after i.v. administration, and the two drugs are pharmacologically equivalent after i.v. administration. After oral administration, ibuterol is adsorbed more rapidly than terbutaline, exhibits an earlier peak plasma concentration, and therefore a shorter duration of effect than oral terbutaline. Interestingly, administration of the pro-drug leads to *increased* conjugation of terbutaline during oral absorption, apparently due to better tissue penetration from the pro-drug.[15] Net improvement in bioavailability is therefore only about 1.6-fold.

After inhalation, ibuterol is about 3 times as effective as terbutaline in inhibition of bronchospasm 5 min after inhalation.[18] Cardiovascular side effects produced by larger doses via this route also were greater for ibuterol. It was suggested that the more pronounced effects of ibuterol are attributable to better tissue penetration,[18] and that may be so. However, since no plasma terbutaline concentrations were measured it might be argued that the enhanced effect is just more rapid absorption of ibuterol, and thus higher terbutaline concentrations at the 5 min

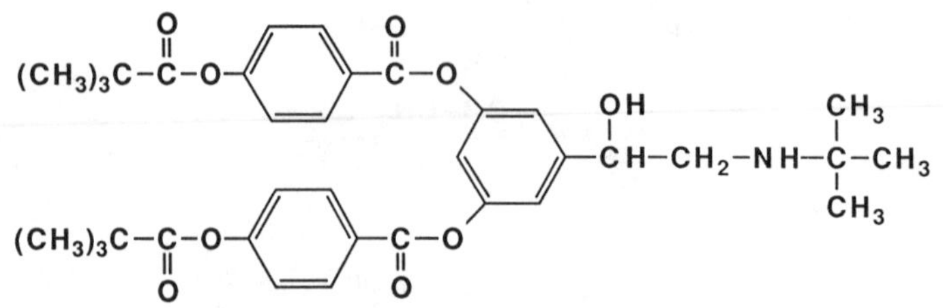

FIGURE 18. The cascade ester terbutaline pro-drug, D 2438.

point of measurement. Other data do show more rapid absorption of ibuterol relative to terbutaline after administration to lung, but at all time points both lung and serum terbutaline concentrations were higher after *terbutaline* administration.[19] It therefore appears that the pro-drug ibuterol does indeed exhibit a greater pulmonary pharmacologic effect or potency than does terbutaline when administered by inhalation.

Isolated perfused lung studies show a 20- to 30-fold greater lung extraction of ibuterol relative to terbutaline, but both ibuterol and its metabolites appear to efflux from lung rapidly upon cessation of drug infusion.[20]

3. Bambuterol

Bambuterol is the *bis-N,N*-dimethylcarbamate of terbutaline (Figure 3). This carbamate pro-drug of terbutaline was developed to provide a compound that would be sufficiently lipophilic to yield good oral absorption and be more resistant to hydrolysis than were fatty acid esters such as ibuterol.[3] Thus, bambuterol produces a sustained release of terbutaline as a result of its slow, primarily extrapulmonary hydrolysis and this derivative can be dosed orally at less frequent intervals than terbutaline.[21] Early clinical studies indicated that both bronchodilator effects and side effects were correlated with terbutaline plasma concentrations.[21] However, it has been suggested that in current clinical trials there appears to be an effect at low doses which is greater than that predicted by plasma concentrations.[22] This ester is not readily metabolized in lung, and inhalation is therefore not an effective route of administration. Though isolated perfused lung studies indicated that bambuterol effluxed from lung quite rapidly, there is also evidence of modest lung biotransformation capability for this compound, and it has been suggested that local release of small quantities of terbutaline in lung may be of significance with respect to the action of this pro-drug.[23]

4. Cascade Ester

A rather unique approach to a terbutaline prodrug is a compound which has been referred to as a cascade ester (Figure 18).[3] The phenolic functions of terbutaline are esterified with *p*-hydroxybenzoic acid, and the -OH of *p*-hydroxybenzoic acid is further esterified with pivalic acid. The hypothesis was that the pivalate ester would initially be hydrolyzed and conjugated during first-pass metabolism, thus protecting the terbutaline -OH, and that the release of terbutaline by hydrolysis of the benzoyl ester link would be delayed. It appears that in dogs the systemic release of terbutaline from this compound is almost as slow as from bambuterol.[3] Reportedly, however, higher esterase activity in humans presents an obstacle to the achievement of such results in man.[24]

Figure 19 illustrates that both bambuterol and the cascade ester are very slowly hydrolyzed in human plasma relative to their half-esters and ibuterol. One does not, therefore, see significant plasma concentration of the monoester of these pro-drugs *in vivo*.

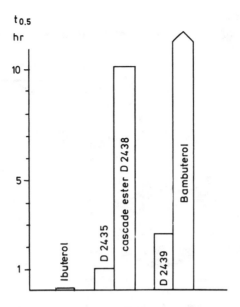

FIGURE 19. Half-lives in human plasma for formation of terbutaline from some ester pro-drugs of terbutaline. D 2435 and D 2439 are the monoesters of the cascade ester D 2438 and bambuterol, respectively. (Reproduced from Olsson, O. A. T. and Svensson, L.-A., *Pharm. Res.*, 1, 19, 1984. With permission.)

B. *N-t*-BUTYLARTERENOL PRO-DRUGS
1. Bitolterol

Bitolterol is the di-*p*-toluoyl ester of *N-t*-butylarterenol (Figure 2). This is a pro-drug which produces a prolonged bronchodilator effect after i.v., aerosol, or intraduodenal administration. It has been claimed that this is a consequence of avid uptake of a major portion of the lipophilic diester by lung, and slow hydrolysis in lung to gradually release the parent drug.[2] Our own isolated perfused lung studies of this drug[25] and the di-*p*-toluoyl ester of isoproterenol[13] (which differs only by an *N*-isopropyl rather than an *N-t*-butyl) show that this definitely is not the case in the rabbit lung. Hydrolysis was found to occur very rapidly in rabbit lung. However, rabbits are known to have esterase activity greater than that of dog or man,[26] so our findings do not necessarily invalidate the hypothesis. Unfortunately, for this foremost example of pulmonary targeting via a pro-drug, we do not have available the definitive data that are available for terbutaline and its pro-drugs. Much of the time-course data available for bitolterol are reported in terms of total radioactivity, and the one published study which appears to support the proposed mechanism for long duration of activity suffers from serious deficiencies in total drug recovery.

In 1976, Tullar et al.[27] reported on a number of pro-drug esters of *N-t*-butylarterenol. Some of these results are reproduced in Table 1. They found that all monoesters had very short duration of action, and that is consistent with previously mentioned experience with terbutaline pro-drugs. Among the di-esters, the di-*p*-toluoyl exhibited more potency and greater duration than the next best, the di-*p*-methoxybenzoyl derivative.

Interestingly, in the case of mixed esters such as *p*-toluoyl and acetyl, or *p*-methoxybenzoyl and acetyl, the *p*-methoxybenzoyl in this case had the longer duration of action.

Bitolterol definitely does exhibit some remarkable pharmacodynamic properties, irrespective of the fact that we do not have the pharmacokinetic data to fully explain them. Minatoya[28]

TABLE 1
Esters of *N-t*-Butylarterenol: Biological Effects in Dogs

R1	R2	Dose (µg/kg)	Bronchodilation		Heart rate	
			Degree	Duration (h)	Degree	Duration (h)
4–CH$_3$C$_6$H$_4$CO–	H	i.v. 10	++	> 3	++	< 0.5
		i.t. 880	++	< 2		
4–CH$_3$OC$_6$H$_4$CO	H	i.t. 800	++	< 2	+	< 0.5
4–CH$_3$C$_6$H$_4$CO–	4–CH$_3$C$_6$H$_4$CO–	i.v. 140	+++	> 5	+	2
		i.d. 280	+++	> 5	+	2
		i.t. 1080	++	> 5	±	< 1
4–CH$_3$OC$_6$H$_4$CO–	4–CH$_3$OC$_6$H$_4$CO–	i.v. 100	+	1	+	< 2
		i.d. 100	+	< 3		
4–CH$_3$C$_6$H$_4$CO–	CH$_3$CO–	i.v. 50	+++	< 1	++	< 0.5
		i.t. 1040	+++	> 1	±	< 1
4–CH$_3$OC$_6$H$_4$CO–	CH$_3$CO–	i.v. 40	+++	> 4	+	2
		i.d. 160	+++	> 5	+	< 3
		i.t. 1000	+++	> 6	±	< 1

Reprinted with permission, from Tullar et al.[27] Copyright (1976) American Chemical Society.

has shown a bronchodilation dose-response comparison of *t*-butylarterenol and bitolterol following i.v. administration to dogs, indicating a 240-fold greater dose of bitolterol to produce equivalent bronchodilator effects. This is in marked contrast to the results with the terbutaline pro-drug ibuterol; in that case, there was no difference in the i.v. dose-response curves for pro-drug and parent drug.

Aerosol administration resulted in more comparable doses of *N-t*-butylarterenol and pro-drug, with the pro-drug producing a lower peak response, but a much more prolonged response.[28] Again, this is in contrast to ibutertol, where 5 min after inhalation ibuterol showed about 3 times as much bronchodilator activity as did terbutaline.

While the bitolterol and *N-t*-butylarterenol aerosol doses are of the same order of magnitude for equivalent bronchodilator response, it should be noted that the aerosol dose of *N-t*-butylarterenol is several hundred-fold larger than that required by i.v. administration. Since administration was intratracheal, it appears that lung efficiently metabolizes *N-t*-butylarterenol.

Another observation from the same paper[28] is that the aerosol dose of bitolterol, administered to lung via tracheal cannula, was at least four times that required intraduodenally and six times that required i.v. to yield the same bronchodilator response. Lung, therefore, appears to show a huge first-pass effect for the pro-drug. Nevertheless, for both i.v. and aerosol administration, duration of effect from administration of bitolterol was some ten times that from *N-t*-butylarterenol.

Shargel and Dorrbecker[2] have suggested that the long duration of bitolterol action results from lung uptake of the intact pro-drug, followed by slow hydrolysis there. This has been the generally accepted mechanism to explain the unique properties of this drug, and it is a most attractive explanation.

Still, there are some pieces which do not comfortably fit the hypothesis. Isolated perfused rabbit lung studies of a closely related di-*p*-toluate ester show both exceptionally rapid lung hydrolysis of the pro-drug and enhanced metabolism of the parent drug.[13] While rabbit lung may be higher in esterase activity, it is difficult to envision that this lung metabolism species difference would extend from exceptionally high metabolism to protection from metabolism. Data comparing lung and blood concentrations in the rat over a 16-h period after i.v. dosing of bitolterol do show an increasing lung/blood radioactivity ratio, but the data are based on total radioactivity measurements.[29]

Alternative explanations which published data have not eliminated include: (1) the possibility that the pro-drug is metabolized in lung to an unknown but potent and long-acting pharmacologic agent (recovery of drug from lung is not complete); (2) the possibility that the pro-drug releases small amounts of the parent drug at sites in lung from which it does not readily efflux; and (3) the possibility that minute amounts of the pro-drug, not reflected by bulk concentrations of pro-drug in lung or plasma, may sequester at specific sites in lung.

It is indeed unfortunate that for this most successful example of pulmonary drug targeting via pro-drugs, we do not have the definitive data with respect to the mechanism for success.

C. OTHER DRUGS

At the time of this writing, we were unaware of published data illustrating either success or failure of pulmonary targeting via pro-drugs for other than the examples already cited. It would appear, however, that there is the potential for applying the pro-drug approach to additional agents, including lipoxygenase inhibitors, steroids, and antibiotics.

Also, we have not addressed the potential use of pro-drugs in which an active moiety is coupled with a nonabsorbable macromolecule; this approach has been treated in a separate chapter in this volume dealing with control of absorption.

REFERENCES

1. **Hussain, A. A. and Truelove, J. E.,** U.S. Patent 3, 868, 461, 1975.
2. **Shargel, L. and Dorrbecker, S. A.,** Physiological disposition and metabolism of [³H] bitolterol in man and dog, *Drug Metab. Dispos.,* 4, 72, 1976.
3. **Olsson, O. A. T. and Svensson, L. -A.,** New lipophilic ester terbutaline prodrugs with long effect duration, *Pharm. Res.,* 1, 19, 1984.
4. **Wilson, A. G. E., Pickett, R. D., Eling, T. E., and Anderson, M. W.,** Studies on the persistence of basic amines in rabbit lung, *Drug Metab. Dispos.,* 7, 420, 1979.
5. **Junod, A. F.,** Accumulation of ¹⁴C-imipramine in isolated perfused rat lungs, *J. Pharmacol. Exp. Ther.,* 183, 182, 1972.
6. **Lullmann, H., Rossen, E., and Seiler, K. -U.,** The pharmacokinetics of phentermine and chlorphentermine in chronically treated rats, *J. Pharm. Pharmacol.,* 25, 239, 1973.
7. **Sloneker, S.,** unpublished data, 1987.
8. **Syce, J. A.,** The Design and Evaluation of Model Prodrugs for Site-Specific Delivery of Drugs to the Lung, Ph.D. dissertation, University of Kentucky, Lexington, 1983.
9. **Felder, T. and Sloneker, S.,** unpublished data, 1987.
10. **Fowler, J. S., Gallagher, B. M., MacGregor, R. R., and Slatkin, D. N.,** Radiopharmaceuticals. XIX. ¹¹C-labeled octylamine, a potential diagnostic agent for lung structure and function, *J. Nucl. Med.,* 17, 752, 1976.
11. **Fowler, J. S., Gallagher, B. M., MacGregor, R. R., and Wolf, A. P.,** Carbon-11 labelled aliphatic amines in lung uptake and metabolism studies: potential for dynamic measurements *in vivo, J. Pharmacol. Exp. Ther.,* 198, 133, 1976.
12. **Mayer, P. R., Lubawy, W. C., McNamara, P. J., and Kostenbauder, H. B.,** Metabolism of isosorbide dinitrate in the isolated perfused rabbit lung, *J. Pharm. Sci.,* 72, 785, 1983.
13. **Brazzell, R. K. and Kostenbauder, H. B.,** Isolated perfused rabbit lung as a model for intravascular and intrabronchial administration of bronchodilator drugs. II. Isoproterenol prodrugs, *J. Pharm. Sci.,* 71, 1274, 1982.
14. **Nyberg, L.,** Pharmacokinetic parameters of terbutaline in healthy man. An overview, *Eru. J. Resp. Dis.,* 65(Suppl. 134), 149, 1984.
15. **Hornblad, Y., Ripe, E., Magnusson, P. O., and Tegner, K.,** The metabolism and clinical activity of terbutaline and its prodrug ibuterol, *Eur. J. Clin. Pharmacol.,* 10, 9, 1976.
16. **Van den Berg, W., Leferink, J. G., Maes, R. A. A., Fokkens, J. K., Kreukniet, J., and Bruynzeel, P. L. B.,** The effects of oral and subcutaneous administration of terbutaline in asthmatic patients, *Eur. J. Resp. Dis.,* 65(Suppl. 134), 181, 1984.

17. **Oosterhuis, B. Braat, M. C. P., Roos, C. M., Wemer, J., and Van Boxtel, C. J.,** Pharmacokinetic-pharmacodynamic modeling of terbutaline bronchodilation in asthma, *Clin. Pharmacol. Ther.,* 40, 469, 1986.
18. **Andersoon, P.,** Bronchospamolytic and cardiovascular effects of ibuterol and terbutaline given intravenously and after inhalation: drug and prodrug compared, *Acta Pharmacol. Toxicol.,* 39, 225, 1976.
19. **Ryrfeldt, A and Bodin, N. -O.,** The physiological disposition of ibuterol, terbutaline and isoproterenol after endotracheal instillation to rats, *Xenobiotica,* 5, 521, 1975.
20. **Ryrfeldt, A and Nilsson, E.,** Uptake and biotransformation of ibuterol and terbutaline in isolated perfused rat and guinea pig lungs, *Biochem. Parmacol.,* 27, 301, 1978.
21. **Holstein-Rathlou, N. -H., Laursen, L. C., Madsen, F., Svendsen, U. G., Gnosspelius, Y., and Weeke, B.,** Bambuterol: dose response study of a new terbutaline prodrug in asthma, *Eur. J. Clin. Pharmacol.,* 30, 7, 1986.
22. **Svensson, L. A.,** Bambuterol—a prodrug-prodrug with built in hydrolysis brake, *Acta Pharm. Suec.,* 24, 333, 1987.
23. **Ryrfeldt, A., Nilsson, E., Tunek, A., and Svensson, L. -A.,** Bambuterol: uptake and metabolism in guinea pig isolated lungs, *Pharm. Res.,* 5, 151, 1988.
24. **Svensson, L. A.,** Sympathomometic bronchodilators: increased selectivity with lung-specific prodrugs, *Pharm. Res.,* 2, 156, 1985.
25. **Small, D. and Kostenbauder, H. B.,** unpublished data, 1985.
26. **Roy, A. C.,** Complement and esterase activity of serums of some common laboratory animals, *Indian J. Med. Res.,* 30, 245, 1942.
27. **Tullar, B. F., Minatoya, H., and Lorenz, R. R.,** Esters of *N-tert*-butylarterenol. Long-acting new bronchodilators with reduced cardiac effects, *J. Med. Chem.,* 19, 834, 1976.
28. **Minatoya, H.,** Studies of bitolterol, di-*p*-toluate ester of *N-tert*-butylarterenol: a new long-acting bronchodilator with reduced cardiovascular effects, *J. Pharmacol. Exp. Ther.,* 206, 515, 1978.
29. **Shargel, L., Dorrbecker, S. A., and Levitt, M.,** Physiological disposition and metabolism of *N-t*-butylarterenol and its di-*p*-toluate ester (bitolterol) in the rat, *Drug Metab. Dispos.,* 4, 65, 1976.

Chapter 5

ABSORPTION, CLEARANCE, AND DISSOLUTION IN THE LUNG

Peter R. Byron and Elaine M. Phillips

TABLE OF CONTENTS

I. INTRODUCTION

Compounds administered to the lung as aerosols can be deposited in different regions as aqueous or nonaqueous solutions or solid particulates. Other chapters have reviewed solute metabolism and/or binding by lung tissues. These chapters presumed that the solute was administered in aqueous solution. Provided, therefore, that the solute was a small enough molecule to pass through lipid membranes at a reasonable rate, it was possible to avoid the consideration of clearance processes which are often associated with the removal of solid particulates from the airways.

In order to estimate correctly the speed with which the lung is cleared of compounds with different physicochemical characteristics, it is necessary to consider the simultaneous processes of absorption, ciliary and phagocytic clearance, and where appropriate, solute dissolution. These processes stand apart from the metabolism and binding properties described in the other chapters, in the sense that absorption, clearance, and dissolution kinetics can, at least in part, be predicted from a knowledge of a compound's physical chemistry and how it was administered. In order to predict the longevity of a compound in the lung after administration by aerosol inhalation, it is necessary to take all of these clearance processes and their kinetics into account. This is the case whether the information is required to predict the pharmacologic duration of action in the lung or the toxicologic implications associated with the inhalation of a slowly dissolving radionuclide.

Figure 1A shows a modification of the lung clearance model presented in 1966 by the Task Group on Lung Dynamics.[1] The model has been modified by removal of the nasopharyngeal compartment (which is not part of the lung) and with respect to the clearance process designated k_2 in which mucociliary clearance is shown correctly from the pulmonary region passing through the tracheobronchial region prior to removal to the gastrointestinal tract. Depending on the aerosol size, concentration, and the breathing regime, different doses will deposit in the tracheobronchial and pulmonary regions of the lung. The symbol f represents the deposition fraction while the subscripts TB and P designate the tracheobronchial and pulmonary compartments, respectively. The tracheobronchial region extends from the trachea to the terminal bronchioles, while the pulmonary region is the area for gas exchange.[1] The clearance processes are frequently exponential in nature and are therefore designated k_1 through k_6 as apparent first-order rate constants. In most cases absorption occurs under sink conditions and the processes k_3 and k_4 are apparently irreversible. Obviously, in some instances (e.g., with inhalation anesthetics) this assumed irreversibility would require modification.

When rapidly absorbed compounds are administered in aqueous solutions at physiologic pH parallel solute removal from the lung by mucociliary clearance can usually be neglected. This case is shown in Figure 1B and the situation is described in detail in the following section. Conversely, when a totally water-insoluble material is administered as solid particulates, then dissolution is impossible and clearance is described by Figure 1C. In practice, no compound exists in which either of the models shown as Figure 1B or 1C are valid in an absolute sense. Nevertheless, simplifications of the larger model provide an excellent framework with which to begin our discussion of the various clearance processes to which different chemical compounds are subject in the lung.

II. ABSORPTION KINETICS

A. METHODOLOGY

Intratracheal insufflation,[2] which was first described in the early 1930s, was a technique widely used to examine the distribution,[3] pharmacologic effect,[4] and clearance[5] of a number of insoluble particulates. The early emphasis was placed on pollutants, carcinogens,[6] and other toxic materials that were present in the workplace. Most of these studies were qualitative in

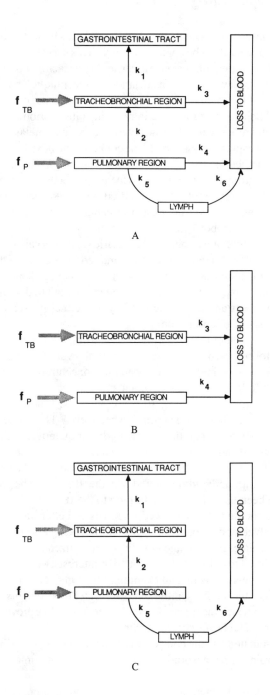

FIGURE 1. Clearance of compounds administered to the respiratory tract in low doses. Metabolism and/or binding are assumed not to occur. In (A), ciliary and lymphatic clearance occur in parallel with absorption from solution while in (B) absorption is much faster than other clearance processes. In (C), this situation is reversed.

nature. Cember et al.[7] examined the distribution and subsequent clearance of barium sulfate particles from rat lungs with the aid of autoradiographs. They were able to generate a plot of dose fraction retained vs. time, and because they considered barium sulfate totally insoluble they attributed the clearance to both mucociliary and phagocytic mechanisms. The Task Group on

Lung Dynamics later observed that many materials regarded as highly insoluble, such as barium sulfate, proved to be quite labile in biological systems.[1] This serves as an example that many of these earlier studies lacked quantitative significance due to factors not well understood at the time by the investigators. Nevertheless, insufflation as a technique of administration allowed scientists to be certain of the instilled dose, even in these early stages.

In 1970, Enna and Schanker[8] refined the intratracheal instillation technique in an effort to estimate absorption rates alone, excluding such variables as drug metabolism, and contribution from the mucociliary transport mechanism. In the course of the next 15 years Schanker's group examined the disappearance of over 50 compounds from the lungs of anesthetized animals. Because many research groups have adopted this technique, Schanker's methodology deserves a brief description. The drug, dissolved in modified Krebs'-Ringer phosphate solution, was injected via plastic tubing inserted into a tracheal cannula in the rat lung. The solution was administered at a point just above the bifurcation of the trachea in a volume of solution approximating 2% of the total lung volume. At specific time intervals after administration, the animal was sacrificed and the lungs excised and examined for amount of drug remaining at that time. The tight fitting cannula prevented the drug from being cleared via the mucociliary escalator. For each compound studied, concentration was varied to determine whether absorption was a saturable process and metabolic stability was either proven or shown to be unimportant relative to the speed of absorption.

In the 1960s and 1970s other research groups were using the isolated, perfused, and saline-filled animal lung to follow the transalveolar transport of a variety of compounds. The drug in solution was either introduced into the plasma and its concentration measured in the alveolar fluid[9,10] or its flux was followed from the alveolar space to the plasma.[11,12] In these cases half-lives were determined from log plots of $[(C_a - C_p)/C_p]$ vs. time where C_a and C_p are the concentrations in the alveolar liquid and plasma, respectively.[13] The isolated perfused lung (IPL) has continued to be a popular preparation, particularly for quantifying the respective permeabilities of the epithelial and endothelial membrane layers.[14] Recently, the isolated perfused lung has been used to study metabolism of bronchodilators[15,16] and work has been published on the absorption rates of compounds administered via the IPL.[17-19] The *in situ* perfused lung preparations[20,21] have been used in a similar fashion to the IPL.

Although all these methods have allowed scientists to better understand the transport of molecules across the alveolar membrane, they fall short in being able to offer any insight on the fate of drugs and particulates entering the lung in an aerosolized form. Research on laboratory animals has been modified to deliver the compound of interest as an aerosol and follow its path by measuring plasma levels, excising and examining the lungs or other organs for content, or tracing its disappearance by gamma scintigraphy. Schanker modified his method by passing an aerosol along a pipe into which the tracheal cannula was fitted, thus preventing clearance by the mucociliary escalator.[22] The beauty of this technique is that neither the animal's coat nor its environment is contaminated and the compound can not be ingested orally. This eliminates the complication of gastrointestinal absorption occuring at the same time as absorption from the respiratory tract.

The refinement of aerosol generation techniques and radioisotopic methods resulted in the first studies of particle deposition and clearance from human lungs in the late 1940s[23-25] in which insoluble material was radiolabeled and administered. Since then, work on the clearance of radiopharmaceuticals from healthy and diseased lung volunteers has grown dramatically. This is often performed now using soluble isotopes to determine absorption kinetics. After aerosolizing the radiopharmaceutical and administration by inhalation, the percent decline in radioactivity in a particular region of the lung is measured by a gamma camera or scintillation probe. Huchon[26] discusses how the clearance is expressed and the various calculations performed to correct for the effect of radioactivity recirculating in the vascular network. More recently, Barrowcliffe et al.[27] have examined the influence of radioactivity in the blood supply on pulmonary clearance calculations.

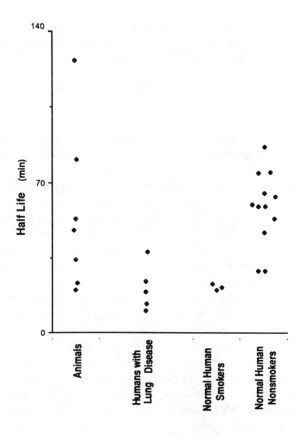

FIGURE 2. Clearance of ^{99m}Tc-diethylaminepentaacetate administered by aerosol to different species of animal and category of human
subjects. Ultrasonication was not used in any of these studies to
generate the aerosol.[22,36-39]

Both jet and ultrasonic nebulizers have been used to generate radioaerosols. However, as
Waldman and co-workers[28] have pointed out, ultrasonic nebulization may destroy the ^{99m}tech-
netium-diethylenetriaminepentaacetate (^{99m}Tc-DTPA) molecule, the most commonly used
radioaerosol. Caution should be used when interpreting data from studies using ultrasonication.[29-31] In their review, O'Brodovich and Coates[32] observe that following the clearance of
^{99m}Tc-DTPA to assess the permeability of the pulmonary epithelium "remains an experimental
investigational tool that is not yet ready for widespread clinical application". This statement is
supported by Figure 2 which shows the clearance of ^{99m}Tc-DTPA administered as an aerosol to
the lungs of various species and human subjects. The data were accumulated from a number of
independent studies and the scatter demonstrates the need to establish a standard protocol when
examining and calculating the clearance of ^{99m}Tc-DTPA from the lungs. Obviously, these are
problems inherent with both aerosol administration and solute instillation as experimental
techniques. Effros and Mason[33] offer a thorough discussion of the attributes and deficiences of
each.

B. FACTORS AFFECTING ABSORPTION KINETICS
1. Chemical Structure

The chemical structure of a compound defines its molecular weight, lipophilicity, melting
point, solubility, and binding characteristics. In other chapters we have seen how the chemical
structure of salbutamol protects it from methylation and how chemical modification of a
compound might improve targeting to the lung. This section examines those physicochemical

properties of compounds that exclusively affect absorption kinetics. The rate of absorption of such compounds as titanium oxide is limited by dissolution. Because dissolution can be an important step in the absorption process it will be considered in a separate section. Binding, metabolism and other forms of chemical transformation which occur in the lung are not discussed here.

a. Molecular Weight

In one of their earliest studies, Enna and Schanker[8] examined the absorption of various molecular weight saccharides and urea. The percentage of dose absorbed in a fixed time interval remained constant over a 100-fold concentration range, suggesting that absorption was occuring by simple diffusion. The plots of log percent unabsorbed vs. time were linear, indicating first-order absorption kinetics. The first-order absorption rate constant, k, decreased with increasing molecular weight. That is, urea (mol wt 60 Da, k = 10.4 h^{-1}) was absorbed much faster than inulin (mol wt 5250 Da, k = 0.024 h^{-1}). Because of the low lipid solubility of these hydrophilic compounds (sucrose, dextran, inulin) Schanker proposed absorption predominantly through aqueous channels (pores) or intercellular spaces in the lipid membrane. In an attempt to explain why the first-order rate constants changed with molecular weight, Schanker hypothesized three different populations of pore sizes. Urea was the smallest compound which could, therefore, pass through all channels, whereas inulin and dextran could only pass through that pore population that had the largest pore size.[8] The opinion that lipid-insoluble compounds passed through intercellular spaces was also held by Theodore et al.,[13] who determined the order of absorption of lipid insoluble compounds to be sucrose > inulin > dextran. The dextran used in their study had a reported molecular weight range of 60,000 to 90,0000 Da.

Schanker continued to examine the absorption of drugs from the rat lung and classified each compound as either lipid soluble or lipid insoluble. However, the classification as it appears in these articles[22,34] is somewhat arbitrary in as much as some compounds with low oil/water partition coefficients are included in the lipid-soluble group because they traverse the lung quickly. Table 1 is a compilation of absorption data determined by Schanker and co-workers for their class of lipid insoluble compounds. Information comes from studies performed in adult rats. Those compounds with molecular weights less than 1000 Da were absorbed at faster rates ($t_{1/2}$ = 90 min) than the larger molecules ($t_{1/2}$ = 3 to 27 h). It is interesting to note that tetraethylammonium (TEA) and mannitol are among the smallest solutes listed in Table 1, but their absorption rate constants are half those of N-acetyl procainamide ethobromide (APAEB) and benzylpenicillin, compounds twice their size. Thus it can be concluded that in a narrow molecular weight range a lipid insoluble drug's absorption rate constant cannot be predicted solely on the basis of molecular weight.

Huchon et al.[35] also tested the hypothesis that clearance from the alveolus to the bloodstream for radiopharmaceuticals depended largely on molecular weight. They studied compounds ranging in molecular weight from 163 to 76,111 Da. Figure 3 shows the relationship between clearance, %/min, and molecular weight for these compounds. The ^{99m}Tc pertechnetate (TcO$_4$) cleared much faster than the ^{111}In transferrin ([^{111}In]TF), however, the clearance of the intermediate six compounds is not strictly ranked according to their molecular weight. Huchon concluded that within a narrow molecular weight range the clearance of radiolabeled solutes is affected by other physicochemical factors in addition to molecular weight.

Effros and Mason[33] generated the log-log plot of solute clearance vs. molecular weight shown in Figure 4. The data were taken from a number of independent studies involving various subjects and methodologies. Absorptive clearance rate constants generally increase with decreasing molecular weight. In this case, some of the scatter can be explained by the inclusion of data collected from different species and the use of different solute administration techniques.[33]

TABLE 1
Absorption of Lipid Insoluble Compounds from Adult Rat Lungs

Compound	MW[a]	$t_{1/2}$[b]	k[c]	Ref.
Guanidine	59	6.3	6.6	208
Urea	60	4.0	10.4	8
Erythritol	122	37.0	1.12	208
TEA[d]	130	63.0	0.660	42
Mannitol	182	60.0	0.693	42
		33.2	1.25[i]	209
PAH[e]	194	41.0	1.01	42
		27.9	1.49[i]	209
		45.0	0.924	37
PAEB[f]	264	70.0	0.594	37
APAEB[g]	306	38.5	1.08	209
Benzylpenicillin	334	33.0	1.3	38
Sucrose	342	87.0	0.479	8
Tc-DTPA[h]	492	30.9	1.35[i]	209
Cyanocobalamin	1,355	180.0	0.231	46
Inulin	5,250	225.0	0.185	8
Dextran	20,000	688.0	0.0604	208
	75,000	1670.0	0.0249	8

[a] Molecular weight (Da).
[b] Half-life (min).
[c] First-order rate constant (h^{-1}).
[d] Tetraethylammonium.
[e] p-Aminohippuric acid.
[f] Procainamide ethobromide.
[g] N-Acetyl procainamide ethobromide.
[h] [99m]Technetium diethylenetriaminepentaacetate.
[i] Calculated from $k = 0.693/t_{1/2}$.

Data extracted from References 8, 37-38, 46, 208–209.

b. Partition Coefficient

Schanker expanded his research on absorption to include compounds of diverse chemical structure.[36-40] Previous studies had reported that solutes penetrated the alveolar wall at rates which increased with the lipid solubility of the compound.[41] Accordingly, the apparent partition coefficient of a number of compounds was determined by measuring the distribution of drug between an aqueous phase (pH 7.4) and an organic phase (chloroform) after shaking the mixture at 23°C for 1 h. Figure 5 shows half-lives plotted as a function of the logarithm of the apparent partition coefficient. The data are taken from Schanker's work.[36,39,40,42] Those compounds having partition coefficients greater than 10^8 are absorbed rapidly, however, there appears to be no continuity for others with partition coefficients less than 10^6.

Given some simplifying assumptions, if the partition coefficients and molecular weights of compounds are taken into consideration simultaneously, the investigator may be more able to estimate which compound will be absorbed most quickly.

In Figure 6, the left-hand donor compartment represents the alveolar space into which drug in solution has been instilled. The narrow barrier of thickness h represents the pulmonary membranes which separate donor from receptor compartments. The latter blood capillary can be thought of most simply as an aqueous compartment with an equivalent pH to that in the alveolar space. In deriving the relationship between molecular weight, partition coefficient, and the first-order rate constant, certain assumptions must be made with regard to this simplified model of absorption across the surface of the lung, among these that the absorption does indeed

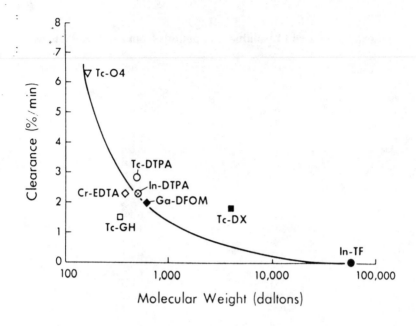

FIGURE 3.   Mean values (%/min) of the respiratory clearance of eight solutes according to their molecular weights (Daltons). Solid line is best fit. (From Huchon, G., et al., *J. Nucl. Med.,* 28 894, 1987. With permission.)

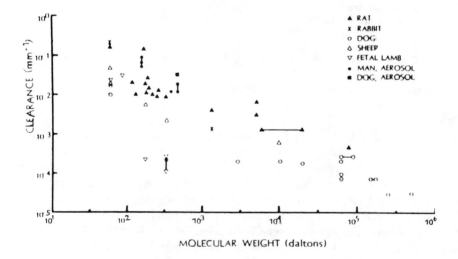

FIGURE 4.   Relationship between solute clearance from the lungs and molecular weight. Bars indicate range of molecular weights or clearance measurements. Clearances generally declined with increasing molecular weight, and were higher in rats and following administration of aerosols. (From Effros, R. M. and Mason, G. R., *Am. Rev. Resp. Dis.,* 127, S59, 1983. With permission.)

ascribe to first-order kinetics, the ratio of $C_1/C_a = C_2/C_p$ is reflected by the partition coefficient, and the concentration gradient across the pulmonary membrane is linear. The rate of change of concentration in the donor compartment with respect to time, t, may then be expressed as

$$dC_a/dt = -kC_a \qquad (1)$$

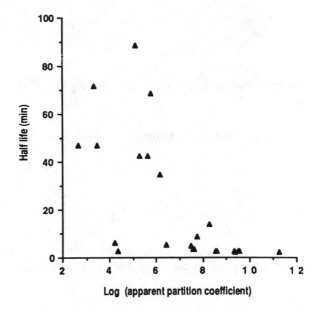

FIGURE 5. Absorption half-lives in the rat lung vs. $\log_{10}$[(chloroform/ aqueous pH 7.4) apparent partition coefficient]$_{23°C}$. Data taken from References 22, 36 to 39 and restricted to solutes with molecular weights <1000 Da.

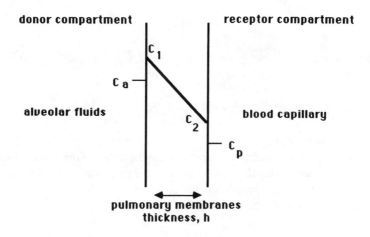

FIGURE 6. A simple model showing transpulmonary diffusion of solutes from the alveolar space to the blood.

where k is the first-order rate constant and C_a is the concentration of drug in alveolar fluid. In diffusional terms, the rate of drug transfer, dM/dt, where M is mass, across the membrane of surface area, S, and thickness, h, may be expressed as a rate of loss from the donor compartment

$$dM/dt = -[SD(C_1 - C_2)]/h \qquad (2)$$

where D is the diffusion coefficient of the drug and C_1 and C_2 are the concentrations of drug in the membrane at the donor compartment and receptor compartment boundaries, respectively. Since these concentrations are experimentally difficult to determine, they can be expressed as a function of the membrane/aqueous partition coefficient, K,

$$K = C_1/C_a = C_2/C_p \tag{3}$$

where C_p is the drug concentration in the blood capillary. Solving Equation 3 for C_1 and C_2 and substituting in Equation 2 yields

$$dM/dt = -[SDK(C_a - C_p)]/h \tag{4}$$

If C_p is assumed to be zero because of the large volume of circulating blood, then Equation 4 reduces to

$$dM/dt = -[SDKC_a]/h \tag{5}$$

If Equation 1 is then expressed in terms of drug amount by dividing by alveolar fluid volume, V (where $C_a = M/V$), then the right-hand sides of Equations 1 and 5 can be set equal to each other to show that

$$-kM = -[SDKM]/hV \tag{6}$$

Assuming that the membrane thickness, alveolar fluid volume, and surface area remain constant, then the first-order rate constant is proportional to the product of the diffusion and partition coefficients.

$$k \propto DK \tag{7}$$

The diffusion coefficient may be represented by the Stokes-Einstein relationship[43] which predicts the diffusion of a solute in a specified solvent as

$$D = RT/[6\pi\eta aN] \tag{8}$$

where η is the viscosity of the solvent, RT is the product of the universal gas constant and absolute temperature, N is Avogadro's number, and a is the radius of the solute molecule. If this relationship is correct, then using the same argument as Byron et al.,[44] it can be shown that the diffusion coefficient of a drug is proportional to the cube root of its molecular weight.[43] Thus, the first-order rate constant may be represented by

$$k \propto K/(MW)^n \tag{9}$$

where MW is molecular weight and n equals 0.33. Because it has been suggested that the Stokes-Einstein relationship does not hold for molecules less than 1000 Da, then the Wilke-Chang equation for diffusivity[45] can be used in place of Equation 8. In this case, Equation 9 would hold for n = 0.56.

Table 2 shows 20 solutes investigated by Schanker's group listed with their molecular weights (mol wt), apparent partition coefficients (K), the values for the ratio, $K/(MW)^n$ (Equation 9) and the experimentally determined first-order rate constants (k_{obs}). Because the compounds used here as examples all have molecular weights less than 1000 Da it is difficult to assess the differences between the use of the Wilke-Chang (n = 0.56) or the Stokes-Einstein (n = 0.33) relationships. The ranking of $K/(MW)^n$ is the same for both n = 0.33 and 0.56 although the predicted dependence of k on molecular weight is reduced somewhat in the latter case. It is

TABLE 2
Relationship Between First-Order Absorption Rate Constants, Solute Molecular Weights and Partition Coefficients

Solute	MW[a]	K[b]	K/(MW)$^{0.33}$	K/(MW)$^{0.56}$	k_{obs}[c]
Antipyrine	188	239,000	41,720	12,731	>41.6
Pentobarbital	226	230,000	37,759	11,052	>41.6
Phenobarbital	232	25,200	4,101	1,193	>41.6
Sulfadimethoxine	310	22,450	3,317	904	>41.6
SMOP[d]	280	14,700	2,247	626	41.6
Isoniazid	137	2,900	563	184	21.9
Chloramphenicol	323	2,460	358	97	21.9
Procaineamide	235	2,000	324	94	13.0
Sulfisoxazole	267	168	26	7.4	12.6
Doxycycline	444	3,769	494	124	5.9
Erythromycin	734	12,578	1,394	312	3.5
Tetracycline	444	1,257	164	41.4	3.0
Benzylpenicillin	334	96	13.8	3.7	1.3
Sulfaguanidine	232	28	4.6	1.3	1.0
Ethambutol	218	12.4	2.0	0.6	1.0
Ouabain	585	37.6	4.5	1.1	0.6
Dihydroouabain	587	8.1	1.0	0.2	0.5
Sulfanilic acid	174	0.2	0.04	0.01	0.9
TEA[e]	130	3.9	0.3	0.25	0.6
PAH[f]	194	0.03	0.01	0.00	0.9

[a] Molecular weight.
[b] Apparent partition coefficient.
[c] Experimentally determined first-order rate constant.
[d] Sulfamethoxypyridazine.
[e] Tetraethylammonium.
[f] p-Aminohippuric acid.

Values for MW, K, k_{obs} taken from References 36 to 39.

clear from the table that despite some improvements in prediction, there are compounds whose absorption rate constants cannot be predicted using this approach. This is probably due to the simplicity of the model which assumes no endocytosis, no membrane sequestration, and no intercellular junctions through which some drugs may pass preferentially. Similar criticism may be aimed at attempts to correlate solute diffusion coefficients with absorption rates in the lung. Often diffusion coefficients are measured in free water[8] which does not accurately reflect the tortuosity of the membrane or, for that matter, the viscous properties of the alveolar fluid. While there may appear to be a relationship between absorption rates and the diffusion coefficient,[46] examination of this parameter alone can be misleading. For example, the diffusion coefficients of mannitol and phenobarbital are roughly equivalent, however, phenobarbital is absorbed at a rate 60 times that of mannitol.[8,37]

Certain chemical structures may well be favored in terms of their absorption rates. Analysis of the chemical structure of the first six compounds in Table 2 reveals that they all contain five- or six-membered rings having at least one nitrogen as a member of the ring. Indeed those compounds having two nitrogens as part of a ring in their structure have observed first-order rate constants greater than 40 h^{-1}. It is quite possible that other structural rules for slow or fast transport may be identified as the number of compounds studied is increased in the future.

Few comparisons can be made between Schanker's work and that of others because partition coefficients are rarely determined when investigating absorption from the lung. Arakawa and Kitazawa[47] studied the absorption of xanthine derivatives using the same technique as Schanker.

TABLE 3
Absorption Half-Lives for Compounds Administered by
Aerosol or Intratracheal Instillation in the Rat Lung

Compound	Aerosol (min)	Instillation (min)
Urea	1.4	4.0
Mannitol	26.5	33.2
		60.0
Procainamide	2.3	3.2
PAH[a]	21.7	45.0
		27.9
		41.3
Guanidine	3.1	6.3
Benzylpenicillin	20.5	33.0
Barbital	0.9	1.4
Erythromycin	6.3	12.0
Amitrole	1.3	2.0
APAEB[b]	34.5	38.5
Salicylic acid	0.7	1.0
Antipyrine	0.3	<1.0

[a]   *p*-Aminohippuric acid.
[b]   *N*-Acetyl procainamide ethobromide.

Data extracted from References 8, 22, 37, 38, 40, 208, 209.

They also measured apparent chloroform/water partition coefficients at 37°C for caffeine, theophylline, and aminophylline, although log plots of percentage of unabsorbed drug vs. time were not rectilinear, and therefore the absorption process was not first-order. Nevertheless, the percent of drug absorbed in 15 s was greatest for caffeine which also had the largest partition coefficient.

c. Permeability Coefficient

The permeability coefficient has also been examined as a parameter by which absorption rates may be estimated. The permeability represents DK/h in Equation 4. It differs from a first-order rate constant ([SDK]/h in Equation 6) in that its calculation requires estimates of the surface area, S, available for solute exchange per volume, V, of alveolar fluid. The problems inherent in determining the apparent permeability coefficient, discussed by Theodore et al.,[13] are often associated with the difficulty of standardizing these terms. It is thus difficult to be able to compare work between independent research groups. This is exemplified by examining the values of permeability coefficients calculated by three research groups for the same solutes.[9-11,13]

2. Administration Technique

Intratracheal instillation and aerosol administration techniques have been discussed previously. Aerosol administration may also be assisted by forced ventilation. The dosage form of the drug delivered to the lung may also be modified by, for example, delivery of the drug in liposomes. It has been observed that these different administration techniques produce variable absorption kinetics, possibly due to alterations in the area of the lung in which the drug deposits.

a. Intratracheal Instillation vs. Aerosol Adminstration

Table 3 is a summary of absorption half-lives for compounds that have been administered to rat lungs by both techniques. Again these data are compiled from the work of Schanker and colleagues.[22,34] In general, it appears that compounds are absorbed twice as fast when given as an aerosol. However, the reason for these increased absorption rates after aerosol administration has not been conclusively proven. Two explanations, which are described below, are commonly advanced although others remain possible. These arguments differ in their fundamental assumptions and the reader should refer to the articles by Effros and Mason[33] and by Brown and Schanker[22] for a more thorough discussion.

Consider a concentration of drug, C, instilled in solution or as a liquid aerosol on the surface of the pulmonary membrane of area, S. Equation 5 can be divided by the fluid volume in which the drug is distributed, V, to yield the change in drug concentration with respect to time as

$$dC/dt = -DSC/Vh \qquad (10)$$

where C (= M/V) is the drug concentration in the fluid lining the airways, D is the diffusion coefficient, and h is the thickness of the membrane. Brown and Schanker believe that the value of V is unaffected by the contribution of instilled carrier fluid because water is supposedly absorbed very rapidly (just as quickly as inhaled liquid aerosol), thereby leaving the drug in a dissolved state on the surface coating of the membrane. Further, they believe that the ratio of S/V is the same for both an instilled solute and one delivered as a liquid aerosol. This belief was based on the observation that the first-order rate constant was unchanged for both a lipid-soluble and lipid-insoluble solute administered from a volume of solution that was increased up to tenfold.[22] Brown and Schanker reasoned that since larger rate constants were observed for aerosolized solutes and since it has been shown that aerosols penetrate to the alveolar region more efficiently than instilled solutions,[48,49] then it must be concluded that the alveolar membrane is more permeable than the membrane of the tracheobronchial region. In other words, the increased rate of absorption of solutes delivered as aerosols is due to the increased permeability of the alveolar as opposed to the bronchial membranes.

Conversely, Effros and Mason propose that the volume of carrier fluid directly affects Equation 10 and postulate that aerosols differ from instillation in that the magnitude of S/V is greater for a solute administered as a liquid aerosol than for an instilled one and is the primary reason for observed increased clearance after aerosol administration. They also argue that if the lung is adequately degassed in certain types of experiments it is likely much of the instillate will reach the alveoli, therefore ruling out the proposed possibility of differences in permeability between the tracheobronchial and alveolar regions. These latter arguments are supported by the data of Byron and Clark,[50,51] who were unable to demonstrate a difference in absorption rate constants between instillation and aerosol administration in the dog.

b. Liposome Encapsulation vs. Free Drug

Liposomes are closed vesicles surrounded by a lipid bilayer. Because of their unique structure they have become candidates to transport solutes that can be encapsulated in their hydrophilic centers or associated with the membrane lipids. Hydrophilic solutes are usually contained in the water-filled core while hydrophobic materials distribute through the phospholipids used to form the bilayers.

When McCullough and Juliano[52] intratracheally administered β-cytosine arabinoside in both the free and encapsulated form to the lungs of rats they observed that the free drug left the lung rapidly ($t_{1/2}$ = 20 min) while the encapsulated drug persisted in the lung ($t_{1/2}$ = 6 h). The log plot of percent total drug vs. time was linear for the free drug but appeared biphasic for the liposomal form. Recently, Dalby and Byron[53] have generated biphasic curves for the *in vitro* release of terbutaline from phosphatidylcholine liposomes while Farr et al.[54] showed prolonged retention of liposome associated ^{99m}Tc label in the lungs following inhalation.

In contrast, Debs et al.[55] investigated the lung uptake of aerosolized free and encapsulated pentamidine in mice. They reported that pentamidine was not cleared during the first 48 h after administration and suggested that pulmonary sequestration had taken place. The pulmonary retention patterns of the free drug were very similar to those of the encapsulated drug. These workers noted that compounds of similar molecular weight are cleared from the lung at a much faster rate and conceded that the drug tissue interactions in the lung are not known. Analysis of the chemical structure of pentamidine reveals multiple positive charged amino groups suggesting the possibility of lung binding. Many factors govern the behavior of liposomes: their size, net surface charge, and the presence of surface proteins. Work has been initiated in examining the surface charge and size characteristics of liposomes in the hopes of optimizing drug delivery to the lungs.[56] The pentamidine example above shows that the performance of these formulations in modifying disposition in the lungs can be expected to be drug specific.

c. Forced Ventilation

In 1976, Egan et al.[57] reported that distension of a portion of the *in vivo* sheep lung by fluid filling resulted in increased clearance of nonelectrolyte solutes. This increased clearance was thought to be due to increased permeability of the membrane caused by stretching the intercellular spaces. Researchers postulated that the same effect would be observed when aerosol administration was assisted by forced ventilation. For example, lung volume may be altered by applying positive end expiratory pressure (PEEP) to the airways, continuous positive airway pressure (CPAP), or negative airway pressure. Intermittent positive pressure breathing (IPPB) is employed to deliver aerosols to humans with obstructed airways.

A number of clinical trials were performed to determine whether IPPB would enhance the pharmacologic effect of salbutamol administered as an aerosol to patients suffering from severe asthma attacks. In 1978, Campbell et al.[58] concluded that IPPB-assisted treatment had no advantage over unassisted salbutamol treatment. More recently, this conclusion was also reached by Fergusson and co-workers.[59] To the contrary, Webber et al.[60] concluded that IPPB-assisted treatment was more efficacious than inhalation of nebulized salbutamol without IPPB. In a nationwide study commissioned by the National Heart, Lung and Blood Institute the effect of IPPB-assisted therapy on patients with chronic obstructive pulmonary disease (COPD) was examined over a period of 3 years. It was reported in an editorial that the results of this investigation "may be regarded as definitive in showing that the regular application of positive pressure to the lungs of stable patients with COPD is of minimal or no therapeutic value".[61]

The conclusions reached in all these investigations were based on the results of experimental techniques that measured macroscopic physiologic parameters such as lung function, heart rate, and exercise capacity. These results give no direct information as to the effect increased lung volume has on the absorption kinetics of solutes across the pulmonary membrane.

In studies involving the clearance of aerosolized ^{99m}Tc-DTPA to assess the permeability of the respiratory epithelium it was recognized that the lung volume at which the studies were carried out affected the rate of solute flux. ^{99m}Tc-DTPA is an appropriate solute to examine the effect of increased lung volume on solute flux because of its hydrophilic nature. Assuming that it is absorbed primarily through aqueous pores (intercellular junctions) in the lipid membrane, then an increase in its flux must be due to altered membrane permeability. In following the clearance of this radioaerosol in ventilated dogs, Rizk et al.[62] found that the clearance was accelerated when PEEP equal to 10 cm water was used. Marks et al.[63] then performed a study to determine the relationship between clearance and increased lung volume in healthy volunteers. Not only did Marks and co-workers measure the clearance of ^{99m}Tc-DTPA while the aerosol was being inhaled by one of the ventilation methods (CPAP and negative pressure), they also continued to follow the clearance of ^{99m}Tc-DTPA after aerosol administration was discontinued in an effort to determine the effect of altered lung volume on materials already deposited in the lung. They concluded that the clearance of ^{99m}Tc-DTPA increased exponentially with increased lung volume. This effect was seen for both positive and negative pressure breathing and the effect was the same during and after aerosol administration. Marks and co-workers attributed the increased clearance to two primary factors. They supported the theory of stretching of intercellular junctions causing increased permeability[64] and they also believed there occurred an increase in available surface area caused by the lung expansion. This reasoning is similar to the speculation of Effros and Mason[33] that during lung inflation the volume of alveolar fluid lining the alveoli would become attenuated. Thus, the ratio of S/V would increase because S would become larger relative to V in Equation 10.

In a similar investigation Nolop and colleagues[65] observed that PEEP increased the clearance of ^{99m}Tc-DTPA in nonsmokers but not in smokers. They also attributed the observed increased clearance to surface area expansion and enhanced permeability due to stretching of intercellular junctions. They rationalized that the clearance of ^{99m}Tc-DTPA in smokers was *not* altered because the intercellular junctions were possibly *already* expanded and would not change with the application of positive pressure. This is somewhat similar to the observation made by Egan who showed that after inflation of a portion of the dog lung, the calculated size of the intercellular junctions (pore radii) remained constant once the lung volume was reduced.[64] It is generally agreed[26,32,66] that increased solute flux under the conditions of forced ventilation is possibly due to a widening of the intercellular junctions, an increase in lung surface area, and changes in the volume of lung fluid and its properties. However, Huchon[26] observes that there are no ultrastructural data available concerning the effect of increased lung volume on these variables. Until such work is performed, contributions to solute flux made by forced ventilation cannot be fully assessed and understood.

III. CLEARANCE

A. MUCOCILIARY TRANSPORT

It has long been recognized that the mucociliary transport system is an important defense mechanism of the lung. In healthy lungs it effectively removes airborne bacteria and insoluble particulates that deposit on the mucus lining. There is evidence that mucociliary dysfunction has been observed in acute and chronic bronchitis,[67-69] cystic fibrosis,[70] and bronchial asthma.[71] Because of this, much work has been performed to examine the components and characteristics of the system. With the increasing use of therapeutic inhalation aerosols, attention has also been directed to the effect drugs have on the mucociliary escalator. Although mucociliary dysfunction has been associated with cigarette smoking,[72] the effects of smoking are not included in this discussion.

The mucociliary escalator extends from the larynx to the terminal bronchioles.[73] It consists of ciliated epithelial cells covered by a layer of respiratory secretions. The manner in which the cilia beat has been thoroughly investigated.[74] In 1934, Lucas and Douglas[75] proposed that the secretions lining the airways consists of two layers: a fluid layer of low viscosity, which surrounds the cilia and a more viscous layer on top, mucus. Mucus is secreted by the goblet cells of the surface epithelium and by the serous and mucus cells in the submucosal glands. Each cell type secretes a range of acid glycoproteins which have viscoelastic properties in aqueous solutions. The chemical composition of airway mucus has been summarized by Lopez-Vidriero.[76]

1. Measurement of Mucociliary Transport

There are two major methods by which mucociliary transport kinetics are determined. A technique developed by Sackner and co-workers[77] in 1973 is an invasive method that determines the velocity of insoluble disks as they travel up the mucociliary escalator. Briefly, Teflon disks of known diameter (approximately 680 μm) are placed on the mucus lining of the airways by administration through a catheter inserted in a bronchofiberscope. Using cinematophotomicrography, a film is made of the disks' helical path up the trachea. By knowing their size, the projection factor,[77] and the filming speed, disk velocities may be calculated. This technique was first performed in anesthetized dogs[77] and has also been carried out in human volunteers.[78,79] A few years later Friedman et al.[80] modified the technique by following the motion of radiopaque Teflon disks with a fluoroscopic image intensifier. This modification made the technique better suited to studies in humans.[81,82]

A second method involves inhalation administration of aerosolized, radiolabeled, insoluble particles whose disappearance from the lung can be followed by radiography. As is the case in absorption investigations, independent research groups have developed their own experimental techniques in order to study mucociliary clearance in this way.[79,83-88] While the method is noninvasive, its efficiency in estimating clearance rates is dependent upon many factors. Among these are particle size and solubility, binding characteristics, inhalation procedures, size and health of the lung and the need to obtain an accurate outline of lung regions prior to performing the study. A primary difference between this and the bronchofiberscopic method is that most often this method gives measurements of the overall mucociliary clearance, not mucociliary velocity. Results from the former are often presented as half-life or clearance rate constants while the latter has dimensions of LT^{-1}. The experimental design of the inhalation studies requires that aerosolized particles are generated with sizes (approximately 5 μm) which should be deposited centrally. Regions of the lung are defined as either peripheral or central, outlined on the gamma camera, and the ratio of percent radioactivity in the central zones to the percent activity in the peripheral zones determined at specific time intervals up to 24 h. Clearance of the insoluble particles within the first 24 h following deposition is normally attributed to the mucociliary transport system because insoluble particles deposited peripherally have retention times much longer than those deposited centrally. Thus a curve of percentage of particles remaining vs. time can be generated, the slope of which provides the clearance rate. One method of analyzing data of this kind to produce a half-life for mucociliary clearance is described by Byron.[89]

Foster and co-workers,[83,90] in addition to measuring whole lung clearance rates, also measured mucus velocities in the trachea and main bronchi by following the path of radiolabeled particles after their deposition from an inhaled aerosol. They outlined a region of the lung from the main bronchi to the trachea and by calibrating the gamma camera they were able to calculate the linear distance through which a bolus of radioactivity passed from the main bronchi to the trachea. Thus, the time required for the bolus to travel a fixed distance allowed the calculation of the mucociliary transport velocity (LT^{-1}).

Santa Cruz et al.,[91] using the bronchofiberscopic method, determined the average mucus velocity in the trachea in 16 nonsmoking volunteers whose average age was 27.4 years. The average mucus velocity, calculated by following the movement of Teflon disks, was 21.5 mm/min (S.D. 5.5 mm/min). In a similar experiment using the same method a few years later, the mean tracheal mucus velocity in young, healthy nonsmokers was reported to be 10.1 ± 3.5 mm/min.[72] Both these studies report much higher average mucus velocities than studies using radioaerosols. Foster and co-workers,[83] using radioaerosols, reported the mean tracheal mucus velocity of 7 healthy nonsmoking volunteers to be 5.5 ± 0.4 mm/min. Similarly, in a study involving 42 healthy, nonsmoking subjects Yeates et al.[85] reported the overall geometric mean tracheal transport rate (MTTR) to be 3.6 mm/min with a coefficient of variation within the population of 75%. Figure 7 is a frequency distribution of the MTTRs from Yeates' study. The scatter seen in these results is much wider than that described by Foster et al.[83] and may be partly explained[92] by intersubject variations in deposition. It is possible that the bronchial deposition patterns of the 1.4 μm particles inhaled by the subjects in the Yeates et al. study[85] showed greater intersubject variation than those of the 4 μm particles inhaled by the subjects in Foster's study (see fractional deposition vs. aerodynamic diameter profiles[89]). However, it should be recognized that the radioaerosol technique contains many variables which are unstandardized between laboratories. The various cameras, software, quenching calculations, and corrections for radioactive decay which are employed in these studies are themselves a source of interlaboratory variation.

123

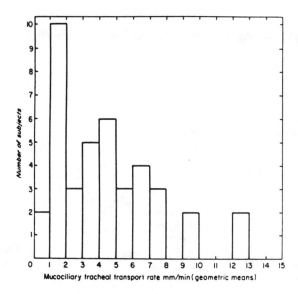

FIGURE 7. Frequency distribution of geometric mean mucociliary transport rates of 42 subjects. (From Yeates, D. B., et al., *J. Appl. Physiol.*, 39, 487, 1975. With permission.)

As far as biological variation is concerned it is difficult to establish a normal mucociliary transport rate for a group of similar individuals, even within a single laboratory. For example, results of mucociliary velocities and clearance tests in a group of bronchial asthmatics showed velocities approximating those of normal subjects in two patients and no observable mucus transport in another five.[90] Nevertheless, decreased mucociliary velocities have been reported in patients with chronic obstructive lung disease[91] and asymptomatic asthmatics.[87] Also, it has been shown that the same individual will give a characteristic clearance pattern if retested.[92] This last fact makes it possible to establish the effect of drugs on mucociliary clearance as long as the same individual is used for both control and test, and that factors such as particle size, breathing pattern, and duration of inhalation are kept constant.

2. Drug Effects
a. Overall Mucociliary Clearance
In many studies the effect of drugs on mucociliary function has been determined by observing the overall mucociliary clearance of an insoluble test aerosol before and after administration of the drug of interest. Table 4 shows the effect of some aerosolized drugs in humans. Adrenergics (isoproterenol, salbutamol) enhance clearance while antiinflammatory steroids (beclomethasone) and cholinergics (ipratropium bromide) have no effect on mucociliary function.[82,86,93,94] Whether the drug has an overall effect can be determined. However, it is often uncertain which component of the mucociliary transport system is affected. Mucociliary transport can be impaired by altering the volume of mucus secretions, the mucus rheology and the ciliary beat frequency.[71] It may be that more than one component is affected simultaneously. For example, a drug might induce mucus secretion and at the same time increase the frequency with which the cilia beat.

b. Volume of Mucus Secretions
As early as the late 1800s scientists were investigating the effects of drugs on mucus secretions.[95] In 1932, Florey et al.[96] were able to show that the tracheal glands in the cat and dog secreted mucus in response to vagal stimulation. More recently, Sturgess and Reid[97] have adopted an organ culture method originally developed by Trowell[98] that allows investigation of

TABLE 4
Effect of Some Aerosolized Drugs on Human Mucociliary Clearance

Drug	Subject	Effect[a]	Ref.
Isoproterenol	Healthy humans	+	90
	Asthmatics	+	90
Epinephrine	Healthy humans	+	84
Isoetharine	Healthy humans	+	83
Salbutamol	Healthy humans	+	69
	Asthmatics	+	69
Beclomethasone	Patients with COLD[b]	0	86
Terbutaline[c]	Patients with chronic bronchitis	+	67
	Patients with bronchial asthma	+	212
	Healthy humans	+	213
Ipratropium bromide	Patients with chronic bronchitis	0	94
	Patients with bronchial asthma	0	82
	Healthy humans	0	93
	Asthmatics	Unpredictable	93
Bethancol	Healthy humans	+	214
Atropine	Anesthetized female patients	–	78
	Healthy humans[d]	–	85
Hyoscine[e]	Elderly patients	–	215

[a] +: increased rate, –: decreased rate, 0: no effect.
[b] Chronic obstructive lung disease.
[c] Drug given subcutaneously.
[d] Drug given i.v.
[e] Drug given orally.

mucus secretion from individual cells excised from the bronchial walls of human cadavers. Tritiated glucose was added to the bronchial explants as a marker for glycoprotein synthesis and secretion. After incubating for 4 h the number of mucus cells discharging radioactivity from the medium was taken as the secretory index (SI). The effect of drug treatment was assessed by comparing the mean SI of six drug-treated explants and six controls. The concentration of drug was varied at least 10-fold and usually ranged from 1 to 100 μg/ml of culture medium. Table 5 is a list of the drugs investigated by Sturgess and Reid and their effect on SI. Sympathomimetics, sympatholytics, and humoral agents had no effect on the explants studied. All the parasympathomimetics increased the SI as a function of dose. The parasympatholytics inhibited the mucus secretion and the degree of inhibition varied widely between specimens. Corticosteroids significantly reduced the SI in only some of the specimens studied while having no effect on the others. Mucolytic agents showed no effect on the volume of mucus secretions. Of the miscellaneous compounds studied, disodium cromoglycate and potassium iodide had no effect while nicotine only affected one of the four specimens studied. Atropine inhibition increased as a function of concentration up to 50 μg/ml. This finding was in agreement with that of Lopez-Vidriero and co-workers.[99] In their discussion, Sturgess and Reid stated that while there was uniformity in response throughout the bronchial tree of one specimen there was a wide variation of response between different specimens. They rationalized that this was due to gland size; the larger the gland size the greater the response to vagal stimulation and the less effective the drug inhibition. They proposed this as an explanation of the poor performance of drugs whose purpose is intended to control hypersecretion in diseased lungs.

TABLE 5
Effect of Drugs on Mucus Secretions

Drug	Effect on secretory index
Parasympathomimetics	Increase as function of dose
Acetylcholine	
Pilocarpine nitrate	
Carbachol	
Parasympatholytics	Decrease as function of dose
Atropine sulfate	
Hyoscine hydrochloride	
Sympathomimetics	No effect
Adrenaline	
Noradrenaline	
Isoprenaline sulfate	
Sympatholytics	No effect
Phenoxybenzamine	
Phentolamine	
Propranolol	
Guanethidine sulfate	
Humoral agents	No effect
Bradykinin	
Mefenamic acid	
Histamine	
Cortocosteroid hormones	Not all subjects affected
Hydrocortisone hemisuccinate	
Betamethasone	
Dexamethasone	
Triamcinolone	
Prednisolone	
Mucolytic agents	No effect
N-Acetyl cysteine	
Vasicine	
Miscellaneous	
Potassium iodide	No effect
Disodium cromoglycate	No effect
Nicotine	Affected 1 in 4 subjects
Sodium salicylate	Decrease as function of dose

From Sturgess, J. and Reid, L., *Clin. Sci.,* 43, 533, 1972. With permission.

c. Mucus Rheology

The mucus lining of the upper airways in healthy humans is usually exposed to water-saturated air due to humidification in the nose. However, the patient with respiratory disease breathes predominantly by mouth and 100% humidification of the upper airways usually does not occur. Richards and Marriott[100] reasoned that decreasing the humidity of inspired air may increase the viscosity of bronchial mucus in diseased lungs. They tested their hypothesis by examining the effect of changes in the humidity of ambient air on the rheological properties of bronchial mucus extracted from the sputum of patients. Their results indicated that a parameter directly related to the residual viscosity of mucus increased as the humidity decreased. Richards and Marriott suggested that a structural change in the mucus took place due to its loss of water as a result of the dry air conditions.

King and Angus[101] have examined the effect of aerosolized atropine, ipratropium, and salbutamol on tracheal mucus in dogs. They reported their results in terms of mucus collection rate, viscoelastic properties, and mucus flux. Because it is unclear whether mucus collection rate and flux represent increases in secretion volume and/or increases in cilia beat frequency, only results concerning the effect of drugs on viscoelastic properties are discussed. Atropine at low doses (0.06 and 0.1 mg) and ipratropium at all doses tested (0.1 to 0.6 mg) did not significantly alter the viscoelastic properties of mucus. Salbutamol at increasing doses (0.1 to 0.6 mg) caused an increase in the ratio of the viscous to the elastic nature of the mucus.

d. Ciliary Beat Frequency

Ciliary beat frequency is a function of the mechanism controlling the ciliated cells and also depends upon the rheological properties of the periciliary fluid and mucus lining. Many studies have investigated the effects of drugs on ciliary activity using a variety of methods.[102-107] However, it is difficult to draw conclusions from results because of complications due to mucus secretion and possible changes in its rheology.

Verdugo et al.[102] examined the effect of isoproterenol on ciliated rabbit cells devoid of mucus secreting cells. Ciliary beat frequency increased proportionately with increasing concentration of isoproterenol (10^{-7} to 10^{-6} M). Propranolol alone did not affect the ciliary beat, but did block the effect of isoproterenol at a concentration of 10^{-7} M. The investigators concluded that the effect of isoproterenol on ciliary beat was due to its specific β-adrenergic properties because its effect was negated by the β-blocker, propranolol.

In addition to studying the effect of isoproterenol, Yanaura et al.[103] also studied the effects of other β-stimulants on ciliary activity. Their results on the stimulating effect of isoproterenol agreed with those of Verdugo et al. Salbutamol was found to be less potent than isoproterenol but did cause an increase in the ciliary beat frequency. Theophylline was equally effective at concentrations 100 times greater than that required for isoproterenol. Propranolol inhibited the action of salbutamol but had no significant influence on theophylline. Yanaura concluded that the action of isoproterenol and salbutamol is probably mediated by $β_2$-adrenoceptors on the ciliated cells. The mechanism of action of theophylline was attributed to its "cilio exciting action" and a contribution to increased mucus production. Van As[104] also observed an increase in ciliary activity due to salbutamol. Increasing concentrations (10^{-8} to 10^{-4} M) of drug produced a log response vs. dose curve in the four trials conducted.

B. PULMONARY ENDOCYTOSIS

There is evidence of some endocytotic activity by almost all alveolar cells.[108-113] In the case of endothelial and epithelial cells this activity would be known as pinocytosis, while for mobile cells such as macrophages and polymorphonuclear leukocytes the process would be called phagocytosis. Pinocytosis, by and through epithelial cells, may represent a clearance pathway which enables some particles and large molecules to reach the interstitium and lymphatics. Phagocytosis by polymorphonuclear leukocytes is also well recognized as part of the inflammatory process in disease. However, because the pulmonary macrophage is abundant even in healthy lung tissue, it is therefore considered to be the most important lung phagocyte. An extensive literature concerns its role in respiratory clearance.

Despite recent advances in experimental techniques, many of the questions concerning respiratory endocytosis raised in 1966 by the Task Group on Lung Dynamics remain unanswered. These questions are reviewed below alongside more recent studies of the various phenomena called endocytosis.

The clearance model described by the Task Group on Lung Dynamics made no allowance for the contribution to particulate clearance by lymphatic drainage. The lymph, of course, can only be reached by crossing the epithelial barrier and, at that time, considerable controversy surrounded the issue of how particles reached the interstitial area, capillaries, and lymph. Although transuranic oxides had been found in alveolar epithelial cells following a single exposure,[114] and there was evidence of other particles being withheld in the alveolar capillary membrane,[115] the Task Group concluded that it was impossible to demonstrate by histological techniques the mechanism by which particles gained access to the interstitium. A few years later

Morrow[116] wrote that there was ample evidence of the existence of a transport pathway from the endothelium of capillaries to the interstitium and lymphatics [117-119] (from the blood). He also summarized the important points for consideration of the lymphatic drainage of inhaled particles as a clearance mechanism[116,120] (from the airways). Since then, clearance of particles from the lung by the lymphatic system has been demonstrated.[121,122] This may proceed via pinocytosis, phagocytosis, or both. However, the contribution to overall clearance is very low.[123,124] Snipes and colleagues[125] studied the clearance of radiolabeled polystyrene microspheres with different particle diameters after these were instilled into the lungs of dogs. Approximately 1.7% of a dose of 3 μm particles were translocated to the tracheobronchial lymph nodes during a 128-d study. The fact that only 0.2% of 7 μm particles and no 13 μm particles were translocated to the lymph nodes may indicate that clearance of these particles via the lymph is a function of particle size. In a subsequent study on the retention of aluminosilicate particles inhaled by dogs, Snipes and co-workers[126] reported that the physical clearance from the lung to the lung-associated lymph nodes (LALN) was independent of the particle size in a much smaller size range (0.7 to 2.8 μm). Even though dose differences certainly exist between these studies, this is one example where the literature indicates a clearance difference between particles with different chemical compositions. The effect of dose or particle burden has been reviewed by Bowden[127] in his article on pulmonary macrophages. He describes a maximum load of particles that saturate the available macrophages,[128,129] making it more likely that particles will cross the epithelium.[130] Transepithelial transport has been demonstrated for a number of particulates.[128,131-133] Although it is possible that particles travel directly across the cytoplasm of type I alveolar cells to gain access to the interstitium,[134] the observation of particle laden macrophages in the interstitium[135,136] also suggests the transepithelial passage of alveolar macrophages containing particles. Bowden supports the theory that as particle burden or dose increases, the free particles cross the epithelial barrier to be engulfed by interstitial macrophages.[137] Interstitial macrophages are said to comprise 1/3 of the total pulmonary macrophage population.[138] Despite the obvious relevance of dose dependency to the administration of aerosolized pharmaceuticals in microparticulates such as microspheres, it is important to recognize that the capacity of the alveolar macrophage system is very large.[139] This is so it can cope with heavily polluted environments and it is unlikely that it could be saturated by a therapeutic aerosol.

The origins and migratory habits of the pulmonary macrophages were unknown to the Task Group. By the early 1970s it was thought possible that they were derived from connective tissue cells, bone marrow, or type II pneumocytes.[108,140-143] Currently, although it is generally agreed that the bone marrow is the predominant site of monocyte production[116,127,144] (macrophages are monocytes), there is continuing debate about the regeneration of the macrophage. van Furth[145] believes that macrophages are exclusively derived from bone marrow, while Volkman[146] believes they proliferate locally. While local proliferation of macrophages is thought by some to be sufficient to maintain their population,[147-149] others have shown that the ability of macrophages to respond to foreign particles is impaired when the supply of monocytes is discontinued.[150] Bowden[127] writes that there is increasing acceptance of the theory that a series of interconnected compartments are involved in the derivation, transport, and response of macrophages.

In 1973, Green[151] wrote that almost every aspect of macrophage migration to the deposited particle and from the pulmonary region is disputed. Although particle-laden macrophages have been observed within minutes of deposition,[48,123,124,129,152] the mechanism that prompts alveolar macrophages to respond to the invasion of foreign particulates has long been studied and almost certainly depends on the nature of the particles. A number of methods of transport of macrophages to deposited particles have been suggested.[116] Findings from recent investigations[153-159] support the hypothesis that inorganic particles that activate complement proteins of alveolar fluid *in vitro* will generate chemoattractants for macrophages at sites of deposition *in vivo*.

It has been established that three stages are involved in phagocytosis: attachment, ingestion, and digestion. Macrophages contain numerous enzyme systems capable of destroying drugs. Green et al.[144] report information on each of the stages of phagocytosis gathered from studies on peritoneal macrophages and polymorphonuclear leukocytes in the hope that pulmonary macrophages function in a similar fashion. Once a particle has been ingested, the macrophage may remain in the lung to digest the particle, exit the lung, or die in the lung releasing its contents. If the macrophage remains in the lung to solubilize and/or metabolize a particle, then it would appear from the data in clearance experiments that the particle had not been removed from the lung. Thus, material remaining to be cleared in some experiments may be phagocytosed and awaiting clearance in pulmonary macrophages. The possibility that ingested material may alter macrophage mobility complicates data interpretation further.

There are two major pathways by which a phagocytosed particle may exit the lung: along the surface of the alveolar and bronchial structures to the mucociliary escalator and through the interstitial spaces and lymphatic channels. The first pathway is thought to be responsible for the initial rapid clearance of insoluble particles in the first 24 h postdeposition period.[144] Morphologic information suggests that particle clearance via the lymphatic channels has a time course of anywhere from 1 to 14 d.[151] The mechanism by which the macrophage travels from the alveoli to the ciliated airway is still not understood. It has been observed that macrophages travel from alveolus to alveolus through the pores of Kohn.[144] Macklin[160] proposed passive transport of macrophages, as if they were particles, by continuous flow of alveolar fluid to the bronchial epithelium. Gross[161] also agreed with the notion of the continuous flow of alveolar fluid and proposed two mechanisms that would make it possible. The combination of the mechanical effect of breathing, and an increase in viscosity of secretions as the respiratory tract was ascended from the alveolar to the bronchial region, would result in the transport of particulates on the surface of the alveolar fluid from the terminal airways to the mucociliary escalator. While the reasoning is open to debate, the existence of a mechanical effect can hardly be denied. Once on the mucociliary escalator, a macrophage must be swept along with other debris unless it is able to define its own fate. The lymphatic pathway, as shown earlier, is not a major clearance route but may be important in the clearance of particles from lung-diseased individuals.

The Task Group recognized that the number, size, shape, and surface reactivity of dust particles affects the extent to which endocytosis occurs.[162-164] Some researchers believe that particle deposition itself alters the alveolar macrophage population[128,129,165-168] and that a relationship between the number of macrophages and the particle load[129] has been demonstrated. It appears that small particles induce a larger number of macrophages than are found with larger particles of identical total weight.[128] Investigators are now trying to establish whether a correlation exists between macrophagic response and lung burden or dose,[167] number of exposures to aerosolized particles, and the interval between exposures. Longer clearance half-lives have been reported for repetitive exposures to aerosolized particles as compared to single exposures.[168-170]

Although many scientists believe endocytosis plays an important role in the removal of insoluble particulates from the lung, complicating factors make it difficult to give absolute estimates of the time required to remove a specific amount of material from the lung by these mechanisms. Of these complicating factors, solubilization is the most important. As previously mentioned, the Task Group on Lung Dynamics recognized that various materials defined as insoluble *in vitro* proved to be soluble in biological systems. Since then, greater emphasis has been placed on the importance of solubilization to the lung clearance process. Once a material has dissolved, absorption becomes possible, the kinetics of which have been described in the previous section.

A further complication concerns data extrapolation from one species to another. Rats and mice have traditionally been used as experimental animals in studies examining long-term clearance of dust particles. Snipes and co-workers[126] have reported significantly different clearance pathways of aluminosilicate particles between the dog, rat, and mouse. In rodents, particles were translocated to the LALN only in the first few days after exposure, while the dogs studied had most of the long-term clearance going to the LALN. These findings were in agreement with those of Thomas[171] and Ferin[172] who examined the long-term clearance of cesium-labeled and titanium oxide particles in dogs and rats, respectively. Other research groups have reported deposition and retention patterns for particles inhaled by dogs to be similar to that seen in humans.[173-176] Therefore, consideration should be given to the validity of the use of rodents in long-term clearance studies.

Pulmonary endocytosis should have a minimal effect on soluble compounds (half-lives <30 min) and those that are delivered to the upper airways. For the less soluble or poorly absorbed compounds reaching the terminal airways, one may expect a fraction of the dose to be phagocytosed. This fraction will depend on the size and number of particles presented, their ability to induce a chemoattractant response, and their frequency of administration. Endocytosis may well play a much greater role in the clearance of therapeutic agents intended to be administered to the lung as sustained release microparticulates and, depending upon the drug target, may well be an event which requires pharmaceutical manipulation.

IV. DISSOLUTION

A. INTRODUCTION

In early studies involving the clearance of insoluble particles (ferric oxide, coal dust, barium sulfate, and others), although dissolution was intuitively known to occur, its contribution to overall lung clearance was considered minimal. The revelation that substances known to be highly insoluble in water dissolved at a finite rate in biological systems, and the prediction by Mercer[177] that long-term retention of relatively insoluble particles in the lung would be governed by the dissolution step, led researchers to examine the importance of solubilization of particles, particularly environmental toxins, that were known to reside in the lung for extended periods. Morrow[116] proposed that information on the role of dissolution could account for the variability seen in the clearance data for a group of insoluble compounds, while in another instance, ferric oxide showed fairly consistent clearance patterns even among different species and for different methods of administration.[5,178]

Unfortunately, little quantitative dissolution data are available for materials administered to the lung *in vivo*. This statement is particularly true for therapeutic agents which are usually administered in much smaller doses than aerosols which present as environmental hazards. Most bronchodilators are rapidly absorbed and for reasons described below, the dissolution process is not considered to be the rate limiting step. This section of the chapter reviews some dissolution models relevant to microparticulates alongside factors which affect dissolution rates *in vitro*. Finally, *in vivo* studies which have examined the clearance of soluble and less soluble forms of various metals are summarized in order to place microparticulate dissolution models in perspective.

B. DISSOLUTION MODELS AND MICROPARTICULATE DISSOLUTION

Figure 8 is a diagrammatic representation of a spherical particle dissolving under conditions in which diffusion across a stationary boundary layer of solvent defines the rate at which dissolution occurs. The magnification shows the concentration profile in the boundary layer which is driven by a compound's solubility, C_s, while there is solid remaining. This model was first described by Noyes and Whitney[179] who used Fick's first law and an assumption of steady-state diffusion in the boundary layer (the concentration gradient is rectilinear) to derive

$$dM/dt = [DS(C_s - C)]/h \qquad (11)$$

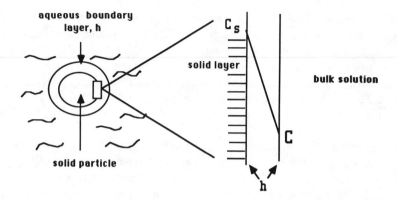

FIGURE 8.   A diagrammatic representation of small particle dissolution. The thickness of the boundary layer, h, often approaches the magnitude of the particle for particles in the size range of interest.

where the rate of mass transfer, dM/dt, is predictable given a knowledge of the solute's diffusion coefficient, D, its surface area, S, solubility, C_s, concentration in the bulk, C, and the boundary layer thickness, h. Under conditions when the concentration in the bulk solvent, C, are less than 5 to 10% of the solubility, C_s, dissolution is said to occur under sink conditions (C → 0, solute removed from the bulk at rates faster than dissolution occurs).

In long-term inhalation exposure studies, where solid particulate aerosols are administered chronically, and solute deposition is high, it is entirely possible that sufficient mass is present in the lung to generate a bulk concentration in lung liquids, C, which approaches the value C_s and causes the existence of dissolution under nonsink conditions. In the circumstances envisaged in this text, however, solute doses administered by inhalation are much smaller than those encountered in these chronic studies and sink conditions are almost certainly maintained. Under these circumstances, Equation 11 reduces to

$$dM/dt = [DSC_s]/h \tag{12}$$

The existence of sink conditions is easily demonstrated by comparing the concentration, C, generated from dissolution of say 0.1 mg of drug in the lung fluid volume of about 100 ml (C = 0.0001 g/100 ml) with a typical bronchodilator solubility, C_s, of 1 g/100 ml. For a wetted solid powder immersed in a solvent, the dissolution rate at time t = 0, $[dM/dt]_{t=0}$, is predictable from Equation 12. It is instructive to recognize how fast dissolution of a fairly soluble micronized powder can be. Typical values for D are of the order 5×10^{-6} cm^2/s (180) in water and are predictable from the Stokes-Einstein[43] and Wilke-Chang[45] relationships. Total surface area, S, for a deposited aerosol is proportional to dose. A 0.1-mg dose of unit density powder, when subdivided into 5 μm diameter smooth, spherical particles has a surface area of 1.2 cm^2 calculated from $S = n4\pi r^2$ where n is the number of spheres (1,527,887) of radius $r = 2.5 \times 10^{-4}$ cm. For a drug with 1% solubility, $C_s = 0.01$ g/cm^3, and if the boundary layer thickness approaches the particle diameter (h = 5×10^{-4} cm), then dissolution rate at time zero

$$[dM/dt]_{t=0} = [DSC_s]/h = 0.12 \text{ mg/s} \tag{13}$$

Thus, if dissolution of this powder occurred at a constant rate, the time taken to dissolve the whole dose (0.1 mg) would be less than 1 s.

In practice, the simplistic approach described above provides unreliable answers for several reasons. Among these reasons are

1. That surface area of the dissolving solid changes with time
2. That powders are rarely monodisperse, spherical, or smooth
3. That extremely small (submicron) solute particles are known to express solubilities greater than those exhibited by larger particles
4. That assigning a value to the diffusive boundary layer thickness, h, is problematic

Because the surface area of a micronized solid can be determined experimentally,[181] assigning a value at time zero in Equation 12 is not really a problem. An experimental determination can be used to compensate for surface irregularities and deviation from sphericity. The fact that area changes with time led to the derivation of the Hixson-Crowell cube root law[182] which is usually expressed as

$$M_o^{1/3} - M^{1/3} = k't \qquad (14)$$

where the difference between the cube roots of the mass of undissolved solute at time zero, M_o, and that at time t, M is equal to the product of a constant k', which is related to the surface area at time zero, and time, t.[179] Equation 14 was derived to describe the dissolution of a monodisperse powder.[183] The added complexity of small particles within a particle size distribution dissolving completely before the dissolution of their larger counterparts has been addressed theoretically by Brooke[184] and theoretically and practically by Cartensen and Musa.[185] With the advent of faster and more powerful computers it has become possible theoretically to generate the surface area term in Equation 12 iteratively as a function of dissolution time for powders which have complex particle size distributions. This approach may be unnecessarily complicated because Mauger et al.[211] recently presented an approximate expression to describe the dissolution profile for multisized drug particles. It is interesting to note in their article that only the mean and S. D. of a particle size population need be known in order to apply these expressions.

As far as the third point (solubility variation with particle size) is concerned, the effect of high surface curvature increasing the escaping tendency of molecules from small particulates (Kelvin effect) is probably unimportant for the majority of the dissolution process occurring from a typically sized aerosol powder.[186] The mass contribution from submicron particulates is small compared to the total mass of polydisperse dissolving powder. Much more significant are the possible changes in solubility induced by physical form.[187] It is important to recognize also that many of the quoted values for drug solubilities in the literature are inaccurate because sufficient care has not been paid to defining the physical form of the material being tested. Furthermore, some low solubility materials may take a considerable time to dissolve and reach solubility equilibrium.[188]

Recently, Mauger and Howard[189] have reviewed the problems associated with assigning a value for the diffusion layer thickness, h, in Equation 12. They point out that a major difference between the Higuchi-Hiestand dissolution model[190,191] and the Hixson-Crowell treatment[182] centers about the magnitude of the diffusion layer thickness. "While the diffusion layer thickness is always the same for all particles of the same size and is comparable to, or greater than, the particle radius for the former, the latter ignores the effective diffusion layer or assumes that it is constant for all particles and remains constant throughout a particle's lifetime."[189] Furthermore, Mauger and Howard point out that although the Huguchi-Hiestand model is more rigorous in assigning values for h which vary with particle radius, it fails to incorporate a quantitative consideration of hydrodynamic effects. These were incorporated by Mauger and Howard by using the Nielsen model[192] which allows for convective effects. For aerosol particles with sizes which, in general, are less than 10 μm, Mauger has shown that the Higuchi-Hiestand and Nielsen models produce coincident predictions for dissolution rates of log-normally distributed powders. In several subsequent publications Mauger's group have tested these theories using carefully segregated, well characterized, micronized powders.[193-195] The Higuchi-Hiestand and

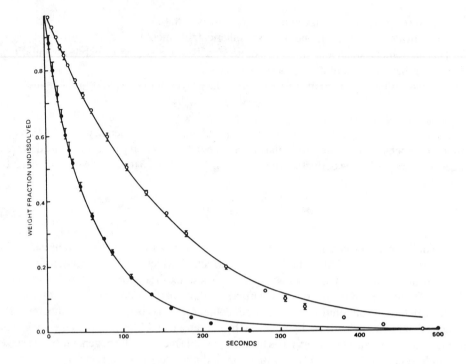

FIGURE 9.   Dissolution profiles for first and second prednisolone fractions. Key: (●) experimental values for fraction 1, with a count median diameter 5.7 µm, solid line calculated using theory; (○) experimental values for fraction 2 with a count median diameter 7.2 µm. (Reproduced by permission of the American Pharmaceutical Association.)

Nielsen models were shown to fit the experimental data well for two prednisolone acetate powders with median size distributions less than 10 µm.[195] Figure 9 is reproduced from their paper to illustrate the speed with which a highly insoluble compound, prednisolone acetate (C_s = 1.5×10^{-5} g/ml), dissolves under sink conditions such as those which may be anticipated in the fluid lining the airways.

C. *IN VIVO* STUDIES

Extensive research has been performed on the toxicologic and pharmacologic effects of toxic metallic compounds which are far less soluble than even lipophilic drugs. These are found in the atmosphere due to incineration, burning of fossil fuels, and the refining of minerals. Many of these studies involve exposing laboratory animals to excessive lung burdens of material and then following its long-term clearance. It should be emphasized that these experimental designs deposit far greater doses in the lung than is the case for a bolus dose of a therapeutic aerosol. This may result in dissolution of high lung burdens occurring more slowly than would be predicted in the previous section under nonsink conditions. Work regarding *in vivo* dissolution is often speculative, based upon clearance data. A few studies are summarized here to represent the general opinion among the scientific community regarding the importance of dissolution of particulates thought to reside for extended periods in the lung.

The clearance of nickel from the lungs has been researched by numerous groups[196-199] because of the incidence of lung cancer among refinery workers. Nickel (Ni) has been instilled into the lungs of rats in either a soluble form ($NiCl_2$) or an insoluble form (Ni_3S_2, NiO). The consensus from these studies is that the insoluble form is solubilized and then transported from the lungs in a pattern similar to the soluble form.

Cadmium is a highly toxic metal that after inhalation could relocate to other organs, specifically the kidney, and cause kidney dysfunction.[200] It has been delivered to the rat lung by aerosolization[200] and intratracheal instillation,[201,202] again in both soluble ($CdCl_2$) and insoluble (CdO) forms. Aihara et al.[201] observed that the soluble form was translocated more rapidly than the less soluble form. A few years earlier, Hadley's group[202] claimed that the CdO was rapidly solubilized, despite its highly insoluble classification by the Task Group. In contrast to these findings Oberdoerster et al.[200] found that the CdO experienced a rapid initial clearance phase while $CdCl_2$ did not, while the long-term half-lives of both cadmium forms were found to be the same. This group concluded that the "apparent dissolution rate of cadmium compounds does not play a major role in the long term clearance of inhaled cadmium from the lung".[200]

The clearance of insoluble and soluble forms of manganese has also been investigated. Researchers observed that while the soluble form ($MnCl_2$) was cleared at a faster initial rate, similar rates of clearance were observed for both forms after the initial period.[203]

Initial rapid solubilization of ^{134}Ce labeled aluminosilicate particles has been observed in clearance studies performed on dogs[126] and in humans.[204-206] Eidson and Mewhinney[210] have shown that up to 2% of the plutonium activity of $^{239}PuO_2$ would dissolve within 2 h after being placed in an *in vitro* system. This datum supports the results of Morrow et al.,[24] who reported an early mean absorption rate of approximately 4% of the initial lung burden of $^{239}PuO_2$, administered as an aerosol to dogs.

V. MODELING OF DRUG RESIDENCE KINETICS

Because of rapid dissolution kinetics, therapeutic doses administered in different aerosol formulations can be assumed to result in the presence of low concentrations of dissolved solutes in the mucus layers lining the airways shortly after inhalation. The fact that these mucus layers are cleared simultaneously by the processes of absorption (Figure 1B) and ciliary clearance (Figure 1C) at similar rates means that both of these processes must be taken into account when predicting drug residence kinetics in the airways. When the rate constants, k_1 through k_6, in Figure 1A are assumed to be apparent first-order, equations have been derived[89] which describe the aerosol dose fraction vs. time profiles in the tracheobronchial (TB) and pulmonary (P) regions. These equations result from solution of differential equations which describe an apparent clearance model. For example, equations consistent with Figure 1A are

$$d(f_{TB})/dt = f_P k_2 - f_{TB}(k_1 + k_3) \tag{15}$$
$$d(f_P)/dt = -f_P(k_4 + k_5 + k_2) \tag{16}$$

The clearance model previously presented by Byron[89] differs somewhat from that shown in Figure 1A and thus the solutions for f_{TB} and f_P vs. the time are also somewhat different from those which would result from the integration of Equations 15 and 16.

The model developed previously allowed for regional deposition of different aerosol dose fractions following mouth inhalation of various particle sizes according to four popular breathing regimes. Predicted pulmonary deposition was dependent on the mode of inhalation and breath holding. Deposition in the ciliated airways was unaffected by breath holding and maximized when aerodynamic diameters were between 5 and 9 μm (slow inhalation) and 3 to 6 μm (fast inhalation). In order to assess the impact of aerosol particle size and inhalation regime upon aerosol residence kinetics, the duration of residence (T) of aerosol was defined arbitrarily as the time taken for the amount of drug in a chosen region to fall to ≤1% of the inhaled dose. Durations were determined in the TB region for completely insoluble and unabsorbed compounds as well as compounds which dissolved and possessed absorption half-lives of 28 min and 14 min in the TB and P compartments, respectively (Figure 1A). Ciliary clearance kinetics with half lives of 44 min for the fast component and 249 min for the slow component were assumed.

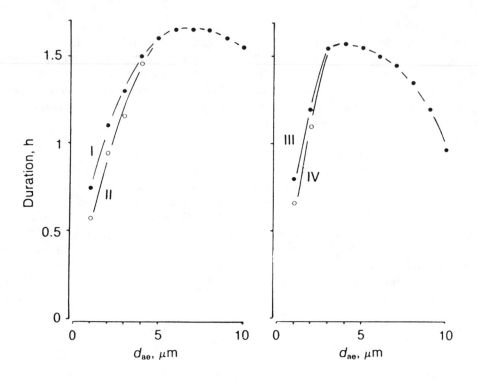

FIGURE 10.   Duration (T, time for f_{TB} to fall to minimum dose fraction = 0.01) vs. aerodynamic diameter d_{ae}, for inhalation modes I to IV. (Reproduced with permission from the American Pharmaceutical Association.)

The model allowed generation of Figure 10 where I through IV are different inhalation modes. In the case of insoluble particulates duration in TB could be extended by depositing material in the pulmonary compartment. For soluble materials, however (Figure 10), maximum duration of residence in TB occurred for aerosol sizes which achieved maximum deposition in the TB compartment. The expected residence times were short and rather insensitive to the mode of inhalation, given the assumptions of normality made for calculating deposition and clearance variables in the model. Duration extention in the TB region could only be extended by deposition of slowly absorbed solutes which were deposited primarily in the pulmonary regions. Under these circumstances, durations were highly dependent upon aerosol size and mode of inhalation. Gonda[207] has recently extended the applications of this model in order to incorporate the release kinetics of drug from the dosage form. Application of these models with approximate values for rate constants k_1 through k_6 in a particular case enable the researcher to gain a reasonable estimate of the drug mass vs. time profiles in the major regions of the lung. These profiles may have toxicologic importance in the case of excipients which are co-administered with drug aerosols as well as therapeutic importance in defining the likely duration of action of drugs acting locally in the respiratory tract.

REFERENCES

1. **Task Group on Lung Dynamics,** Deposition and retention models for internal dosimetry of the human respiratory tract, *Health Phys.,* 12, 173, 1966.
2. **Kettle, E. A. and Hilton, R.,** Technique of experimental Pneumoconiosis, *Lancet,* 1, 1190, 1932.

3. **Taplin, G. V., Grevior, J. S., and Drusch, H.,** Pulmonary retention of fine particles administered by intratracheal insufflation and inhalation, *Ann. West. Med. Surg.,* 4, 391, 1950.
4. **Mohanty, G. P., Roberts, D. C., King, E. J., and Harrison, C. V.,** Effects of feldspar, slate and quartz on lungs of rats, *J. Pathol. Bacteriol.,* 65, 501, 1953.
5. **Gibb, F. R. and Morrow, P. E.,** Alveolar clearance in dogs following inhalation of an iron 59 oxide aerosol , *J. Appl. Physiol.,* 17, 429, 1962.
6. **Pylev, L. N.,** Induction of lung cancer in rats by intratracheal insufflation of carcinogenic hydrocarbons, *Acta Unio Int. Contra Cancrum,* 19, 688, 1962.
7. **Cember, H., Hatch, T. F., Watson, J. A., and Grucci, T. B.,** Pulmonary penetration of particles administered by intratracheal insufflation, *Arch. Ind. Hyg. Occup. Med.,* 10, 24, 1954.
8. **Enna, S. J. and Schanker, L. S.,** Absorption of saccharides and urea from the rat lung, *Am. J. Physiol.,* 222, 409, 1972.
9. **Taylor, A. E. and Garr, K. A., Jr.,** Estimation of equivalent pore radii of pulmonary capillary and alveolar membranes, *Am. J. Physiol.,* 218, 1133, 1970.
10. **Taylor, A. E., Guyton, A. C., and Bishop, V. S.,** Permeability of the alveolar membrane to solutes, *Circ. Res.,* 16, 353, 1965.
11. **Wangensteen, O. D., Wittmers, L. E., Jr., and Johnson, J. A.,** Permeability of the mammalian blood-gas barrier and its components, *Am. J. Physiol.,* 216, 719, 1969.
12. **Wangensteen, D. and Yankovich, R.,** Alveolar epithelium transport of albumin and sucrose: concentration difference effect, *J. Appl. Physiol.: Resp. Environ. Exercise Physiol.,* 47, 846, 1979.
13. **Theodore, J., Robin, E. D., Gaudio, R., and Acevedo, J.,** Transalveolar transport of large polar solutes, *Am. J. Physiol.,* 229, 989, 1975.
14. **Effros, R. M., Mason, G. R., Silverman, P., Reid, E., and Hukkanen, J.,** Movement of ions and small solutes across endothelium and epithelium of perfused rabbit lungs, *J. Appl. Physiol.,* 69, 100, 1986.
15. **Ryrfeldt, A. and Nilsson, E.,** Uptake and biotransformation of ibuterol and terbutaline in isolated perfused rat and guinea pig lungs, *Biochem. Pharmacol.,* 27, 301, 1978.
16. **Ryrfeldt, A., Nilsson, E., Tunek, A., and Svensson, L. A.,** Bambuterol: uptake and metabolism in guinea pig isolated lungs, *Pharm. Res.,* 5, 151, 1988.
17. **Niven, R. W. and Byron, P. R.,** Solute absorption from the airways of the isolated rat lung. I. The use of absorption data to quantify drug dissolution or release in the respiratory tract, *Pharm. Res.,* 5, 574, 1988.
18. **Byron, P. R., Roberts, N. S. R., and Clark, A. R.,** An isolated perfused rat lung preparation for the study of aerosolized drug deposition and absorption, *J. Pharm. Sci.,* 75, 168, 1986.
19. **Charles, J. M., Abou-Donia, M. B., and Menzel, D. B.,** Absorption of paraquat and diquat from the airways of the perfused rat lung, *Toxicology,* 9, 59, 1978.
20. **Effros, R. M., Mason, G. R., Reid, E., Graham, L., and Silverman, P.,** Diffusion of labelled water and lipophilic solutes in the lung, *Microvasc. Res.,* 29, 45, 1985.
21. **Pitt, B. R., Cole, J. S., Davies, P., and Gillis, C. N.,** Rapid increases in respiratory epithelial permeability occur after intratracheal instillation of PMA, *J. Appl. Physiol.,* 63, 292, 1987.
22. **Brown, R. A. and Schanker, L. S.,** Absorption of aerosolized drugs from the rat lung, *Drug Metab. Dispos.,* 11, 355, 1983.
23. **Wilson, I. B. and LaMer, V. K.,** The retention of aerosol particles in the human respiratory tract as a function of particle radius, *J. Ind. Hyg. Toxicol.,* 30, 265, 1948.
24. **Morrow, P. E., Gibb, F. R., and Gazioglu, K. M.,** A study of particulate clearance from the human lungs, *Am. Rev. Resp. Dis.,* 96, 1209, 1967.
25. **Taplin, G. V., Poe, N. D., and Greenberg, A.,** Lung scanning following radioaerosol inhalation, *J. Nucl. Med.,* 7, 77, 1966.
26. **Huchon, G. J.,** Respiratory clearance of solutes, *Bull. Eur. Physiopathol. Resp.,* 22, 495, 1986.
27. **Barrowcliffe, M. P., Otto, C., and Jones, J. G.,** Pulmonary clearance of 99m Tc-DTPA: influence of background activity, *J. Appl. Physiol.,* 64, 1045, 1988.
28. **Waldman, D. L., Weber, D. A., Oberdorster, G., Drago, S. R., Utell, M. J., Hyde, R. W., and Morrow, P. E.,** Chemical breakdown of Technetium-99m DTPA during nebulization, *J. Nucl. Med.,* 28, 378, 1987.
29. **Elwood, S. K., Kennedy, S., Belzberg, A., Hogg, J. C., and Pare, P. D.,** Respiratory mucosal permeability in asthma, *Am. Rev. Resp. Dis.,* 128, 523, 1983.
30. **Oberdorster, G., Utell, M. J., Morrow, P. E., Hyde, R. W., and Weber, D. A.,** Bronchial and alveolar absorption of inhaled ^{99m}Tc-DTPA, *Am. Rev. Resp. Dis.,* 134, 944, 1986.
31. **Oberdorster, G., Utell, M. J., Weber, D. A., Ivanovich, M., Hyde, R. W., and Morrow, P. E.,** Lung clearance of inhaled 99m Tc-DTPA in the dog, *J. Appl. Physiol.,* 57, 589, 1984.
32. **O'Brodovich, H. and Coates, G.,** Pulmonary clearance of 99m Tc-DTPA: a noninvasive assessment of epithelial integrity, *Lung,* 165, 1, 1987.
33. **Effros, R. M. and Mason, G. R.,** Measurements of pulmonary epithelial permeability *in vivo, Am. Rev. Resp. Dis.,* 127, S59, 1983.

34. **Schanker, L. S., Mitchell, E. W., and Brown, R. A., Jr.,** Species comparison of drug absorption from the lung after aerosol inhalation or intratracheal injection, *Drug Metab. Disp.,* 14, 79, 1986.
35. **Huchon, G. J., Montgomery, A. B., Lipavsky, A., Hoeffel, J. M., and Murray, J. F.,** Respiratory clearance of aerosolized radioactive solutes of varying molecular weight, *J. Nucl. Med.,* 28, 894, 1987.
36. **Lanman, R. C., Gillilan, R. M., and Schanker, L. S.,** Absorption of cardiac glycosides from the rat respiratory tract, *J. Pharm. Exp. Ther.,* 187, 105, 1973.
37. **Enna, S. J. and Schanker, L. S.,** Absorption of drugs from the rat lung, *Am. J. Physiol.,* 223, 1227, 1972.
38. **Burton, J. A. and Schanker, L. S.,** Absorption of antibiotics from the rat lung, *Proc. Soc. Exp. Biol. Med.,* 145, 752, 1974.
39. **Burton, J. A. and Schanker, L. S.,** Absorption of sulfonamides and antitubercular drugs from the rat lung, *Xenobiotica,* 4, 291, 1974.
40. **Burton, J. A., Gardiner, T. H., and Schanker, L. S.,** Absorption of herbicides from the rat lung, *Arch. Environ. Health,* 29, 31, 1974.
41. **Normand, I. C. S., Oliver, R. E., Reynolds, E. O. R., and Strang, L. B.,** Permeability of lung capillaries and alveoli to nonelectrolytes in the fetal lamb, *J. Physiol. (London),* 219, 303, 1971.
42. **Hemberger, J. A. and Schanker, L. S.,** Pulmonary absorption of drugs in the neonatal rat, *Am. J. Physiol.,* 234, C191, 1978.
43. **Sten-Knudsen, O.,** Passive transport processes, in *Membrane Transport in Biology. I. Concepts and Models,* Giebisch, G., Tosteson, D. C., and Ussing, H. H., Eds., Springer-Verlag, Berlin, 1978, 53.
44. **Byron, P. R., Guest, R. T., and Notari, R. E.,** Thermodynamic dependence of interfacial transfer kinetics of nonionized barbituric acid derivatives in two phase transfer cell, *J. Pharm. Sci.,* 70, 1265, 1981.
45. **Wilke, C. R. and Chang, P.,** Correlation of diffusion coefficients in dilute solutions, *Am. Inst. Chem. Eng. J.,* 1, 264, 1955.
46. **Schanker, L. S. and Burton, J. A.,** Absorption of heparin and cyanocobalamin from the rat lung, *Proc. Soc. Exp. Biol. Med.,* 152, 377, 1976.
47. **Arakawa, E. and Kitazawa, S.,** Studies on the factors affecting pulmonary absorption of xanthine derivatives in the rat, *Chem. Pharm. Bull.,* 35, 2038, 1987.
48. **Brain, J. D., Knudson, D. E., Sorikin, S. P., and Davis, M. A.,** Pulmonary distribution of particles given by intratracheal instillation or by aerosol inhalation, *Environ. Res.,* 11, 13, 1976.
49. **Brain, J. D. and Valberg, P. A.,** Deposition of aerosol in the respiratory tract, *Am. Rev. Resp. Dis.,* 120, 1325, 1979.
50. **Byron, P. R. and Clark, A. R.,** Drug absorption from inhalation aerosols administered by positive pressure ventilation. I. Administration of a characterized solid disodium fluorescein aerosol under a controlled respiratory regime to the beagle dog, *J. Pharm. Sci.,* 74, 934, 1985.
51. **Clark, A. R. and Byron, P. R.,** Drug absorption from inhalation aerosols administered by positive pressure ventilation. II. Effect of disodium fluorescein aerosol particle size on fluorescein absorption kinetics in the beagle dog respiratory tract, *J. Pharm. Sci.,* 74, 939, 1985.
52. **McCullough, H. N. and Juliano, R. L.,** Organ selective action of an antitumor drug: Pharmacologic studies of liposome encapsulated B-cytosine arabinoside administered via the respiratory system of the rat, *JNCI,* 63, 727, 1979.
53. **Dalby, R. N. and Byron, P. R.,** Liposome formation following actuation of lecithin containing metered dose inhalers, *J. Pharm. Sci.,* 76, S262, 1987.
54. **Farr, S. J., Kellaway, I. W., Parry-Jones, D. R., and Woolfrey, S. G.,** 99m-Technetium as a marker of liposomal deposition and clearance in the human lung, *Int. J. Pharm.,* 26, 303, 1985.
55. **Debs, R. J., Straubinger, R. M., Brunette, E. N., Lin, J. M., Lin, E. J., Montgomery, A. B., Friend, D. S., and Papahadjopoulas, D. P.,** Selective enhancement of pentamidine uptake in the lung by aerosolization and delivery in liposomes, *Am. Rev. Resp. Dis.,* 135, 731, 1985.
56. **Abra, R. M., Hunt, C. A., and Lau, D. T.,** Liposome disposition *in vivo.* VI. Delivery to the lung, *J. Pharm. Sci.,* 73, 203, 1984.
57. **Egan, E. A., Nelson, R. M., and Olver, R. E.,** Lung inflation and alveolar permeability to nonelectrolytes in the adult sheep *in vivo, J. Physiol. (London),* 269, 409, 1976.
58. **Campbell, I. W., Hill, A., Middleton, H., Momen, M., and Prescott, R. J.,** Intermittent positive pressure breathing, *Br. Med. J.,* 1, 1186, 1978.
59. **Fergusson, R. J., Carmichael, J., Rafferty, P., Willey, R. F., Crompton, G. K., and Grant, I. W. B.,** Nebulized salbutamol in life threatening asthma: is IPPB necessary?, *Br. J. Dis. Chest,* 77, 255, 1983.
60. **Webber, B. A., Shenfield, G. M., and Patterson, J. W.,** A comparison of three different techniques for giving nebulized albuterol to asthmatic patients, *Am. Rev. Resp. Dis.,* 109, 293, 1974.
61. **Anon.,** IPPB trial group: IPPB in COPD, *Chest,* 86, 341, 1984.
62. **Rizk, N. W., Luce, J. M., Hoeffel, J. M., Price, D. C., and Murray, J. F.,** Site of deposition and factors affecting clearance of aerosolized solute from canine lungs, *J. Appl. Physiol.,* 56, 723, 1984.

63. **Marks, J. D., Luce, J. M., Lazar, N. M., Wu Naog-Su, J., Lipavsky, A., and Murray, J. F.,** Effect of increases in lung volume on clearance of aerosolized solutes from human lungs, *J. Appl. Physiol.,* 59, 1242, 1985.

64. **Egan, E. A.,** Response of alveolar epithelial solute permeability to changes in lung inflation, *J. Appl. Physiol. Resp. Environ. Exercise Physiol.,* 49, 1032, 1980.

65. **Nolop, K. B., Braude, S., Royston, D., Maxwell, D. L., and Hughes, J. M. B.,** Positive end expiratory pressure increases pulmonary clearance of inhaled 99m Tc-DTPA in nonsmokers but not in healthy smokers, *Bull. Eur. Physiopathol. Resp.,* 23, 57, 1987.

66. **Barrowcliffe, M. P. and Jones, J. G.,** Solute permeability of the alveolar capillary barrier, *Thorax,* 42, 1, 1987.

67. **Mossberg, B., Strandberg, K., Philipson, K., and Camner, P.,** Tracheo-bronchial clearance and Beta-adrenoceptor stimulation in patients with chronic bronchitis, *Scand. J. Resp. Dis.,* 57, 281, 1976.

68. **Camner, P., Mossberg, B., and Philipson, K.,** Tracheobronchial clearance and chronic obstructive lung disease, *Scand. J. Resp. Dis.,* 54, 272, 1973.

69. **Lafortuna, C. L. and Fazio, F.,** Acute effect of inhaled salbutamol on mucociliary clearance in health and chronic bronchitis, *Respiration,* 45, 111, 1984.

70. **Wanner, A.,** Effect of ipratropium bromide on airway mucociliary function, *Am. J. Med.,* 81(Suppl. 5A), 23, 1986.

71. **Dunnill, M. S.,** The pathology of asthma with specific reference to changes in the bronchial mucosa, *J. Clin. Pathol.,* 13, 27, 1960.

72. **Goodman, R. M., Yergin, B. M., Landa, J. F., Golinvaux, M. H., and Sackner, M. A.,** Relationship of smoking history and pulmonary function tests to tracheal mucous velocity in nonsmokers, young smokers, ex-smokers and patients with chronic bronchitis, *Am. Rev. Resp. Dis.,* 117, 205, 1978.

73. **Whelan, A. J. and Rutland, J.,** Drugs which influence cough, mucus, and ciliary function, in *Drug Use in Respiratory Disease,* Wilson, J. D., Ed., Williams & Wilkins, Baltimore, 1987, 47.

74. **Fulford, G. R. and Blake, J. R.,** Mucociliary transport in the lung, *J. Theor. Biol.,* 121, 381, 1986.

75. **Lucas, A. M. and Douglas, L. C.,** Principles underlying ciliary activity in the respiratory tract, *Arch. Otolaryngol.,* 20, 518, 1934.

76. **Lopez-Vidriero, M. T.,** Airway mucus: production and composition, *Chest,* 80(Suppl.), 799, 1981.

77. **Sackner, M. A., Rosen, M. J., and Wanner, A.,** Estimation of tracheal mucous velocity by bronchofiberscopy, *J. Appl. Physiol.,* 34, 495, 1973.

78. **Annis, P., Landa, J., and Lichtiger, M.,** Effects of atropine on velocity of tracheal mucus in anesthetized patients, *Anesthesiology,* 44, 74, 1976.

79. **Camner, P.,** Production and use of test aerosols for studies of human tracheobronchial clearance, *Environ. Physiol. Biochem.,* 1, 137, 1971.

80. **Friedman, M., Stott, F. D., Poole, D. O., Dougherty, R., Chapman, G. A., Watson, H., and Sackner, M. A.,** A new roentgenographic method for estimating mucous velocity in airways, *Am. Rev. Resp. Dis.,* 115, 67, 1977.

81. **Mezey, R. J., Cohn, M. A., Fernandez, R. J., Januszkiewicz, A. J., and Wanner, A.,** Mucociliary transport in allergic patients with antigen-induced bronchospasm, *Am. Rev. Resp. Dis.,* 118, 677, 1978.

82. **Bell, J. A., Bluestein, B. M., Danta, I., and Wanner, A.,** Effect of inhaled ipratropium bromide on tracheal mucociliary transport in bronchial asthma, *Mt. Sinai J. Med.,* 51, 215, 1984.

83. **Foster, W. M., Langenback, E., and Bergofsky, E. H.,** Measurement of tracheal and bronchial mucus velocities in man: relation to lung clearance, *J. Appl. Physiol. Resp. Environ. Exercise Physiol.,* 48, 965, 1980.

84. **Foster, W. M., Bergofsky, E. H., Bohning, D. E., Lippmann, M., and Albert, R. E.,** Effect of adrenergic agents and their mode of action on mucociliary clearance in man, *J. Appl. Physiol.,* 41, 146, 1976.

85. **Yeates, D. B., Aspin, N., Levison, H., Jones, M. T., and Bryan, A. C.,** Mucociliary tracheal transport rates in man, *J. Appl. Physiol.,* 39, 487, 1975.

86. **Fazio, F. and Lafortuna, C. L.,** Beclomethasone dipropionate does not affect mucociliary clearance in patients with chronic obstructive lung disease, *Respiration,* 50, 62, 1986.

87. **Thomson, M. L. and Short, M. D.,** Mucociliary function in health, chronic obstructive airway disease and asbestosis, *J. Appl. Physiol.,* 26, 535, 1969.

88. **Thomson, M. L., Pavia, D., and McNicol, M. W.,** A preliminary study of the effect guaiphenesin on mucociliary clearance from the human lung, *Thorax,* 28, 742, 1973.

89. **Byron, P. R.,** Prediction of drug residence time in regions of the human respiratory tract, *J. Pharm. Sci.,* 75, 433, 1986.

90. **Foster, W. M., Langenback, E. G., and Bergofsky, E. H.,** Lung mucociliary function in man: Interdependence of bronchial and tracheal mucus transport velocities with lung clearance in bronchial asthma and healthy subjects, *Ann. Occup. Hyg.,* 26, 227, 1982.

91. **Santa Cruz, R., Landa, J., Hirsch, J., and Sackner, M. A.,** Tracheal mucus velocity in normal man and patients with obstructive lung disease: effects of terbutaline, *Am. Rev. Resp. Dis.,* 109, 458, 1974.

92. **Albert, R. E., Lippmann, M., Peterson, H. T., Berger, J., Sanborn, K., and Bohning, D.,** Bronchial deposition and clearance of aerosols, *Arch. Intern. Med.,* 131, 115, 1973.

93. **Francis, R. A., Thompson, M. L., Pavia, D., and Douglas, R. B.,** Ipratropium bromide: mucociliary clearance rate and airway resistance in normal subjects, *Br. J. Dis. Chest,* 71, 173, 1977.

94. **Pavia, D., Bateman, J. R. M., Sheahan, N. F., and Clarke, S. W.,** Effect of ipratropium bromide on mucociliary clearance and pulmonary function in reversible airways obstruction, *Thorax,* 34, 501, 1979.

95. **Calvert, J.,** Effect of drugs on the secretion from tracheal mucous membrane, *J. Physiol.,* 20, 158, 1896.

96. **Florey, H. W., Carleton, H. M., and Wells, A. O.,** Mucus secretion in the trachea, *Br. J. Exp. Pathol.,* 13, 269, 1932.

97. **Sturgess, J. and Reid, L.,** An organ culture study of the effect of drugs on the secretory activity of the human bronchial submucosal gland, *Clin. Sci.,* 43, 533, 1972.

98. **Trowell, O. A.,** The culture of mature organs in a synthetic medium, *Exp. Cell Res.,* 16, 118, 1959.

99. **Lopez-Vidriero, M. T., Costello, J., Clark, T. J. H., Das, I., Keal, E. E., and Reid, L.,** Effect of atropine on sputum production, *Thorax,* 30, 543, 1975.

100. **Richards, J. H. and Marriott, C.,** Effect of relative humidity on the rheologic properties of bronchial mucus, *Am. Rev. Resp. Dis.,* 109, 484, 1974.

101. **King, M. and Angus, G. E.,** Effect of aerosolized bronchodilators on viscoelastic properties of canine tracheal mucus, *Chest,* 80(Suppl.), 851, 1981.

102. **Verdugo, P., Johnson, N. T., and Tam, P. Y.,** B-Adrenergic stimulation of respiratory ciliary activity, *J. Appl. Physiol. Resp. Environ. Exercise Physiol.,* 48, 868, 1980.

103. **Yanaura, S., Imamura, N., and Misawa, M.,** Effects of B-adrenoceptor stimulants on the canine tracheal ciliated cells, *Jpn. J. Pharmacol.,* 31, 951, 1981.

104. **Van As, A.,** The role of selective B-adrenoceptor stimulants in the control of ciliary activity, *Respiration,* 31, 146, 1974.

105. **Blair, A. M. J. N. and Woods, A.,** The effects of isoprenaline, atropine and disodium cromoglycate on ciliary motility and mucous flow measured *in vivo* in cats, *Br. J. Pharmacol.,* 35, 379, 1969.

106. **Iravani, J. and Melville, G. N.,** Mucociliary function in the respiratory tract as influenced by drugs, *Respiration,* 31, 350, 1974.

107. **Lee, W. I. and Verdugo, P.,** Laser light scattering spectroscopy: a new application in the study of ciliary activity, *Biophys. J.,* 16, 1115, 1976.

108. **Moore, R. D. and Schoenberg, M. D.,** The response of the histiocytes and macrophages in the lungs of rabbits injected with Freund's adjuvant, *Br. J. Exp. Pathol.,* 45, 488, 1964.

109. **Casarett, L. J. and Milley, P. S.,** Alveolar reactivity following inhalation aerosols, *Health Phys.,* 10, 1003, 1964.

110. **Karrer, H. E.,** Electron microscopic study of the phagocytosis process in lung, *J. Biophys. Biochem. Cytol.,* 7, 357, 1960.

111. **Hapke, E. J. and Pederson, H. J.,** Cytoplasmic activity in type I pulmonary epithelial cells induced by macroaggregated albumin, *Science,* 161, 580, 1968.

112. **Sanders, C. L., Jackson, T. A., Adee, R. R., Powers, G. J., and Wehner, A. P.,** Distribution of inhaled metal oxide particles in pulmonary alveoli, *Arch. Intern. Med.,* 127, 1085, 1971.

113. **Low, F. N. and Sampaio, M. M.,** The pulmonary alveolar epithelium as an entodermal derivative, *Anat. Rec.,* 127, 51, 1957.

114. **Morrow, P. E. and Casarett, L. J.,** *Inhaled Particles and Vapours,* Pergamon Press, Oxford, 1961, 157.

115. **Gross, P. and Hatch, T.,** *Arch Gewerbepathol. Gewerbehyg.,* 19, 660, 1962.

116. **Morrow, P. E.,** Alveolar clearance of aerosols, *Arch. Intern. Med.,* 131, 101, 1973.

117. **Boyd, R. D. G., Hill, J. R., Humphreys, P. W., Normand, I. C. S., Reynolds, E. O. R., and Strang, L. B.,** Permeability of lung capillaries to macromolecules in fetal and newborn lambs and sheep, *J. Physiol.,* 201, 567, 1969.

118. **Chinard, F. P.,** Exchange across the alveolar-capillary barrier, in *The Pulmonary Circulation and Interstitial Space,* Fishman, A. P. and Hecht, H. H., Eds., University of Chicago Press, Chicago, 1969.

119. **Chien, S., Sinclair, D. G., Chang, C., Peric, B., and Dellenback, R. J.,** Simultaneous study of capillary permeability to several macromolecules, *Am. J. Physiol.,* 207, 513, 1964.

120. **Morrow, P. E.,** The Lymphatic Drainage of the Lungs in Dust Clearance, paper presented at the New York Academy of Science International Conference on Coal Worker's Pneumoconiosis, New York, September 13 to 17, 1971.

121. **Bowden, D. H., and Adamson, I. Y. R.,** Pathways of cellular efflux and particulate clearance after carbon instillation to the lung, *J. Pathol.,* 143, 117, 1984.

122. **Leak, L. V.,** Lymphatic removal of fluids and particles in the mammalian lung, *Environ. Health Perspect.,* 35, 55, 1980.

123. **Sorokin, S. P. and Brain, J. D.,** Pathways of clearance in mouse lungs exposed to iron oxide aerosols, *Anat. Rec.,* 118, 581, 1975.

124. **Brain, J. D., Godleski, J. J., and Sorokin, S. P.,** Quantification, origin, and fate of pulmonary macrophages, in *Respiratory Defense Mechanisms, Part II,* Brain, J. D., Proctor, D. F., and Reid, L., Eds., Marcel Dekker, New York, 1977.

125. **Snipes, M. B., Chavez, G. T., and Muggenberg, B. A.,** Disposition of 3-, 7-, and 13-μm microspheres instilled into lungs of dogs, *Environ. Res., 33,* 333, 1984.

126. **Snipes, M. B., Boeker, B. B., and McClellan, R. O.,** Retention of monodisperse or polydisperse aluminosilicate particles inhaled by dogs, rats and mice, *Toxicol. Appl. Pharmacol.,* 69, 345, 1983.

127. **Bowden, D. H.,** Macrophages, dust and pulmonary diseases, *Exp. Lung Res.,* 12, 89, 1987.

128. **Adamson, I. Y. R. and Bowden, D. H.,** Dose response of the pulmonary macrophagic system to various particulates and its relationship to transepithelial passage of free particles, *Exp. Lung Res.,* 2, 165, 1981.

129. **Brain, J. D.,** The effects of increased particles on the number of alveolar macrophages, in *Inhaled Particles III,* Vol. 1, Walton, W. H., Ed., Unwin Bros., London, 1971, 205.

130. **Adamson, I. Y. R. and Bowden, D. H.,** Effects of irradiation on macrophagic response and transport of particles across the alveolar epithelium, *Am. J. Pathol.,* 106, 40, 1982.

131. **Bowden, D. H. and Adamson, I. Y. R.,** The role of cell injury and the continuing inflammatory response in the generation of silicotic pulmonary fibrosis, *J. Pathol.,* 144, 149, 1984.

132. **Brody, A. R., Hill, L. H., Adkins, B., and O'Connor, R. W.,** Chrysotile asbestos inhalation in rats: deposition pattern and reaction of alveolar epithelium and pulmonary macrophages, *Am. Rev. Resp. Dis.,* 123, 670, 1981.

133. **Bowden, D. H. and Adamson, I. Y. R.,** Bronchiolar and alveolar lesions in the pathogenesis of crocidolite induced pulmonary fibrosis in mice, *J. Pathol.,* 147, 257, 1985.

134. **Lauweryns, J. M. and Baert, J. H.,** Alveolar clearance and the role of the pulmonary lymphatics, *Am. Rev. Resp. Dis.,* 115, 625, 1977.

135. **Tucker, A. D., Wyatt, J. H., and Undery, D.,** Clearance of inhaled particles from alveoli by normal interstitial drainage pathways, *J. Appl. Physiol.,* 35, 719, 1973.

136. **Spector, W. G.,** Pulmonary fibrosis due to chemicals and particles, *Ann. N. Y. Acad. Sci.,* 221, 309, 1974.

137. **Crapo, J. D., Barry, B. E., Gehr, P., Bochofen, M., and Weibel, E. R.,** Cell numbers and cell characteristics of the normal human lung, *Am. Rev. Resp. Dis.,* 126, 332, 1982.

138. *Lehnert, B. E., Valdez, Y. E., and Holland, L. M.,* Pulmonary macrophages: alveolar and interstitial populations, *Exp. Lung Res.,* 9, 177, 1985.

139. **Bowden, D. H. and Adamson, I. Y. R.,** Adaptive response of the pulmonary macrophagic system to carbon. I. Kinetic studies, *Lab. Invest.,* 38, 422, 1978.

140. **Pinkett, M. O., Cowdrey, C. R., and Nowell, P. C.,** Mixed hematopoietic and pulmonary origin of alveolar macrophages as demonstrated by chromosome markers, *Am. J. Pathol.,* 48, 859, 1966.

141. **Brain, J. D.,** Free cells in the lungs: symposium on pulmonary responses to inhaled materials, an evaluation of model systems, *Arch. Intern. Med.,* 126, 477, 1970.

142. *Brunstetter, M. A., Hardie, J. A., Schiff, R., Lewis, J. P., and Cross, C. E.,* The origin of pulmonary macrophages, *Arch. Intern. Med.,* 127, 1064, 1971.

143. **Godleski, J. J. and Brain, J. D.,** The origin of alveolar macrophages in mouse radiation chimeras, *J. Exp. Med.,* 136, 630, 1972.

144. **Green, G. M., Jakab, G. J., Low, R. B., and Davis, G. S.,** Defense mechanisms of the respiratory membrane, *Am. Rev. Resp. Dis.,* 115, 479, 1977.

145. **van Furth, R.,** The origin and turnover of promonocytes, monocytes and macrophages in normal mice, in *Mononuclear Phagocytes,* van Furth, R., Ed., Davis, Blackwell, 1970, 151.

146. **Volkman, A.,** Disparity in origin of mononuclear phagocyte populations, *J. Reticuloendothelial. Soc.,* 19, 249, 1976.

147. **Sawyer, R. T.,** The significance of local resident pulmonary alveolar macrophage proliferation to population renewal, *J. Leukocyte Biol.,* 39, 77, 1986.

148. **Sawyer, R. T.,** The cytokinetic behavior of pulmonary alveolar macrophages in monocytopenic mice, *J. Leukocyte Biol.,* 39, 89, 1986.

149. **Evans, M. J., Shami, S. G., and Martinez, L. A.,** Enhanced proliferation of pulmonary alveolar macrophages after carbon instillation in mice depleted of blood monocytes by Strontium-89, *Lab. Invest.,* 54, 154, 1986.

150. **Bowden, D. H. and Adamson, I. Y. R.,** Alveolar macrophage response to carbon in monocyte-depleted mice, *Am. Rev. Resp. Dis.,* 126, 708, 1982.

151. **Green, G. M.,** Alveolobronchiolar transport mechanisms, *Arch. Intern. Med.,* 131, 109, 1973.

152. **Brain, J. D.,** Clearance of Particles from the Lungs: Alveolar Macrophages and Mucus Transport, Doctoral thesis, Harvard University, Cambridge, MA, 1966.

153. **Warheit, D. B., Overby, L. H., George, G., and Brody, A. R.,** Pulmonary macrophages are attracted to inhaled particles through complement activation, *Exp. Lung Res.,* 14, 51, 1988.

154. **Olenchock, S. A., Mull, J. C., Major, P. C., Peach, M. J., Gladish, M. D., and Taylor, G.,** *In vitro* activation of the alternative pathway of complement by settled grain dust, *J. Allergy Clin. Immunol.,* 62, 295, 1978.

155. **Wilson, M. R., Gaumer, H. R., and Salvaggio, J. R.,** Activation of the alternative complement pathway and generation of chemotactic factors by asbestos, *J. Allergy Clin. Immunol.,* 60, 218, 1977.
156. **Saint-Remy, J. M. R. and Cole, P.,** Interactions of chrysotile asbestos fibers with the complement system, *Immunology,* 41, 431, 1980.
157. **Warheit, D. B., Hill, L. H., and Brody, A. R.,** *In vitro* effects of crocidolite asbestos and wollastonite on pulmonary macrophages and serum complement, *Scanning Electron Microscopy II,* 919, 1984.
158. **Yano, E., Takeuch, A., Yukiyamo, Y., and Brown, R. C.,** Chemotactic factor generation by asbestos: fibre type differences and the effect of leaching, *Br. J. Exp. Pathol.,* 65, 223, 1984.
159. **Hill, J. O., Rothenberg, S. J., Kanapilly, G. M., Hanson, R. L., and Scott, B. R.,** Activation of immune complement by fly ash particles from coal combustion, *Environ. Res.,* 28, 113, 1982.
160. **Macklin, C. C.,** Pulmonary sumps, dust accumulations, alveolar fluid and lymph vessels, *Acta Anat.,* 23, 1, 1955.
161. **Gross, P.,** The mechanism of dust clearance from the lung, a theory, *Am. J. Clin. Pathol.,* 23, 116, 1953.
162. **Robertson, O. H.,** Phagocytosis of foreign matter in the lung, *Physiol. Rev.,* 21, 112, 1941.
163. **Fenn, W. O.,** The phagocytosis of solid particles, *J. Gen. Physiol.,* 3, 439, 575, 1921.
164. **Schoenberg, M. D., Gilman, P. A., Mumaw, V., and Moore, R. D.,** Proliferation of the reticuloendothelial system and phagocytosis, *Exp. Mol. Pathol.,* 2, 126, 1963.
165. **Bingham, E., Pfitzer, E. A., Barkley, W., Radford, E. P.,** Alveolar macrophages: reduced numbers in rats after prolonged inhalation of lead sequinoxide, *Science,* 162, 1297, 1962.
166. **Rasche, B. and Ulmer, W. T.,** Reactions of alveolar phagocytes to aerosols during short term exposures to dust, in *Inhaled Particles and Vapours II,* Davis, C. N., Ed., Pergamon Press, Oxford, 1967, 243.
167. **Lehnert, B. E. and Morrow, P. E.,** Characteristics of alveolar macrophages following the deposition of a low burden of iron oxide in the lung, *J. Toxicol. Environ. Health,* 16, 855, 1985.
168. **Ferin, J.,** Emphysema in rats and clearance of dust particles, in, *Inhaled Particles,* Vol. 3, Walton, W. H., Ed., Gresham Press, Old Woking, England, 283.
169. **Morrow, P. E., Gibb, F. R., and Leach, L. J.,** The clearance of uranium dioxide dust from the lung following single and multiple inhalation exposures, *Health Phys.,* 12, 1217, 1966.
170. **Downs, W. L., Wilson, H. B., Sylvester, G. E., Leach, L. J., and Maynard, E. A.,** Excretion of uranium by rats following inhalation of uranium dioxide, *Health Phys.,* 13, 445, 1967.
171. **Thomas, R. G.,** An interspecies model for retention of inhaled particles, in *Assessment of Airborne Particles,* Mercer, T. T., Morrow, P. E., and Stober, W., Eds., Charles C Thomas, Springfield, IL, 1972, 405.
172. **Ferin, J.,** Effect of particle content of lung on clearance pathways, in *Pulmonary Macrophage and Epithelial Cells,* Sanders, L., Schneider, R. P., Dagle, G. E., and Ragan, H. A., Eds., National Technical Information Center, 1977, 414.
173. **Cuddihy, R. G., Brownstein, D. G., Raabe, O. G., and Kanapilly, G. M.,** Respiratory tract deposition of inhaled polydisperse aerosols in beagle dogs, *J. Aerosol Sci.,* 4, 35, 1973.
174. **Fish, B. R.,** Inhalation of uranium aerosols by mouse, rat, dog and man, in *Inhaled Particles and Vapours,* Davis, C. N. Ed., Pergamon Press, Oxford, 1961, 151.
175. **Waligora, S. J.,** Pulmonary retention of zirconium oxide (95 Nb) in man and beagle dogs, *Health Phys.,* 20, 89, 1971.
176. **Wolff, R. K., Kanapilly, G. M., DeNee, P. B., and McClellan, R. O.,** Deposition of 0.1 μm chain aggregate aerosols in beagle dogs, *J. Aerosol Sci.,* 12, 119, 1981.
177. **Mercer, T. T.,** On the role of particle size in the dissolution of lung burdens, *Health Phys.,* 13, 1211, 1967.
178. **Albert, R. E.,** The clearance of radioactive particles from the human lung, in *Inhaled Particles and Vapours II,* Davies, C. N., Ed., Pergamon Press, Oxford, 1967, 361.
179. **Martin, A.,** Diffusion and dissolution, in *Physical Pharmacy: Physical Chemical Principles in the Pharmaceutical Sciences,* Martin, A., Swarbrick, J., and Cammarata, A., Eds., Lea & Febiger, Philadelphia, 1983, 400.
180. **Stout, P. J. M., Khaoury, N., Mauger, J., and Howard, S.,** Evaluation of a tube method for determining diffusion coefficients for sparingly soluble drugs, *J. Pharm. Sci.,* 75, 65, 1986.
181. **Swintosky, J. V., Riegelman, S., Higuchi, T., and Busse, L. W.,** Studies on pharmaceutical powders and the state of subdivisions. I. The application of low-temperature nitrogen adsorption isotherms to the determination of surface areas, *J. Am. Pharm. Assoc.,* 38, 210, 308, 1949.
182. **Hixson, A. and Crowell J.,** *Ind. Eng. Chem.,* 23, 923, 1931.
183. **Niebergall, P., Milosovich, G., and Goyan, J.,** Dissolution rate studies. II. Dissolution of particles under conditions of rapid agitation, *J. Pharm. Sci.,* 52, 236, 1963.
184. **Brooke, D.,** Dissolution profile of log-normal powders: exact expression, *J. Pharm. Sci.,* 62, 795, 1973.
185. **Carstensen, J. and Musa, M.,** Dissolution rate patterns of log-normally distributed powders, *J. Pharm. Sci.,* 61, 223, 1972.
186. **Martin, A.,** Solublity and distribution phenomena, in *Physical Pharmacy: Physical Chemical Principles in the Pharmaceutical Sciences,* Martin, A., Swarbrick, J., and Cammarata, A., Eds., Lea & Febiger, Philadelphia, 1983, 302.

187. **Vidgren, M. T., Vidgren, P. A., and Paronen, T. P.,** Comparison of physical and inhalation properties of spray dried and mechanically micronized disodium cromoglycate, *Int. J. Pharm.,* 35, 139, 1987.

188. **Mufson, D., Triyanond, K., Zarembo, J. E., and Ravin, L. J.,** Cholesterol solubility in model bile systems: implications in cholelithiasis, *J. Pharm. Sci.,* 63, 327, 1974.

189. **Mauger, J. and Howard, S.,** Model systems for dissolution of finely divided (multisized) drug powders, *J. Pharm. Sci.,* 65, 1042, 1976.

190. **Higuchi, W. I., and Hiestand, E. N.,** Dissolution rates of finely divided drug powders I, *J. Pharm. Sci.,* 52, 67, 1963.

191. **Higuchi, W. I., Rowe, E. L., and Hiestand, E. N.,** Dissolution rates of finely divided drug powders II, *J. Pharm. Sci.,* 52, 162, 1963.

192. **Nielsen, A.,** Diffusion controlled growth of a moving sphere. The kinetics of crystal growth in potassium perchlorate precipitation, *J. Phys. Chem.,* 65, 46, 1961.

193. **Howard, S. A., Mauger, J. W., and Phusanti, L.,** Dissolution profiles for multisized prednisolone acetate suspensions, *J. Pharm. Sci.,* 66, 557, 1977.

194. **Howard, S. A., Mauger, J. W., Khwangsopha, A., and Lee, P.,** Separation of multisized drug suspensions into narrow distributions by centrifugal elutriation, *J. Pharm. Sci.,* 67, 673, 1978.

195. **Mauger, J. W., Howard, S. A., and Amin, K.,** Dissolution profiles for finely divided drug suspensions, *J. Pharm. Sci.,* 72, 190, 1983.

196. **English, J. C., Parker, R. D. R., Sharma, R. P., and Oberg, S. G.,** Toxicokinetics of nickel in rats after intratracheal administration of a soluble and insoluble form, *Am. Ind. Hyg. Assoc. J.,* 42, 486, 1981.

197. **Finch, G. L., Fisher, G. L., and Hayes, T. L.,** The pulmonary effects and clearance of intratracheally instilled Ni_3S_2 and TiO_2 in mice, *Environ. Res.,* 42, 83, 1987.

198. **Valentine, R. and Fisher, G. L.,** Pulmonary clearance of intratracheally administered $^{63}NiCl_2$ in strain A/J mice, *Environ. Res.,* 34, 328, 1984.

199. **Carvalho Machado, S. M., and Ziemer, P. L.,** Distribution and clearance of ^{63}Ni administered as $^{63}NiCl_2$ in the rat: intratracheal study, *Arch. Environ. Contam. Toxicol.,* 11, 245, 1982.

200. **Oberdoerster, G., Baumert, H. P., Hochrainer, D., and Stoeber, W.,** The clearance of cadmium aerosols after inhalation exposure, *Am. Ind. Hyg. Assoc. J.,* 40, 443, 1979.

201. **Aihara, M., Sharma, R. P., and Shupe, J. L.,** Short term disposition of soluble versus insoluble forms of cadmium in rat lung after intratracheal administration: an autoradiographic assessment, *Toxicology,* 36, 109, 1985.

202. **Hadley, J. G., Conklin, A. W., and Sanders, C. L.,** Rapid solubilization and translocation of ^{109}CdO following pulmonary deposition, *Toxicol. Appl. Pharmacol.,* 54, 156, 1980.

203. **Drown, D. B., Oberg, S. G., and Sharma, R. P.,** Pulmonary clearance of soluble and insoluble forms of manganese, *J. Toxicol. Environ. Health,* 17, 201, 1986.

204. **Bailey, M. R., Fry, F. A., and James, A. C.,** Pulmonary retention of inhaled particles in man in *Radiological Protection Bulletin,* Vol. 43, p. 13-20, 1981, National Radiological Protection Board.

205. **Bailey, M. R., Fry, F. A., and James, A. C.,** The long term clearance kinetics of insolible particles from the lung, *Ann. Occup. Hyg.,* 26, 273, 1982.

206. **Bailey, M. R., Hudgson, A., Smith, H., Strong, J. C., and Savory, A. J.,** *In vitro* and *in vivo* dissolution characteristics of monodispersed labeled aluminosilicate particles, in *Aerosols in Science, Medicine and Technology — Physical and Chemical Properties of Aerosols,* Stober, W. and Hochrainer, D., Eds., Schmallenburg, Berlin, 1980, 265.

207. **Gonda, I.,** Drugs administered directly into the respiratory tract: modeling of the duration of effective drug levels, *J. Pharm. Sci.,* 77, 340, 1988.

208. **Schanker, L. S. and Hemberger, J. A.,** Relation between molecular weight and pulmonary absorption rate of lipid insoluble compounds in neonatal and adult rats, *Biochem. Pharmacol.,* 32, 2599, 1983.

209. **Brown, R. A. and Schanker, L. S.,** Sex comparison of pulmonary absorption of drugs in the rat, *Drug Metab. Disp.,* 11, 392, 1983.

210. **Eidson A. F. and Mewhinney J. A.,** *In vitro* dissolution of respirable aerosols of industrial uranium and plutonium mixed-oxide nuclear fuels, *Health Phys.,* 45, 1023, 1983.

211. **Mauger, J. W., Brooke, D., and Damewood, E. Z.,** Dissolution profile for multisized drug particles: new approximate expression, *J. Pharm. Sci.,* 66, 553, 1977.

212. **Mossberg, B., Strandberg, K., Philipson, K., and Camner, P.,** Tracheobronchial clearance in bronchial asthma: response to beta-adrenoceptor stimulation, *Scand. J. Resp. Dis.,* 57, 119, 1976.

213. **Camner, P., Strandberg, K., and Philipson, K.,** Increased mucociliary transport by adrenergic stimulation, *Arch. Environ. Health,* 31, 79, 1976.

214. **Chopra, S. K.,** Effect of atropine on mucociliary transport velocity in anesthetized dogs, *Am. Rev. Resp. Dis.,* 118, 367, 1978.

215. **Pavia, D. and Thomson, M. L.,** Inhibition of mucociliary clearance from the human lung by hyoscine, *Lancet,* 1, 449, 1971.

Chapter 6

AEROSOL FORMULATION, GENERATION, AND DELIVERY USING NONMETERED SYSTEMS

Peter R. Byron

TABLE OF CONTENTS

I. METERED VS. NONMETERED SYSTEMS

Devices which can be used to generate inhalation aerosols fall into two main categories: those which purport to meter the drug dose provided to the patient and those which do not. Because the formulation of metered dose inhalers or MDIs presents the pharmaceutical scientist with some unique challenges, these devices are described separately in another chapter. The present chapter attempts to come to grips with the principles of operation of continuous aerosol generators and their use in the treatment of human disease. These devices, of which nebulizers are the most common example, are used widely by pharmacologists involved with drug testing in animals and are increasingly seen as a useful adjunct to MDI therapy in humans. Despite the implication in the chapter title that nebulizers provide an unknown dose, they can be used conveniently by researchers who seek to establish the dosimetry of compounds delivered to the lungs. This step is a necessity in the development phase for a new drug entity and should be performed prior to the formulation and design of metered dose units. While the majority of this chapter is concerned with the use of continuous aerosol generators to administer drugs in a therapeutic setting, two sections (II.C and V.C) address the subject of assigning a value for "dose to the lung" applicable to a drug development protocol.

Some of the advantages and disadvantages of nonmetered systems such as portable nebulizers are listed in Table 1. In view of the fact that aerosols are presently inhaled mostly by breathing-impaired patients, the predominant factor dictating the use of a nebulizer over an MDI is patient preference. Nebulizers offer the possibility of tidal inhalation and exhalation (as opposed to deep inhalation and breath-hold, phased with actuation for optimal MDI usage). However, in view of the fact that some new compounds may be administered to lung-normal patients (for systemic delivery perhaps), this factor is drug and disease specific. From a technological point of view, the possibility of administering much larger doses by employing continuous aerosol inhalation is the nebulizer's most appealing advantage. Disadvantages, on the other hand, are many; the level of patient education is critical if hygiene is to be maintained and, because of the complexity associated with these devices, much of the control remains in the hands of the patient. The wide variety of available devices and their different specifications makes misuse a likely occurence.

II. ESTIMATING DOSIMETRY

Only a basic understanding of the factors affecting aerosol deposition in the lung is necessary in order to realize that neither continuous generators nor so-called "metered dose inhalers" really control the drug dose reaching the airways of the lung. It is true that the MDI limits the amount a patient can inhale from a single actuation of the inhaler, but in neither this case, nor that of the nebulizer, will all of the aerosolized material reach and deposit in the lung. While it is not the intention to review deposition in detail (see Chapter 1), the importance of defining dosimetry in terms of drug mass requires that a simple mass-based deposition model be presented here as a precursor to later arguments to be used in this and the next chapter.

A. STABLE AEROSOLS INHALED BY NORMAL HUMANS

When discussing the different categories of generation and delivery device, it is helpful to keep a simple model of aerosol deposition in mind. Aerosol size distribution is the single most important variable in defining the site of droplet or particle deposition in the patient; in short, it will determine whether drug targeting succeeds or fails. From a pharmaceutical point of view, the most important parameter is usually the mass median aerodynamic diameter (MMAD) of an aerosol. This is the aerodynamic diameter above and below which 50% of the mass resides. Aerodynamic diameter is the diameter of a unit density sphere which behaves in air in the same way as the droplet or particle in question. In the frequent event that MMAD is determined by

TABLE 1
Advantages and Disadvantages of Nonmetered Aerosol Delivery Devices

Advantages	Disadvantages
1. Large respirable dose	1. Complexity
2. Patient preference[a]	2. Expense and portability
3. Water is usually the solvent[b]	3. Hygiene maintainence
4. Patient coordination is not usually a problem	4. Devices and techniques are nonstandardized

[a] In the home; in public places, smaller devices like MDIs are usually preferred.
[b] Propellant and excipient toxicity is not an issue.

fractionating the aerosol according to droplet size and then analyzing drug content in each of the fractions, then the term reflects the size above and below which 50% of the drug mass resides.[1] Because the concentration of drug may be different in small and large droplets, this is not necessarily the same as the MMAD of the aerosol itself. Nevertheless, it is this drug MMAD which matters here because this will define how the drug mass will deposit in the lung.[2] It is important when reading the literature to realize that the mass median diameter is often about three to four times larger than either the count or number mean or median diameters.[3] The number median, for example, is the diameter above and below which 50% of the number of droplets resides. The latter value is smaller than the MMAD because a single 10 μm sphere has 1000 times the mass of one with a diameter of 1 μm. Articles in the medical literature and device manufacturers frequently state count mean diameters to describe the output of different devices which make the aerosols sound much better for inhalation than they really are.[4] Diameters other than aerodynamic are sometimes also quoted. The difference between actual and aerodynamic diameters, d_{ae}, which are related through the density and shape of the particle or droplet, is given for spheres with diameters greater than ≈ 1 μm by

$$d_{ae} = (\text{actual diameter}) \cdot (\text{density})^{1/2} \tag{1}$$

where density is expressed in gcm^{-3}. This relationship is less important for aqueous aerosols than it is for aerosolized pharmaceutical powders where densities are often in the range of 1 to 2 gcm^{-3}.[5] Readers should review a simple text on particle size analysis[3] in order to clarify their understanding of these points. Provided an aerosol is log-normally distributed and the geometric standard deviation is known, it is possible to relate the different mean and median diameters analytically. Even so, because therapeutic aerosols often deviate from log-normality and sometimes display polymodal distributions, it is better to measure the MMAD itself rather than try to calculate it from some other value.[6]

Different aerosol size distributions may be expected to deposit preferentially in different regions of the respiratory tract. Aerosols inhaled through the nose have different deposition patterns to those inhaled orally.[7] In Figure 1, oral inhalation by normal subjects is assumed because this is the more frequent mode of inhalation. Fractional deposition (in terms of particle or droplet mass) is shown for monodisperse, stable aerosols. The data in support of Figure 1 are derived from human exposure to radiolabeled dust aerosols with subjects inhaling and exhaling tidally.[7,8] If the horizontal axis on Figure 1 were labeled "mass median aerodynamic diameter" so that polydisperse aerosols were considered,[9] the curves indicating deposition in the lung may be reduced in height, indicating less efficient deposition, but the maxima would remain at the same diameters.[10] In normal subjects, deposition in the pulmonary or alveolar compartment is optimal for aerosols with aerodynamic diameters around 2 to 3 μm provided inhalation is slow (20 to 30 l/min).[7,11] Maximum deposition in the tracheobronchial regions occurs with slightly

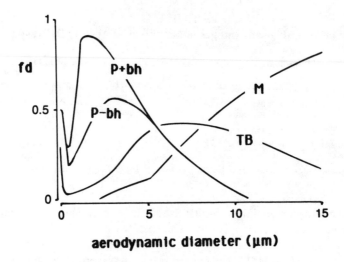

FIGURE 1. Simulated fractional mass deposition, fd, vs. aerodynamic diameter (μm) in oropharynx or mouth (M), tracheobronchial region (TB), and pulmonary region with (P + bh) and without breath-hold (P – bh). Deposition is for stable monodisperse aerosols inhaled by normal humans breathing tidally with inspiratory flow rates ≈22 l/min. Polydisperse aerosols produce similar curves with lower maxima when mass median aerodynamic diameter is plotted on the horizontal axis. (Reproduced with permission of the American Pharmaceutical Association.)

larger particles, although mucociliary clearance can remove material quite quickly from this region (Chapter 6).

B. BREATHING PATTERN AND DISEASE

The curve maxima in Figure 1 shift on both axes if the breathing pattern is changed. With faster inhalation, smaller aerosols usually deposit higher in the respiratory tract (tracheobronchial deposition is enhanced) than would be the case if inhalation were slow. In part this is due to increased turbulence. The tracheobronchial or conducting airways extend down to the terminal bronchioles.[9] Constriction of the tracheobronchial airways is responsible for most of the breathing difficulty in reversible asthma. Unlike the pulmonary region, these airways have smooth muscle in their walls. It is obvious that aerosol deposition in an asthmatic individual will be different from that in a normal subject. Partly due to turbulence in constricted airways but also because the aerosol cannot penetrate well into poorly ventilated areas, deposition tends to occur more centrally in patients than it does in normal subjects.[12] Also, intersubject variations in deposition are much larger in the diseased population. This variability in aerosol deposition, which the pathophysiology of asthma creates,[12] obliterates many of the finer differences resulting from aerosol size changes and breathing pattern. Even so, the trends shown in Figure 1 remain broadly true. Aerosol particles with larger aerodynamic diameters have an increased tendency to collide with surfaces in their paths and separate by impaction in the upper airways. Smaller particles (which form more stable aerosols) tend to separate largely by sedimentation in the small, peripheral airways provided the airflow takes them there. The upper curve in Figure 1 shows an estimate of the increased deposition in the lung periphery resulting from breath-holding after inhalation.[11] If small particles (≈2 μm; Figure 1) do not reach the periphery, where the sedimentation distances become small enough for them to deposit during a breath-holding pause, then they are more likely to be exhaled.[1,13] In the bronchoconstricted asthmatic, when airway narrowing is substantial, some small enhancement in deposition due to settling may be expected in the upper airways as a result of breath-holding.

C. PRINCIPLES OF DOSE ESTIMATION

Presumably, the drug formulator and product designer wish to deliver a known dose more or less reliably to the lungs of a patient. If we assume at this stage that it is possible to generate several tidal volumes of homogeneously distributed aerosol and make this available at the subject's mouth, in principle it is then possible for the formulator to estimate the dose administered to the lungs. Several basics should be standardized and have known values. These are

1.   Drug concentration in air
2.   Aerosol size distribution (drug MMAD and a measure of polydispersity)
3.   The subject's breathing pattern (rate and frequency of inspiration, duration of breath-hold, and inhaled volume)

Then, let us assume that a well-trained, "lung-normal" subject inhales at a known rate, say 20 to 30 l/min, and breath-holds for a chosen interval. Assume further that he or she inhales a tidal volume of aerosol equal to 3 l on 4 separate inhalations. If the aerosol size is known, then it is usually possible to choose an appropriate deposition model and assign a value to mass fractional deposition, fd (Figure 1). This may be in the whole lung (TB + P; Figure 1) or a portion of it, as described in an earlier chapter, whichever is considered to be most important. The product of the aerosol concentration and inhaled volume then provides an estimate of the drug mass inhaled which, when multiplied by fd, gives the estimated dose deposited. While some of the deficiencies of this approach are discussed later in Section V.C, it is apparent that the aerosol formulator and device designer must work closely together *to produce a combination which delivers drug in aerosolized form with an appropriate concentration and particle size distribution so as to optimize its mass deposition in the respiratory tract.* The aerosol concentration and size distribution which matters is the one which the patient sees at his or her oro- or nasopharynx, and is not necessarily the one which was determined perhaps 1 m of tubing before reaching the patient. Although it is difficult to achieve, the ideal aerosol should be presented to the patient as a stationary, stable cloud of particles or droplets suspended in air.

III. DYNAMICS OF INHALATION AEROSOLS

An understanding of three important phenomena which affect aerosol size and concentration are required prior to explaining the performance characteristics of different devices. An understanding of particle or droplet impaction, sedimentation, and solvent evaporation or condensation kinetics is essential to the design of successful administration systems. These three phenomena (impaction, sedimentation, and the size changes induced by evaporation or condensation) stand out from others in aerosol physics (thermophoresis, photophoresis, and particle diffusion, for example) as being the primary mechanisms by which aerosolized medicaments separate and/or change their particle size distributions most rapidly within delivery systems. Each topic is described briefly in turn.

A. DROPLET OR PARTICLE IMPACTION

Aerosol segregation on the basis of the inertial properties of the dispersed phase is important not only to explain deposition in the upper airways (Chapter 1), but also to understand some of the principles by which inhalation devices function and, in some cases, fail to function. It is necessary to gain a simple understanding of the process (which is also used as the principle of operation for cascade impactors) sufficient to be able to say when droplet impaction is or is not likely to occur. Figure 2 is a schematic showing aerosol passage within a circular tube of internal diameter, W. The large droplet is shown leaving the airflow and impacting while the smaller one deviates with the airflow. In order to simplify the theory, the distance from the end of the tube

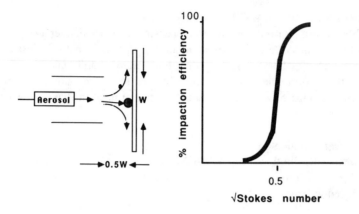

FIGURE 2. Diagrammatic representation of particle impaction as an aerosol stream impinges on a horizontal plate in its path. Impaction efficiency is often approximately 50% when √(Stokes' number) = 0.5.

to the impaction surface is held equal to 1/2 the width of the tube, W, and is thus equal to the maximum distance a particle or droplet traveling down its center must deviate from the airflow in order to collide with the surface in its path. Figure 2 also shows a typical plot of impaction efficiency as a function of the dimensionless Stokes' number, Stk, which, for unit density spheres >1 μm in diameter, in air at 1 atm and 20°C, can be written in the centimeter-gram-second system as:

$$Stk = V\ d^2/(0.00165\ W) \tag{2}$$

where V is the linear velocity of the airflow and d is droplet diameter. Because √Stk is often ≈0.5 (Stk = 0.25) for a 50% probability of impaction occurring (Figure 2), it is a simple matter to calculate the approximate linear velocity at which a droplet of known diameter will impact in an arrangement like that shown in Figure 2. If, for example, W were 1 cm and d = 5 μm (or 5 × 10⁻⁴ cm) then the critical velocity for a 50% chance of impaction would be

$$V_{50\%} \approx \frac{0.25 \times 0.00165 \times 1}{(5 \times 10^{-4})^2} \approx 1650\ cm/s \tag{3}$$

or 16.5 m/s. In order to increase impaction of smaller droplets in this set up, greater velocities are necessary. Alternatively, the value of 0.5 × W (the distance the droplet needs to deviate from the airflow) can be made smaller. Calculations of this type are relevant to baffle design in jet nebulizers and particle deposition from MDIs. They can also be used to explain why impaction is only a major mechanism of deposition in the upper airways of the lung where the linear airflow velocities remain high.

B. SEDIMENTATION

Table 2 shows sedimentation velocities of unit density spheres in still air at 20°C. The values only attain meaning when used in conjunction with aerosol residence times in containers of known dimensions. Consider, for example, an aerosol flowing horizontally at 5 l/min along a 30 cm tube with an internal diameter equal to 2 cm. The linear airflow velocity is given by (volume flow rate)/(area) or (5000 cm³ min⁻¹)/1 π cm² = 1592 cm   min⁻¹. The residence time in 30 cm of tubing (30 cm/1592 cm min⁻¹ = 0.0188 min) is thus 1.13 s. Because a 10-μm sphere can settle 0.35 cm in this residence time, about 18% of 10 μm spheres will be deposited in the tube during the passage of the aerosol. This percentage is a function of droplet size and can be

TABLE 2
Sedimentation Velocities of Unit Density Spheres in
Dry Air at 20°C and 1 atm Pressure

Aerodynamic diameter (μm)	Sedimentation velocity (cm/s)
2.0	0.013
4.0	0.050
6.0	0.111
8.0	0.197
10.0	0.306
20.0	1.212

estimated quite simply from the ratio of distance settled in the residence time to the internal diameter of the tubing. Although these arguments neglect to account for turbulent mixing, they can be extended to their logical conclusions which are frequently found in practice to be correct. There are three main results of passing polydispersed aerosols in our size range of interest (Figure 1) along tubes. The segregation induced by the sedimentation process ensures that the aerosol flowing from the tubing outlet has (1) decreased concentration, (2) a smaller median diameter, and (3) decreased "polydispersity". The relative magnitude of all these segregation effects becomes smaller as the aerosol droplet or particle size is reduced at the inlet to the tube because the aerosol becomes "more stable" and is less likely to sediment quickly. The "polydispersity" of the aerosol distribution refers to the magnitude of the spread of the particle size distribution. It is frequently characterized numerically as the geometric standard deviation (GSD) of log-normally distributed aerosols.[3] Some of these effects are shown in our work designed to determine drug absorption kinetics after characterized aerosol administration to dogs.[14,15] As they were generated, the aerosols of three median sizes were all significantly polydispersed (GSD ≈ 2). After passage along the tubes required for administration by positive pressure ventilation, however, segregation caused the larger aerosols (3.5 and 4 μm MMAD) to tend toward monodispersity (GSD = 1.3). This effect was much less for the smallest aerosol (1.0 μm MMAD) which was administered after passage through the same apparatus, with a GSD equal to 1.6.[15]

C. EVAPORATION AND CONDENSATION

Therapeutic aerosols are unstable in two major respects. First, they contain droplets or particles which are too large to stay in suspension for long. Second, they contain volatile or hygroscopic materials which cause aerosol size changes to occur as a function of time, temperature, aerosol dilution, and droplet or particle content. The thermodynamics and kinetics of this latter subject are too complex to consider in detail here, even when single particles or droplets are considered. In simple terms, and as far as therapeutic aerosols are concerned, two questions are of importance:

1.   How *fast* can evaporation or condensation alter the particle size distribution of an aerosol?
2.   How *much* can they change the size distribution (if they occur fast enough)?

The enormous surface:volume ratio presented by typical medicinal aerosols requires that we think of water as a volatile material and thus, a reasonable answer to the first question is "fast enough to worry about". The calculated lifetime of a 10-μm water droplet at 25°C and 80% relative humidity is only ≈0.6 s[16] and a breath of aerosol usually takes several seconds to inhale.[1] Furthermore, and with obvious relevance to MDIs, some of the solvents and propellants used in therapeutic aerosols are more volatile than water. Thus, as a rule of thumb, we can often assume that aerosols adjust their size distributions extremely quickly. To answer the second question, droplets will grow or shrink until their solvent vapor pressures are in equilibrium with the environment. Different droplet "environments" may display a wide range of temperatures but rarely contain fluorocarbon or ethanol vapors in significant concentrations. While ingredients like these *should* be lost rapidly and completely, we will see the complexity of the subject in the following chapter, when we observe that inadequate heat transfer to supercooled propellant droplets ultimately slows and governs the rate at which the size of MDI generated aerosols can shrink to the respirable range.

Because atmospheric air, compressed air, and the air in the lung contain water vapor, the behavior of aqueous aerosols can vary as a function of the environmental humidity. Pure water aerosols will obviously tend to evaporate at all relative humidities less than 100%. At constant temperature, aqueous aerosols containing dissolved salts have a particular relative humidity with which they exist in equilibrium. At this relative humidity, which is roughly predictable from a consideration of Raoult's law and a psychrometric chart,[17] they show no tendency to grow or shrink. However, systems which are isotonic with blood are very dilute and tend to evaporate as they pass in dilution air from a nebulizer to the patient. The opposite occurs with some hypertonic solution and dry powder aerosols.[1] These often display hygroscopic growth in the humid environment of the lung.[1,18] The relative humidity in the lung is in excess of 99% at 37°C.[2] This relative humidity would be that measured over a solution of isotonic saline at the same temperature. Water-soluble drugs administered as hypertonic solutions or solids, therefore, tend to grow rapidly as they pass through the humid environment of the respiratory tract.[18,19] The size they try to attain during inhalation is defined theoretically by the aqueous droplet size which would contain a drug concentration isotonic with blood. These concentrations are often of the order of 1 to 5% showing that the growth tendency of a typical hygroscopic solid is to take on board about 20 to 100 times its own mass of water (employing hypertonic aerosols to enhance deposition in the lung has been advocated recently in the literature[20]). Because the diameter of a droplet is proportional to the cube root of its volume (and ignoring density considerations), a 20-fold growth in mass would correspond to an approximate growth ratio of (equilibrium diameter at lung humidity)/(dry particle diameter) $\approx 20^{1/3}$ or 2.7. In practice during inhalation, ratios less than those predicted at equilibrium are operative because the process is dynamic. Nevertheless, this discussion shows the importance of paying careful attention to the various humidities which can be encountered in administration systems as well as the hygroscopic tendencies of some solid materials.

IV. AEROSOL GENERATION

There are two major types of nonmetered inhalation device which are used largely for the treatment and prevention of respiratory disease. These are jet or ultrasonic nebulizers. In practice, neither of these have been well accepted for the delivery of therapeutic agents for systemic purposes. Systemic administration potential clearly exists, however, given the wide acceptance of this route for the administration of drugs of abuse. Inhalation offers rapid absorption opportunities for compounds which require fast onset. Furthermore, the anatomical arrangements of the major vessels are such that they could usefully be employed to target absorbed compounds to the heart.

Mainly over the last decade, the design and construction of devices has been improved in order to enhance the drug doses which can be delivered successfully to the breathing-impaired. The main improvements have been to increase the output of respirable aerosol. This has been achieved in two ways: first, by increasing total output concentrations and secondly, by reducing droplet or particle sizes emitted by nebulizers. Because of recent improvements in aerosol dust-generator design and the usefulness of these latter devices for animal experimentation and

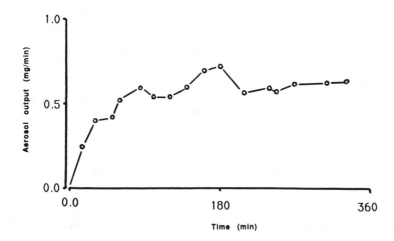

FIGURE 3. Mass of micronized disodium fluorescein powder emitted per minute as dry powder aerosol from a Model 3400 fluidized bed aerosol generator (TSI, St Paul, MN)[14] supplied with dry air at 10 l/min. Aerosol concentrations approach constancy after approximately 3 h when conveyed powder input to the fluid bed is balanced by aerosol ouput from the generator.

toxicity testing, the following discussion includes three major device categories. These are discussed in turn alongside some of the accessories which are commonly used with them: (1) dry powder generators, (2) air-blast nebulizers, and (3) ultrasonic nebulizers.

A. DRY POWDER GENERATORS

Dust generators have long been in existence, the most famous of which is probably the Wright Dust-Feed Apparatus.[21] However, these generators have historically been difficult to adapt to pharmaceutical studies. More recently, fluidized bed technology has improved to such an extent that generators are now available commercially which are capable of deaggregating powder charges and providing these as dispersions of powders in air.[14,22] The dispersed dust can often be shown to possess the same size characteristics as the powder with which the bed was supplied.[22] Thus, it is possible to micronize pharmaceutical powders, pass these into a bed of metal beads which are fluidized by dry air or gas which causes the beads to appear to "boil", and utilize the aerosol formed by the deaggregating action of the bed. Provided the bed is fed with powder continuously, a steady state is reached between powder input and aerosol output which demands that the aerosol output remain at a constant concentration (Figure 3). Steady-state concentrations of respirable aerosol (<5 μm aerodynamic diameter), which can approach 1 mg/l under some circumstances, are several times higher from these devices than those which can be produced by other generators.[14] The high concentrations are important for reasons described below. The devices themselves and their utilization have been described in more detail elsewhere.[14,22] They are manufactured and marketed by TSI (St. Paul, MN).

Performance of inhalation dosimetry and toxicity studies usually requires dose ranging and is often severely limited by the maximum available aerosol concentration emitted by the chosen generator. This is especially true for pharmaceutical studies where it is important that the stability of the administered compound is maintained during aerosol generation. Condensation generators, for example, require vaporization of the chemical agent prior to its condensation as a high concentration aerosol.[23] Such a procedure is usually unacceptable in pharmaceutical trials.[24] The selection of a generator which provides the greatest output concentration is important for two main reasons. First, and most important, respiratory (as opposed to systemic) toxicity is extremely difficult to detect, yet it remains important, even in phase I studies of new compounds, to assess a margin of safety and efficacy. High aerosol doses can often only be administered by repetitive inhalation. Second, because absorption after aerosol administration can sometimes be so rapid, the true dose residing in the lung is more often represented by the steady state existing between input (deposition) and output (absorption). In short, if it takes hours to administer the dose, then the dose residing in the lung must be calculated with a knowledge of clearance kinetics. For these reasons, therefore, it is important to be aware of pharmaceutically acceptable aerosol generation methods which provide increased respirable aerosol concentrations.

B. AIR-BLAST NEBULIZERS

Many of the "air-blast" or "jet" nebulizers which are available commercially were not designed specifically for the purpose of delivering drugs. It is helpful to appreciate this fact especially when attempting to select a unit for a particular purpose. The major markets for many years have been in support of air conditioning units for various purposes and, in the medical arena, in support of respiratory therapists. Practicing therapists derive from several sources depending largely upon the design of the health services they serve. However, the main use of nebulizers by therapists in the past has been to prevent dehydration of the patient's lungs with a variety of assisted breathing devices. Some of the older "nebulizers" would therefore more aptly be described as "humidifiers": their design having been mainly concerned with water output rather than droplet size.

More recently, and especially in Europe, nebulizers are being used increasingly for the delivery of antiasthmatic medication at home. They can be used to deliver a much higher dose of drug than MDIs. Provided they are used correctly, most of the aerosol output is usually <5 μm in aerodynamic diameter and lung penetration is good. If a typical nebulizer were used to deliver salbutamol solution for inhalation (3 ml of an 0.83 mg/ml solution are usually placed in the nebulizer cup) then approximately 12% of the dose or, in this case, 300 μg could be expected to reach the lungs of the patient.[25] If we assume (somewhat incorrectly) that the performance of all MDIs is similar, this is >10 times the amount reaching the lung from 2 puffs of an MDI metering salbutamol at 100 μg per dose because much of the metered dose fails to reach the lungs.[26] To administer this dose, the nebulizer must be operated continuously and repetitive inhalation is required. Some studies indicate little difference in efficacy when the same bronchodilator is administered in both ways (nebulizer vs. MDI[27]), although this statement should be qualified and restricted at present to β-adrenergic bronchodilators. It is likely that the indicator of efficacy (forced expiratory volume in 1 s; FEV_1), which is conventionally used for comparison of these drugs and their dosage forms, is insufficiently sensitive to changes in dose and regional deposition to be able to detect a difference between the two treatment modes. This problem is exacerbated by large intersubject variations in lung performance tests shown by asthmatic patients. It is likely that differences between the nebulizer and MDI will be detectable in the future for different drug classes, administered to groups of patients with reduced intersubject variation in lung dynamics.

The preference of the patient is a key factor involved in the choice between devices like MDIs and nebulizers. The latter can overcome some of the difficulties of administering drugs to poorly coordinated, debilitated, or very young patients. In some cases, especially in the U.S., nebulizers are used in a breath actuated mode to deliver aerosolized materials by intermittent positive pressure breathing (IPPB). Once again, there is little evidence of clinical advantage in the case of β-adrenergic compounds and devices are more complex, expensive, and require additional training. In other instances, bronchodilators have been administered via in-line nebulizers attached to positive pressure ventilators used in life support systems.

Figure 4 shows the operating principle of air-blast nebulizers. A jet of high velocity gas (usually air or oxygen) is passed, either tangentially (4A) or coaxially (4B) over the top of a liquid feed capillary. While it is possible for the liquid to be pumped at a chosen rate,[6,28] under normal

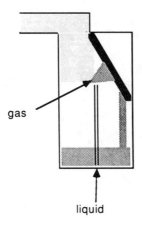

gas

liquid

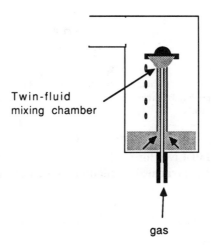

Twin-fluid
mixing chamber

gas

FIGURE 4. The two principle designs of air-blast
nebulizer. (A) Tangential airflow; (B) coaxial flow. The
latter has two jets separated by a twin fluid mixing chamber;
the lower (air) jet is smaller than the upper spray jet.

circumstances, liquid is drawn from the tube due to the rapidly expanding cone of air which
creates a negative pressure in the vicinity of its exit (the Bernoulli effect). The rate of liquid feed
is thus related to the gas supply rate and this, in turn, is a function of the applied gas pressure and
the diameter of the airjet (Figure 5). As the liquid leaves the supply tube in filaments, it is broken
into aerosol droplets by the high velocity gas.[29] The vast majority of the energy input (the air
supply) in these fluid mills goes into accelerating the liquid. Only a small proportion of it is used
to create fresh surface. The majority of the liquid mass produced during this primary atomization
process is in the form of large nonrespirable droplets.[30] For aqueous aerosols, many have
diameters >20 μm. Thus, a large proportion (>97%) of the total droplet mass impacts on various
internal surfaces of the nebulizer and returns to the reservoir for recirculation. When the volume
flow rates (l/min; Figure 5) through the airjet are converted to linear velocities, these often
approach the speed of sound (≈344 m/s). It is not surprising, therefore (Equations 2 and 3), that
the impaction efficiency of the large droplets approaches 100%. Table 3 illustrates this point and

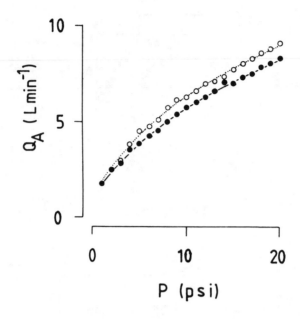

FIGURE 5. Air flow rate, QA, vs. operating pressure, P, in psi (gauge), for Bird micronebulizer (O) and Acorn Mark II nebulizer (O). (Reproduced with permission from the American Pharmaceutical Association.)

TABLE 3
Absorption Half-Lives for Compounds Administered by Aerosol or Intratracheal Instillation in the Rat Lung

Compound	Aerosol (min)	Instillation (min)
Urea	1.4	4.0
Mannitol	26.5	33.2
		60.0
Procainamide	2 3	3.2
PAH[a]	21.7	45.0
		27.9
		41.3
Guanidine	3.1	6.3
Benzylpenicillin	20.5	33.0
Barbital	0.9	1.4
Erythromycin	6.3	12.0
Amitrole	1.3	2.0
APAEB[b]	34.5	38.5
Salicylic acid	0.7	1.0
Antipyrine	0.3	<1.0

[a]   *p*-Aminohippuric acid.
[b]   *N*-Acetyl procainamide ethobromide.

Data extracted from References 8, 22, 37, 38, 40, 208, 209.

shows the aerosol output of two jet nebulizers modified to enable control over the liquid supply rate[6] and operated with an applied air pressure of 20 psig (gauge pressure 138 kPa). The internal design of the Bird micronebulizer, the least efficient of the two, is more like that shown in Figure

4A while the Acorn Mark II has a coaxial fluid supply (liquid drawn up around the gas input) like that shown in 4B. Most of the more recent nebulizers have this coaxial design which often turns out to be more efficient. The reason for the improvement in efficiency can be found in the twin-fluid mixing chamber which occurs prior to the main jet which increases the proportion of smaller droplets (Figure 4B) emitted from the main orifice. Most available devices operate best with flows >8 l/min.[31] These flows often correspond to applied pressures ≥20 psig (Figure 5). When purchasing small compressors, therefore, two sensible specifications require first that units are capable of maintaining this pressure and second that they can provide it at a flow of at least 8 l/min. Many portable units available in the U.S. especially those which plug into car cigarette lighters and/or with chargeable batteries, are incapable of meeting these specifications.

Because of the large throughput of air in these devices there is a continuous preferential loss of solvent which induces a drop in reservoir temperature of several degrees[32] during the initial 5 to 10 min operating period until a new heat balance is established. The magnitude of the effect on the output is difficult to predict and depends on variables such as the heat capacity and transfer characteristics of the nebulizer walls, the ambient temperature, and the humidity and temperature of the input air.[32] The aerosol output changes as a function of time in several ways. First, and most important, the reservoir concentration increases as a function of operating time. This causes a progressive increase in aerosol drug concentration (mass of drug per unit volume of air). Theoretically, this increase will continue until the solute concentration in the reservoir reaches the drug solubility. At this point, the aerosol concentration could become constant but the more likely occurrence is device malfunction due to crystals forming in the liquid supply tube. In practice, most bronchodilator drugs are very hydrophilic and nebulizer solutions are formulated at concentrations well below their solubilities. Because of this, and the fact that reservoir volumes are usually small (often as little as 3 ml), the end of nebulizer output is usually typified by erratic aerosol output which coincides with a small (≈0.5 ml) dead volume of concentrated solution which adheres to the internal walls of the device and refuses to return to the empty reservoir. The changes in aerosol size are usually insignificant.[31,33] The second time-dependent change in output is also predictable. Once the reservoir has cooled and the aerosol output allowed to mix with ambient air, the relative humidity of the mixture is invariably less than the aqueous vapor pressure exhibited by the droplets such that the output aerosol from these devices tends to evaporate and become smaller in size and more "respirable" as the device is spaced further from the patient.

C. ULTRASONIC NEBULIZERS

Although ultrasonic generators are not presently used widely for drug therapy, a number of companies are improving and developing these devices which have higher output concentrations than most air-blast nebulizers. Drug administration via a conventional nebulizer often takes 10 min or more. Ultrasonic nebulizers offer either increased drug doses reaching the lung in a fixed period or a decreased duration over which medication must be inhaled. An example can be found in current requirements to increase the delivery of antiallergic drugs like cromolyn sodium for prophylactic purposes.[4] A schematic, which illustrates the operation of the ultrasonic FISOneb is shown in Figure 6. In nebulizers such as this, the dispersing force is mechanical energy produced by a piezoelectric crystal vibrating in an electric field produced by an electronic high frequency oscillator. It is easier for a patient to switch such a device on and off rather than a blast nebulizer. In the latter devices, the initial droplet size produced at the nozzle is large and the output must be well baffled. In ultrasonic generators, however, a frequency is chosen which almost literally shakes the molecular aggregates apart. A large vertical pressure gradient is created in the liquid above the transducer which creates a geyser. If some extremely large drops (which rapidly fall back into the reservoir) are ignored, then ultrasonic generators *initially* produce a higher concentration of aerosol of a smaller particle size than is generated at the jet of conventional nebulizers. Mass median diameters of 6 to 7 μm are often reported at

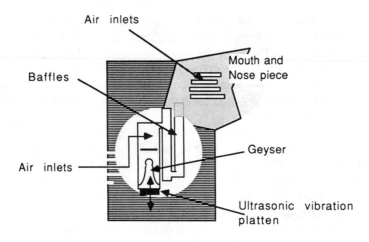

FIGURE 6. An ultrasonic nebulizer. The liquid reservoir forms a geyser under the influence of 1–2 MHz vibration. Droplets are removed in an airstream via a rather ineffective baffle system to the patient's oropharynx.

concentrations which are frequently 10 times greater than those emitted at the output of air-blast devices. While this suggests that these devices will assume increasing importance, there are several important points concerning ultrasonic generators which should be emphasized:

1. Although the droplet size is related to the frequency of oscillation and the surface tension and density of the formulation,[34,35] it is relatively insensitive to the parameter changes which can realistically be achieved. This tends to result in the designer being stuck with an output droplet size which is larger than ideal (>5 μm; mass median diameters of aerosols emitted from well-baffled air-blast nebulizers are usually <5 μm).
2. Because of the alternative energy source in these devices there is no compulsory dilution with high velocity input air (Figure 6). The disadvantage of this is that moderately large (5 to 10 μm) aerosol droplets are extremely difficult to remove by baffles. The calculation of impaction efficiency which occurs earlier in this chapter demonstrates how quickly these droplets need to move in order to be removed on baffles.
3. The reservoir temperature in these devices rises rapidly and has been associated with chemical breakdown of radiolabeled DTPA aerosols which are frequently used for diagnostic purposes.[36] Keeping the reservoir cool is not easy and this has obvious implications for the stability of pharmaceuticals.[37]
4. One point which is related to stability concerns both ultrasonic and air-blast nebulizers. Patients are inclined to leave solutions in the reservoir of nebulizers to avoid waste. Thus, microbiological contamination, chemical stability, and solvent evaporation all become issues. The practice can be minimized by packaging drug solutions as unit doses and emphasizing the need for strict hygiene in the preparation of all types of nebulizer prior to use.

V. FORMULATION AND CHARACTERIZATION

A. GOALS AND INGREDIENTS

In the event that a compound were to be administered as a dry powder aerosol, it may be sufficient to micronize and aerosolize, for example, in a fluidized-bed device as described previously. While there may be reasons to control the physical form and size of a powder for use in such a device, and even to coat the powder in some circumstances, there are presently no drugs

TABLE 4
Solution Formulation Ingredients Other than Drugs in Nonpressurized Products for Aerosol Inhalation[53]

Purpose	Ingredient
Solvent	Water[a]
	Glycerol
Stabilizer[b]	Acetone sodium bisulfate
	Sodium metabisulfate
	Disodium edetate
	Ascorbic acid
	Citric acid
	Hydrochloric acid
	Sodium hydroxide
	Sulfuric acid
	Nitrogen[c]
Preservative	Parahydroxybenzoic acid
	Benzalkonium chloride
	Chlorbutanol
	Phenol
Tonicity adjustment	Sodium chloride
Flavoring agent	Sodium saccharin

[a] Two of the latest compounds being used for inhalation, ribavirin and pentamidine isethionate, are supplied as pure lyophilized powders for reconstitution in water for injection.
[b] Some of these compounds act as both buffer salts and antioxidants. Strong acids and bases such as HCl and NaOH are only used as pH adjusters to achieve values for pH within 2–3 U of neutrality.
[c] Vials purged with nitrogen to minimize oxidation risk.

which employ this technology. Because liquid formulations for use with different nebulizers predominate, this section is devoted to some fairly simple solution formulations which are similar in goals and design to parenteral formulations. Table 4 lists the chemical compounds other than drugs, which are presently included in solutions for nebulization and marketed in the U.S. If the drug is ignored for a moment, these "excipients" fall into five main categories:

1. Solvents
2. Stabilizing agents
3. Antimicrobial preservatives
4. Tonicity adjusters
5. Flavoring agents

Because the drugs in these formulations are administered in solution form, the formulator can only seek to control the dose reaching the airways and possibly the way in which it is deposited. The formulator has no control over drug release once deposition has occurred, even though disposition and binding within lung tissue should be a function of molecular structure (pentamidine is a compound which exhibits enhanced retention in the lung;[38] see also Chapter 5). Because of this lack of control, one of the primary goals of the nebulizer solution formulator is to keep the formulation as simple as possible. In this sense, the solutions are again similar to injectables. Many of the "formulation rules" are indeed identical.[39] Any additives which are "required" should have their concentrations minimized. There is no value in adding excipients with possible toxicologic consequences without good reason.

In all cases of liquid aerosol generation, the dose of solvent administered to the airways is often more than two orders of magnitude larger than that of the drug. Because of this, water is the solvent of choice. Cosolvents which reduce the dielectric constant of the medium are sometimes used to increase drug solubility.[39] Glycerol or propylene glycol are possible cosolvents for this purpose. Their use creates a variety of changes in the output from a nebulizer, all of which need to be taken into account.[29,30] Formulations with large fractions of these cosolvents have altered viscosity, density, surface tension, and vapor pressure. These physical properties of the solution define many of the output characteristics of nebulizers.[1,30,40,41] Increased viscosity, for example, decreases output (mass of formulation emitted as aerosol per unit time).

Nebulizers are usually designed for use with simple aqueous solutions. Because their output is also dependent upon operating conditions and the efficiencies of different jet and baffle designs, the consequences of incorporating cosolvents in a formulation must be evaluated carefully with respect to the changes they produce in the respirable output. It is usually true to say that doubling the concentration of drug in the reservoir of a nebulizer containing water as the solvent will double the drug concentration in air and thus double the respirable dose per inhalation. If the means of doubling this reservoir concentration is to incorporate, say, 50% glycerol in the formulation, it is possible that the nebulizer output may fall, increase by a factor less than two or remain unchanged. The empirical relationships which exist in the literature are not sufficiently developed to be able to predict the exact outcome of this type of formulation change. Ethanol[40] has also been proposed as a more volatile, low viscosity cosolvent in inhalation solution formulations in order to minimize some of these problems. Because it evaporates at a rate which does not depend upon relative humidity, it could potentially be used to counterbalance some of the hygroscopic tendencies of propylene glycol and glycerol at high relative humidities as well as modifying the kinematic viscosity of these formulations. The introduction of a solvent, however, which is neither pharmacologically nor toxicologically inert, requires that dosing limitations are due to the drug and not the solvent. It is not prudent to formulate an aerosol in such a way that the maximum dose is dictated by an excipient and not the drug!

The inclusion of stabilizing agents (buffer salts, antioxidants, and chelating agents) is dictated for nebulizer solutions in a similar fashion to those described for injectables.[39] Thus, an optimum pH must be selected for drug stability; if a buffer is chosen, it should not catalyze breakdown. Antioxidants and metal-ion chelating agents may be required in optimum concentrations. If oxidative breakdown is a problem, ampule or vial packaging may be performed under purge with an inert gas such as nitrogen. Two anti-infective compounds which are fairly new to the inhalation scene (pentamidine for treatment of *Pneumocystis carinii* infection in AIDS and ribavirin for respiratory syncytial virus infections) are both packaged as lyophilized powders for reconstitution with water for injection immediately prior to administration by aerosol.[33,42]

One issue relating to stability which is unique to aerosol formulations concerns the physical and/or chemical stability of the drug during the nebulization process itself. ^{99m}Technetium labeled DTPA (a chelate) is known to break down to the more rapidly absorbed pertechnetate ion at temperatures which are commonly experienced in the nebulization cups of ultrasonic nebulizers.[36] This leads to erroneous estimates of pulmonary epithelial permeability when the aerosol is administered as a diagnostic tool to determine its retention time in the lung (Chapter 6). With implications for proteins and peptides as products of biotechnology is the fact that the high shear forces involved in air-blast nebulizers are capable of inducing conformational changes in these molecules. This may result, for example, in physical changes such as molecular aggregation with varying effects on the biological properties of these molecules. Because some proteins physically denature (change their conformations) at liquid-gas interfaces, it is possible that these phenomena may be affected by the inclusion of surfactants in formulations. Surfactant effects are themselves a problem in air-blast devices, however. The process of foam build-up within the nebulizer reservoir occurs in a fashion similar to that in a washing machine which contains too much detergent. The subject of foam stability is an interesting one which lies beyond the scope of this chapter. Nevertheless, foaming problems are multifactorial. They are functions of the formulation, the exact surfactant and its concentration, the nebulizer design, and all of its operating conditions.

The inclusion of antimicrobial preservatives in multidose packages should probably be frowned upon for any new formulations. Sterile unit dose packaging with appropriate cleaning and microbial control of the aerosol generating devices is preferred. The fact that adverse effects related to some of these compounds are so difficult to detect has probably less to do with their toxicity and/or irritancy and more to do with the resilience of the lung when confronted with environmental assaults. This last point, however, is very important. If a sound pharmaceutical reason exists for incorporating a new compound in an aerosol formulation, reports of its toxicity when administered by other routes should not always preclude its trial. Toxicity to preservatives has been reported on occasions following the use of multidose injectables.[43] This fact alone has not prevented, and should not prevent, their inclusion in aerosols.

Biological issues such as bitter taste and bronchial hyperreactivity require the use of flavor-masking agents such as saccharin and tonicity adjustment with sodium chloride or other biocompatible salts. Because of the inevitability of some naso- and oropharyngeal deposition during inhalation, the formulator must be aware of the need to mask the taste and smell of drugs which display these problems. Also, hypertonic solutions and acids and bases at the extremes of pH can be used as aerosols to induce bronchoconstriction in reactive individuals. However, what is permissible is highly dependent on the patient group being treated. The best example of this can be found in the observation that a nonasthmatic individual may show no response to histamine given by aerosol at doses which are orders of magnitude greater than those required to cause severe discomfort in an asthmatic patient. In individuals with hyperreactive airways, therefore, it is more important to remain close to isotonicity and pH neutrality than in other subject groups.[44] While the formulator would be unwise to deviate from these norms unnecessarily, because the phenomenon of bronchoconstriction is further related to the intended dose of the formulation, it is foolish to make one rule to fit all circumstances.

B. SIZE AND CONCENTRATION DETERMINATION

These variables are defined by the formulation, the aerosol generating device and its operating conditions, and any related delivery equipment. If the patient's own respiratory dynamics are ignored for a moment, aerosol size and concentration broadly define the drug dose deposited in the lung. Devices themselves have improved considerably in the last 5 years and some comparative information on the size of aerosol produced by the different generators is available in the literature.[31,35] While this particle size data is usually internally consistent (within any one publication), it is often difficult to compare values between laboratories. There are two reasons for this problem. First, measuring techniques often differ and operating conditions, even for similar aerosol generating units, are varied between institutions. Second, and most important, the speed with which aerosol size distributions can change due, for example, to evaporation and impaction, requires that similar sampling procedures and plumbing are used to enable data comparability to be feasible. Sampling methodologies and plumbing arrangements are usually inadequately described in the medical literature. Because of this, it is often difficult, if not impossible, to reproduce experimental aerosol data. New investigators, therefore, have little choice but to perform a series of comparisons of different aerosol generators themselves prior to optimizing the performance of one or two of them with their formulation.

Particle size and concentration of the aerosolized formulation (the latter in terms of drug mass per unit volume of air) should be measured at a point where the aerosol would enter the patient. Thus, the mouthpiece of a hand-held nebulizer is appropriate or perhaps the inside of an oxygen hood in the event that, for example, ribavirin aerosol is delivered to a hood placed over an infant's head (Figure 7). If it is necessary for experimental reasons to sample the aerosol elsewhere, then every effort should be made to determine the loss of drug and particle size changes in additional tubing and reservoirs which are required to deliver aerosol to the patient. It is only by

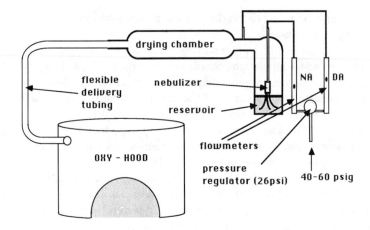

FIGURE 7. The "Small Particle Aerosol Generator Mk II" (ICN Pharmaceuticals, Inc., Costa Mesa, CA) shown diagrammatically connected to an oxygen-hood as used in practice to treat neonatal respiratory syncytial virus infections. (From Byron, P. R., et al., *Resp. Care,* 33, 1011, 1988. With permission.)

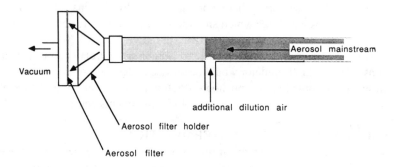

FIGURE 8. A simple sampling arrangement which can be used in practice to determine aerosol concentrations from nebulizers. The amount of drug collected on the filter and surfaces of the sampling apparatus is determined by chemical analysis. The airflow from the nebulizer is determined prior to aerosol collection by some form of flow meter. Dilution air is introduced because the flow rate induced by the vacuum is usually greater than that from the nebulizer.

systematically studying the dependence of aerosol size and drug concentration on formulation, device design, and operating variables that we will see improvements in inhalation drug therapy.

Figure 8 shows a simple but effective means of sampling the aerosol output from a nebulizer in order to determine the concentration in air. It is presumed in this figure that the input air supply (say in l/min) required to run the generator is known. It is also important to recognize that gas-flow meters which are usually calibrated relative to atmospheric pressure cannot be placed in the high pressure line supplying the nebulizer without recalibration (they provide the wrong answers). The vacuum (Figure 8) must not be allowed to evacuate the nebulizer chamber and thus change the latter's operating conditions. To avoid the difficulties associated with adjusting the vacuum flow rate to demand precisely the same flow as that used to drive the generator, it can demand several times the air supply rate of the nebulizer and take all of this output, plus additional room "make-up" air, onto the filter arrangement as shown. While other options are possible, the selection of a low resistance, high-efficiency filter, in a wide-mouthed holder, enables drug in the filter and holder to be assayed after collection for a known duration.[6] This

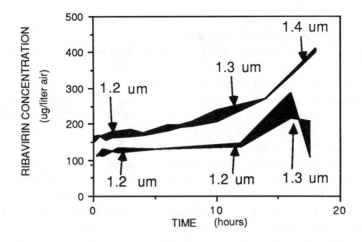

FIGURE 9. Ribavirin aerosol concentration vs. time profile for an 18 h period of aerosol generation in the SPAG (Figure 7).[33] Data are presented as the range of experimental values determined on different occasions. Upper curves derive from samples withdrawn from the drying chamber. Lower curves show concentrations in the oxyhood when it is housed in a drafty environment. Nebulizer airflow was 7 l/min while drying airflow was 8.5 l/min. Aerosol sizes shown on the curve are values for MMAD determined by cascade impaction. Experiments commenced with a reservoir volume equal to 300 ml and a ribavirin concentration of 20 mg/ml. After 18 h, the drug concentration was around 66 mg/ml, with a minimal volume remaining to be nebulized. (From Byron, P. R., et al., *Resp. Care,* 33, 1011, 1988. With permission.)

drug mass, divided by the air volume leaving the nebulizer during a fixed time interval, provides the "concentration available to the patient". Figure 9 shows an example of how the ribavirin concentration in an oxygen hood changes as a function of time of aerosol generation in the apparatus shown in Figure 7. The Small Particle Aerosol Generator (SPAG; Figure 7) which is marketed for use with the antiviral, ribavirin, in the U.S., is a modified "collison" generator which was first described in the 1930s.[45] The generator is a high output device which successfully generates an extremely small and relatively stable aerosol.

There are many methods available for particle and droplet size determination. While some newer techniques are under development which utilize high speed optical data collection, only two techniques are presently useful in the context of sizing the aerosols discussed in this chapter. Because the aerosols in question are usually polydispersed according to an unknown function,[6,19] it is important to either try to size the whole of the generator output or to ensure that a sample is collected isokinetically without segregating the distribution in favor of either the smaller or larger droplets.[3,14] Cascade impaction[3,19,46] is an invasive technique which collects and fractionates an aerosol dependent upon its aerodynamic particle size distribution. Forward light scattering (usually employing a Particle Size Analyzer, Malvern Instruments, Inc., Southborough, MA) is a noninvasive technique which provides an estimate of volume median diameter and some index of polydispersity. Neither of these techniques is ideal and thus determining the particle size of the aerosol can be a problem.

Cascade impaction can be performed with a calibrated instrument (the calibration should be checked on commercially available devices[19]) to determine the *aerodynamic* particle size distribution. For a stable aerosol, this is the method of choice. After drug analysis on each stage, it provides values for the fraction of drug in each of the impactor's known aerodynamic size ranges.[19] For an unstable aerosol, which air-blast nebulizers generate, smaller droplets take longer than the larger ones to separate from the airstream in an impactor. Thus, if conditions within the impactor cause the aerosol to evaporate as it passes through the stages, the aerosol will appear to be smaller than it actually was when it entered the device. The problem is usually less important when the aerosol is increasing in size as it passes through. Nevertheless, growth and shrinkage of therapeutic aerosols are known to occur within the residence time required for separation into size fractions.[1] Because the impactor draws air at a fixed volume flow rate (usually defined by a critical orifice below its smallest stage), it is common that diluent air is drawn down the impactor and mixed with the aerosol itself. If this diluent air has a different relative humidity and/or temperature to that of the gas phase of the aerosol, then the aerosol will change its size distribution within the cascade impactor.

Light scattering measurements can be made in a small enough time frame to overcome these problems of aerosol instability. Furthermore, measurements can be made without segregating the droplet distribution. The problem in forward light scattering is sizing the output from fluorocarbon propelled systems because of rapid transient variations in the refractive index of the gas phase containing the particles or droplets. This is not a problem with aqueous aerosols. Also, because this method provides a value for the volume median diameter (VMD) of the aerosol, the density of aqueous droplets tends to unity, and the same droplets are usually spheres, the VMD can reasonably be interpreted as being equivalent to mass median diameter. Despite these statements, two main problems remain with this method. First, a function of some sort must be forced through data for scattered light intensity vs. forward scattering angle (aerosol droplets in a laser beam scatter light according to their sizes). This requires some assumptions to be made concerning the form of the particle size distribution even while this remains as an unknown. Secondly, it is difficult to calibrate these devices, and even when calibration is performed, the techniques recommended by the suppliers are not well related to aerosol measurements.

In summary, cascade impaction suffers from a tendency to allow size changes prior to segregating droplets. Nevertheless, it does provide a useful aerodynamic measure of particle size distribution which can be compared between devices and formulations. Figure 9 shows the values for MMAD for ribavirin and how they changed with time and increasing aerosol concentration from the SPAG (Figure 7).[33] Sampling airflow rates in the cascade impactor used in these experiments avoided the use of diluent air mixing with the aerosol. When this can be arranged, the aerodynamic sizes provided by the cascade impactor are reliable and make the device the method of choice. More importantly, the impactor can be used to assess how an aerosol is distributed (polymodal distributions are often seen). Light scattering, on the other hand, offers a useful means of determining a median diameter for aqueous aerosols provided the instrument calibration is reliable.[31] Both methods can be used in concert to provide valuable information on the size distributions of therapeutic aerosols produced by the nonmetered delivery devices discussed here.

C. DETERMINING THE DOSE OF A THERAPEUTIC AEROSOL

For the reasons above, as well as the preferential solvent loss from air-blast nebulizers (Figure 9), it is difficult to make an absolute estimate of the concentration and size of an aqueous inhalation aerosol. This point is especially true when a nebulizer is employed which cannot supply the airflow rate demanded during the patient's inhalation. Virtually none of the hand-held air-blast nebulizers which are commercially available are able to supply much more than 10 l/min when operated at safe pressures.[31] Devices such as the SPAG (Figure 7), however, supply aerosol at a rate greater than that demanded during inhalation. The usual arrangement for hand-held nebulizers is shown in Figure 10. With an airflow around 8 l/min, dilution air must flow at between 12 and 22 l/min if the patient is to inhale at an acceptable rate of 20 to 30 l/min. Often the rate of inhalation may be even higher than this.[47] Thus, the true aerosol concentration inhaled is under the control of the patient and is highly dependent upon the degree to which he or she has been trained to use the device. Depending upon the arrangement used, the patient may exhale into room air; more often, however, he or she exhales through the head-space of the device, thus

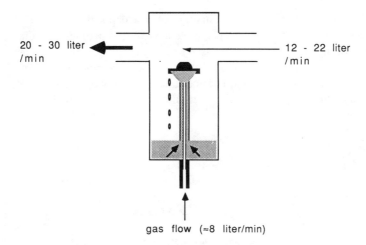

20 - 30 liter
/min

12 - 22 liter
/min

gas flow (≈8 liter/min)

FIGURE 10. A nebulizer as used in practice. Dilution air flows in addition to the
nebulizer supply to make up the patient's inspiratory flow rate. Exhalation can also
take place through the head of the device.

expelling aerosol during exhalation from the port used for addition of the dilution air. Depending
on the humidity in the room and the nature of the formulation being nebulized, this dilution air
may or may not serve to reduce the size of the aerosol droplets significantly during inhalation.

With this level of uncertainty concerning the true droplet size and concentration inhaled by
the patient, the approach described previously to estimate the dose delivered to the lung can only
be used to gain an approximate answer. If, for example, most of the output from a particular
nebulizer were 1 to 5 μm in aerodynamic diameter and continuous breathing from a large
reservoir by a well-trained, lung-normal subject were assumed, the total lung deposition per
breath, given a breath-holding pause, could be crudely approximated by assuming a deposition
fraction, fd ≈ 0.8 (total deposition throughout the lung, see Figure 1) and tidal volume, TV ≈ 3
l, so that:

$$\text{Mass deposited} = \text{aerosol concentration} \times 0.8 \times 3 \text{ liters} \qquad (4)$$

To make this equation function correctly in the circumstances shown by Figure 10, the aerosol
concentration flowing from the device must be multiplied by an additional ratio or dilution
factor, DF = (airflow through jet)/(total airflow to patient) so that

$$\text{Mass deposited} = \text{aerosol concentration} \times \text{fd} \times \text{TV} \times \text{DF} \qquad (5)$$

In practice, as new compounds with new therapeutic purposes are administered by aerosol
inhalation, the present situation where the true dose to the lung is a subject for educated
guesswork is becoming increasingly untenable. It is necessary for new generation compounds
to have known activities and toxicities which are related to the dose deposited and not a guess
of the "dose inhaled" as at present. Newman[48,49] has reviewed the literature and reported a wide
variation (approximately 0 to 20%) in the percentage of an instilled dose (the mass of drug placed
in the nebulizer reservoir) reaching the lungs from nebulizers. Newman et al.[50] have pioneered
the quantification of therapeutic aerosol dosimetry using gamma scintigraphic techniques.
These techniques are well described in the literature[48,51,52] and, with the widespread availability
and sophistication of the newer gamma cameras (3-D tomography as well as 2-D scintigraphy
are now available at many major centers), there is little excuse for continuing to perform inexact
inhalation aerosol administration when the true doses can be determined. Aqueous systems

particularly lend themselves to *in vivo* estimations of dose deposition, because of the ease with which compounds such as ^{99m}Tc-DTPA can be added to a formulation as a radioactive marker. The deposition of the marker can then be used to estimate quantitatively the deposition of the drug itself. By using these techniques alongside pharmacodynamic and pharmacokinetic evaluations in trained subjects, it should be possible to correctly optimize the delivery of drugs to the lung by studying the performance of formulation-device combinations as complete drug delivery systems.

REFERENCES

1. **Byron, P. R., Davis, S. S., Bubb, M. D., and Cooper, P.,** Pharmaceutical implications of particle growth at high relative humidity, *Pest. Sci..*, 8, 521, 1977.
2. **Gonda, I. and Byron, P. R.,** Perspectives on the biopharmacy of inhalation aerosols, *Drug Dev. Ind. Pharm.*, 4, 243, 1978.
3. **Reist, P. C.,** *Introduction to Aerosol Science,* Macmillan, New York, 1984, 11.
4. **Rhind, G. B. and Sudlow, M. F.,** Effect on spirometry of distilled water and cromoglycate solutions nebulized by a small portable ultrasonic generator, *Respiration,* 51, 86, 1987.
5. **Swintosky, J. V., Riegelman, S., Higuchi, T., and Busse, L. W.,** Specific surface area and average particle size of some drugs determined by the BET method, *J. Am. Pharm. Assoc. (Sci. Ed.),* 38, 210, 1949.
6. **Hickey, A. J. and Byron, P. R.,** Effect of solution flow rate on the output of two modified commercially available jet nebulizers, *J. Pharm. Sci.,* 76, 338, 1987.
7. **Gonda, I.,** A semiempirical model of aerosol deposition in the human respiratory tract for mouth inhalation, *J. Pharm. Pharmacol.,* 33, 692, 1981.
8. **Lippmann, M.,** Regional deposition of particles in the human respiratory tract, in *Handbook of Physiology,* Sect. 9: *Reactions to Environmental Agents,* American Physiological Society, Bethesda, MD, 1977, 213.
9. **Task Group on Lung Dynamics,** Deposition and retention models for internal dosimetry of the human respiratory tract, *Health Phys.,* 12, 173, 1966.
10. **Gonda, I.,** Study of the effects of polydispersity of aerosols on regional deposition in the respiratory tract, *J. Pharm. Pharmacol.,* 33, 52p, 1981.
11. **Byron, P. R.,** Prediction of drug residence times in regions of the human respiratory tract following aerosol inhalation, *J. Pharm. Sci.,* 75, 433 and 1207, 1986.
12. **Laube, B. L., Swift, D. L., Wagner, H. N., Norman, P. S., and Adams, K. G.,** The effect of bronchial obstruction on central airway deposition of a saline aerosol in patients with asthma, *Am. Rev. Resp. Dis.,* 133, 740, 1986.
13. **Davies, C. N.,** The deposition and distribution in the lungs of inhaled particles, in *Respiratory Protection — Principles and Applications,* Ballantyne, B. and Schwabe, P.H., Eds., Chapman & Hall, London, 1981, 65.
14. **Byron, P. R. and Clark, A. R.,** Drug absorption from inhalation aerosols administered by positive pressure ventilation. I. Administration of a characterized solid disodium fluorescein aerosol under a controlled respiratory regime to the beagle dog, *J. Pharm. Sci.,* 74, 934, 1985.
15. **Clark, A. R. and Byron, P. R.,** Drug absorption from inhalation aerosols administered by positive pressure ventilation. II. Effect of disodium fluorescein aerosol particle size on fluorescein absorption kinetics in the beagle dog respiratory tract, *J. Pharm. Sci.,* 74, 939, 1985.
16. **Byron, P. R.,** Some future perspectives for unit dose inhalation aerosols, *Drug. Dev. Ind. Pharm.,* 12, 993, 1986.
17. **Felder, R. M. and Rousseau, R. W.,** *Elementary Principles of Chemical Processes,* 2nd ed., Wiley Interscience, New York, 1986, 368.
18. **Morrow, P. E.,** Factors determining hygroscopic aerosol deposition in airways, *Physiol. Rev.,* 66, 330, 1986.
19. **Gonda, I., Kayes, J. B., Groom, C. V., and Fildes, F. J. T.,** Characterization of hygroscopic inhalation aerosols, in *Particle Size Analysis,* Stanley-Wood, N.G. and Allen, T., Eds., Wiley Heyden, Ltd., London, 1981, 31.
20. **Persons, D. D., Hess, G. D., and Scherer, P. W.,** Maximization of pulmonary hygroscopic aerosol deposition, *J. Appl. Physiol.,* 63, 1205, 1987.
21. **Wright, B. M.,** A new dust feed mechanism, *J. Sci. Instrum.,* 27, 12, 1950.
22. **Marple, V. A., Liu, B. Y. H., and Rubow, K. L.,** A dust generator for laboratory use, *Am. Ind. Hyg. Assoc. J.,* 39, 26, 1978.
23. **Mercer, T. T.,** Production and characterization of aerosols, *Arch. Int. Med.,* 131, 39, 1973.

24. **Byron, P. R. and Hickey, A. J.,** Spinning disk generation and drying of monodisperse solid aerosols with output concentrations sufficient for single breath inhalation studies, *J. Pharm. Sci.,* 76, 60, 1987.
25. **Lewis, R. A., Cushley, M. J., Fleming, J. S., and Tattersfield, A. E.,** Is a nebulizer less efficient than a metered dose inhaler and do pear shaped extension devices work?, *Am. Rev. Resp. Dis.,* 25, 94, 1982.
26. **Newman, S. P., Pavia, D., Moren, F., Sheahan, N. F., and Clarke, S. W.,** Deposition of pressurized aerosols in the respiratory tract, *Thorax,* 36, 52, 1981.
27. **Jenkins, S. C., Heaton, R. W., Fulton, T. J., and Moxham, J.,** Comparison of domiciliary nebulized salbutamol and salbutamol from a metered dose inhaler in stable chronic airflow limitation, *Chest,* 91, 804, 1987.
28. **Liu, B. Y. H. and Lee, K. W.,** An aerosol generator of high stability, *Am. Ind. Hyg. Assoc. J.,* 36, 861, 1975.
29. **Gordon, G. D.,** Mechanism and speed of breakup of drops, *J. Appl. Phys.,* 30, 1759, 1959.
30. **Byron, P. R.,** Pulmonary targeting with aerosols, *Pharm. Tech.,* 11, 42, 1987.
31. **Clay, M. M., Pavia, D., Newman, S. P., and Clarke, S. W.,** Factors influencing the size distribution of aerosols from jet nebulizers, *Thorax,* 38, 755, 1983.
32. **Mercer, T. T., Tillery, M. I., and Chow, H. Y.,** Operating characteristics of some compressed air nebulizers, *Am. Ind. Hyg. Assoc. J.,* 29, 66, 1968.
33. **Byron, P. R., Phillips, E., and Kuhn, R.,** Ribavirin administration by inhalation: Aerosol generation factors controlling drug delivery to the lung, *Resp. Care,* 33, 1011, 1988.
34. **Lang, R. J.,** Ultrasonic atomization of liquids, *J. Acoust. Soc. Am.,* 34, 16, 1962.
35. **Mercer, T. T., Goddard, R. F., and Flores, R. L.,** Output characteristics of three ultrasonic nebulizers, *Ann. Allergy,* 26, 18, 1968.
36. **Waldman, D. L., Weber, D. A., Oberdorster, G., Drago, S. R., Utell, M. J., Hyde, R. W., and Morrow, P. E.,** Chemical breakdown of technetium-99m DTPA during nebulization, *J. Nucl. Med.,* 28, 378, 1987.
37. **Gale, A. E.,** Drug degeneration during ultrasonic nebulization, *J. Aerosol Sci.,* 16, 265. 1985.
38. **Debs, R. J., Straubinger, R. M., Brunette, E. N., Lin, J. M., Lin, E. J., Montgomery, A. B., Friend, D. S., and Papahadjopoulos, D. P.,** Selective enhancement of pentamidine uptake in the lung by aerosolization and delivery in liposomes, *Am. Rev. Resp. Dis.,* 135, 731, 1987.
39. **DeLuca, P. P. and Boylan, J. C.,** Formulation of small volume parenterals, in *Pharmaceutical Dosage Forms: Parenteral Medications,* Avis, K.E., Ed., Marcel Dekker, New York, 1984, chap. 5.
40. **Davis, S. S., Elson, G., and Whitmore, J.,** Physicochemical studies on aerosol solutions for drug delivery. II. Water-propylene glycol-ethanol systems, *Int. J. Pharm.,* 1, 85, 1978.
41. **Davis, S. S.,** Physicochemical studies on aerosol solutions for drug delivery. I. Water-propylene glycol systems, *Int. J. Pharm.,* 1, 71, 1978.
42. **Corkery, K. J., Luce, J. M., and Montgomery, A. B.,** Aerosolized pentamidine for treatment and prophylaxis of *Pneumocystis carinii* pneumonia: an update, *Resp. Care,* 33, 676, 1988.
43. **Turco, S. and King, R. E.,** *Sterile Dosage Forms,* 2nd ed., Lea & Febiger, Philadelphia, 1979, 55.
44. **Smith, C. M., Anderson, S. D., and Black, J. L.,** Methacholine responsiveness increases after ultrasonically nebulized water but not after ultrasonically nebulized hypertonic saline in patients with asthma, *J. Allergy Clin. Immunol.,* 79, 85, 1987.
45. **May, K. R.,** The collison nebulizer: description, performance and application, *Aerosol Sci.,* 4, 235, 1973.
46. **Allen, T.,** *Particle Size Measurement,* 2nd ed., Chapman & Hall, London, 1974, 56.
47. **Newman, S. P., Pavia, D., and Clarke, S. W.,** Improving the bronchial deposition of pressurized aerosols, *Chest,* 80(Suppl.), 909, 1981.
48. **Newman, S. P.,** Therapeutic aerosols, in *Aerosols and the Lung: Clinical and Experimental Aspects,* Clarke, S.W. and Pavia, D., Eds., Butterworths, London, 1984, 197.
49. **Newman, S. P.,** Aerosol deposition considerations in inhalation therapy, *Chest,* 88(Suppl.), 152S, 1985.
50. **Flavin, M., MacDonald, M., Dolovich, M., Coates, G., and O'Brodovich, H.,** Aerosol delivery to the rabbit lung with an infant ventilator, *Paediatr. Pulm.,* 2, 35, 1986.
51. **Newman, S. P.,** Production of radioaerosols, in *Aerosols and the Lung: Clinical and Experimental Aspects,* Clarke, S.W. and Pavia, D., Eds., Butterworths, London, 1984, 71.
52. **Boudreau, R. J. and Loken, M. K.,** Techniques for measuring regional pulmonary blood flow and ventilation, in *Pulmonary Nuclear Medicine,* Loken, M.K., Ed., Appleton & Lange, Norwalk, CT, 1987, 7.
53. *Physician's Desk Reference,* 42nd ed., Medical Economics, Oradell, NJ, 1988.

Chapter 7

AEROSOL FORMULATION, GENERATION, AND DELIVERY USING METERED SYSTEMS

Peter R. Byron

TABLE OF CONTENTS

I. INTRODUCTION

Treatment of asthma has improved considerably in recent years with the discovery of potent compounds which prevent or alleviate some of the symptoms. While many of these compounds are effective orally, formulation-device combinations have been developed which facilitate their delivery direct to the airways. This "local" aerosol administration to the site of action is one of the simpler cases of drug targeting. Typically, the blood levels of drug that are achieved during inhalation administration are much less than those following oral dosing. Using albuterol as an example, 2 to 4 mg in a tablet is equivalent in terms of bronchodilation to 90 to 180 μg by metered dose inhaler (MDI). Oral dosing produces plasma levels in the 5 to 15 ng/ml range,[1,2] while inhalation therapy produces levels which are <<1 ng/ml[3,4] and are difficult to assay even though a substantial proportion of each metered dose is usually swallowed and absorbed through the gastrointestinal tract.[5,6] Concentrations which are required to do the job at the site of action (airway smooth muscle) are similar to plasma levels after oral therapy (around 10 ng/ml),[3] showing the ease with which small aerosol doses can generate effective drug concentrations in the small fluid volumes lining the airways. While this example makes drug delivery to the lung sound appealing, there are many technical difficulties associated with this route of administration. It is these difficulties and, where possible, their solutions in the form of different metered inhalation devices and the formulations which they contain, which form the subject material for this chapter.

MDIs and dry powdered generators (DPGs) which are currently available are complete drug delivery systems. That is, they meter, aerosolize, and, in some cases, partly control how the patient inhales the chosen dose of drug. They can be perceived from two different viewpoints. From the patient's point of view, these devices appear to be much simpler than nebulizers and are certainly much smaller. They are easier to carry and to conceal. Furthermore, privacy can be maintained more readily during self-medication. Hygiene is usually less of a problem than it is with nebulizers and metering mechanisms endow patients with an awareness of how much medication they have inhaled. From the pharmaceutical scientist's point of view, MDIs and DPGs are more complex and pose greater technical challenges than do nebulizers. If they are correctly formulated, however, they do a reliable job of dispensing medication in the form of a reproducible aerosol. Thus, pharmacologic response vs. time profiles are reproducible following inhalation of a metered dose by a given subject population,[7,8] provided subjects have been correctly trained in the use of the device.[9,10] Nebulizers offer much less reproducibility, partly because of the variable ways in which they are used and partly due to the fact that a particular drug solution may be nebulized in several different devices. Again, from the scientist's perspective, marketing a "self-contained" MDI which is sealed and effectively tamperproof is much more appealing than an aqueous solution which can be contaminated and inhaled in inappropriate doses. In short, pharmaceutical quality assurance and control imposed during the manufacture of an MDI is more effective in defining the clinical outcome than that which is presently imposed on the manufacture of a nebulizer solution.

Both unit dose and multidose DPGs are also drug metering devices. In their case, however, the energy for powder dispersion or aerosolization originates from the patient's own inspiration. Because they contain dry powder in a variety of different packaging materials, they can present storage problems (humidity, for example). Also, encapsulated dry powders are clearly not as tamperproof as a drug contained in an MDI. The major advantage of DPGs lies in the ease with which inhalation and aerosol generation are coordinated. Their recent growth in popularity (there are several new additions to the original "Spinhalers") is related more to the regulatory problems which presently beset the chlorofluorocarbons (CFCs) than it is to their possessing obvious clinical advantages. These problems are connected with destruction of the ozone layer surrounding the earth which is believed to be related to CFC production and accumulation in the atmosphere.[11] In the U.S., CFCs are used mostly as refrigerants and as volatile solvents in

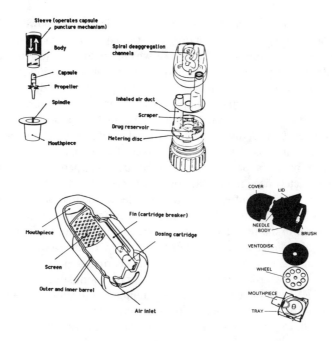

FIGURE 1.   Four metered dry powder generators. Clockwise from top left: Fison's Spinhaler™, Astra's Turbohaler™, Glaxo's Diskhaler™, and Glaxo's Rotahaler™. The Turbohaler and the Diskhaler are multidose units.

polystyrene foam manufacture (their use as general aerosol propellants has been banned since 1978). The contribution of MDIs, in which they are still permitted, to CFC escape and accumulation is a fraction of 1% of total production. Nevertheless, from a clinical point of view, if DPGs can be made bioequivalent (in terms of drug delivery to the lung) to MDIs, they have an obvious toxicologic advantage over their pressurized counterparts. If drug administration can be accomplished in air as opposed to propellant vapor, dosing limitations which may be imposed upon MDIs due to propellant inclusion may be relaxed in the case of DPGs.

II. TYPES OF UNIT DOSE AEROSOL

A. DRY POWDER GENERATORS (DPGs)

Some locally active compounds are available for inhalation administration using either an MDI or a dry powder inhaler. Figure 1 shows some typical devices which are described briefly in the legend. These should ideally aerosolize a fixed dose of previously micronized powder. This is usually packaged as the required unit dose capsules, although in some cases it may be mixed with inert diluents like lactose. The device recently launched by Astra Pharmaceuticals, the Turbohaler™, was the first dry powder generator with multidose capability. The patient can reprime this device by twisting a grip on its base. The powder in this case is metered by volume from the reservoir which contains an equivalent number of doses as that found in an MDI. A new Diskhaler™ has recently been launched by Glaxo which contains eight doses of albuterol in each disposable disk. The storage of this device is less sensitive to environmental humidity because each individual dose is blisterpacked until, just prior to inhalation, both sides of the blister are punctured by lifting the lid of the Diskhaler. More multidose devices may be expected in the future. When capsules are used for dose metering, these are broken within the device and mechanical deaggregation of the powder achieved by various techniques.[12,13] This is accompanied by a small risk of the patient inhaling some hard gelatin fragments from the capsule itself. In general terms, these devices not only dispense aerosol without propellant gases, they also overcome the coordination problem associated with MDIs. Despite powder micronization to diameters <5 μm, however, unit doses of drug are still required which are far in excess of that deposited in the lung. There are two main reasons why this is so. First, to activate these devices, patients must inhale rapidly (≥60 l/min). When particles are inhaled rapidly, they have increased inertia and are more likely to impact in the back of the throat. Second, deaggregating a powder with a median size around 100 μm is a simple matter compared to performing the same job on one of 5 μm. It could usefully be borne in mind that the smallest particle we can easily see with the naked eye is about 30 μm across. Micronized powders adhere strongly to most surfaces they come into contact with, most especially themselves. These adhesion forces are difficult to predict, reduce, to overcome and the energy input from the patient's inhalation is usually insufficient to completely deaggregate the powder charge.[14] Third, and to some extent because of the variability with which different patients inhale, the degree of deaggregation may be expected to show large variations[15] alongside the dose of drug reaching the lung. These variations are shown in the recent work by Vidgren et al.,[16] who document deposition of a laboratory packaged, radiolabeled formulation of cromolyn sodium from a Spinhaler (Figure 1), ranging from just under 20% to about 50% of the dose in normal subjects. While these deposition data are impressive, earlier articles would suggest that <10% normally reaches the lung from this particular device.[17,18] Different devices have different aerosolization efficiencies.[19] From the manufacturer's point of view, accurately dispensing very small doses of micronized solid drugs is a problem in itself. Cromolyn sodium as Intal used to be mixed with a lactose diluent. This overcame some powder dispensing problems as well as enabling easier deaggregation (the lactose was present in a much larger particle size than the drug itself). In order to avoid occasional clinical problems with the inert diluent, the pure drug is now packaged into capsules. To make this possible, a technique was developed which allowed the formation of large, loosely packed floccules which could be dispensed and packaged accurately, while retaining ease of deaggregation. Vibration can be a factor affecting the stability of dosage forms like these, and also because the presence of water is critical in the deaggregation process, the selection of packaging materials and the patient's adherence to advice on storage are very important.

B. METERED DOSE INHALERS (MDIs)

Many of the topics covered in the previous chapter on nonmetered aerosols are also relevant to a discussion of their metered counterparts. This statement is especially true for the sections on the dynamics of inhalation aerosols and their mechanisms of formation. The reader should study those sections, especially where reference is made to the factors governing inertial impaction and evaporation; additional information on these subjects is only presented here to explain aerosol behavior which is unique to MDIs.

Figure 2 is a diagrammatic representation of an MDI and actuator. All inverted metering valves in these systems meter liquid volume and require that they are covered with liquid when being used. Some are more prone to "lose prime" on standing the container upright than others, by virtue of different design features.[20] Metered volumes can be as high as 150 μl, although with smaller volumes (25 or 50 μl is common), less evaporation is ultimately required and the propellant dose to the patient is minimized.[14] In some of the earlier formulations, cosolvents such as ethanol were blended with CFCs in order to produce solutions of hydrophilic drugs in MDIs.[21] Because these solution systems usually have lower vapor pressures, atomization can be less efficient and subsequent evaporation slower.[22] The end result is a larger aerosol. In most cases, therefore, the drug is suspended in "micronized" form in a high vapor pressure hydrophobic blend of liquid CFCs containing different, but usually unquoted, concentrations of hydrophobic surfactants to stabilize the suspension. Obviously, these must be shaken before use. The propellant blends in these suspension systems usually have gauge vapor pressures in the range of 3 to 4 atm (4 to 5 atm absolute). Although it is possible to formulate solution systems with similar pressures, there are several problems to be overcome before these become available.[23]

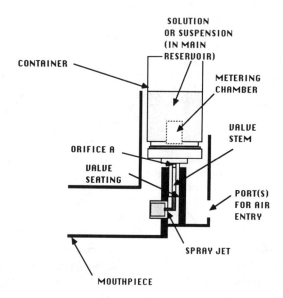

FIGURE 2. Diagrammatic representation of a typical pressurized metered dose inhaler.

III. AEROSOL GENERATION AND DRUG DELIVERY FROM MDIs

CFC propellant blends usually have densities of the order of 1.4 g cm^{-3}, although the exact value will vary with temperature and the blend employed. Propellant vapor pressure is also a function of the system temperature and performance can be affected markedly if the device is stored or operated in an inappropriate environment. The process of actuating an MDI produces an aerosol spray of propellant droplets from the spray nozzle. Depression of the valve stem forces the orifice, A, into contact with the contents of the metering chamber (at this point the junction between the main reservoir and the chamber is sealed, Figure 2). The contents of the chamber expand into the valve stem, displacing air through the spray jet, followed closely by the formulation which oftens tends to "explode" into droplets on the other side of the nozzle. Because the relative sizes of A and the spray jet can influence spray characteristics, the correct combination is important (the jet, not the size of the orifice, A, should determine the rate of spray formation).

The duration of the spray depends upon metering volume, diameters of A and the spray jet (Figure 2), vapor pressure, and the nature of the formulation. The majority of the droplets emitted at the spray jet, however, are once again quite large. Volume median diameters in the 30 to 50 μm range are common and only a small fraction of the metered volume is emitted as smaller "satellite" droplets.[15] The initial size of the CFC droplets are somewhat smaller than those emitted when aqueous sprays are created at similar pressures because the CFCs have lower surface tensions and are inclined to explode after passing through the jet. Were it not for rapid evaporation, we could expect about 1% of the output to be respirable and penetrate the lung. In reality, about 10% can reach the airways from presently marketed MDIs without extension devices[24] when the devices are used correctly (patients must exhale, then inhale slowly while coordinating their inspiration with device actuation, and then employ a breath-holding pause[9,10]). The problems which prevent greater penetration are associated with impaction, sedimentation, and evaporation (Figure 3). Typical propellant droplets exit the spray jet at high linear velocities (25 to 50 m/s),[25] which, if actuation is straight into the oral cavity, is sure to result in high oropharyngeal losses due to impaction. While lower vapor pressure formulations have reduced expulsion velocities, the primary droplet size is then increased. In addition, low vapor pressure

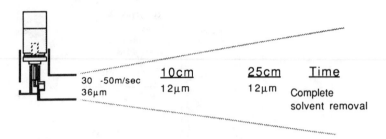

FIGURE 3. The course of events following actuation of an MDI. The flume is expelled at high velocities from the spray jet consisting of fairly large droplets. Time and heat are required for complete propellant evaporation to occur.

propellants do not evaporate as completely or as rapidly as is actually required.[26] While CFC 12 and 114 have very low boiling points (-29.8° and +4.1°C, respectively), CFC 11 is a liquid at room temperature (boiling point = +23.7°C). The latter propellant is incorporated at ≈25% in many commercial products and in these, droplet emission from the spray jet is followed by a rapid loss of >75% of droplet mass. Because the volume of a spherical droplet is proportional to the cube of its diameter, 75% loss should result in a reduction in mean size from say, 40, to approximately 25 μm. Mean droplet sizes 10 to 25 cm from the jet have been reported to be around 14 μm,[27] indicating nearer to 95% loss of propellants, but, in order to effect complete evaporation and leave surfactant coated micronized drug suspended in air, heat and time are required to remove the now supercooled, low volatility CFC 11 and surfactant which remains as a concentrated solution. During this final evaporation process further droplet losses occur due largely to sedimentation. Measurements of final mass median diameters have been reported some 5 s after actuation which are consistent with the size of micronized powders originally placed in the suspensions (values <5 μm).[28,29]

In many concentrated nonaqueous suspension products, single propellant droplets containing more than one drug particle are frequently emitted. This creates particle aggregates in the output after propellant evaporation, even when these have not been present in the original suspension. The problem becomes more severe as the drug concentration is increased.[30,31] As an example of the magnitude of the effect, four 10 μm spheres as an aggregate might be expected to possess an aerodynamic diameter of about 15 μm. Gonda[30] has indicated that aggregation based growth in aerodynamic diameter is a problem at drug in suspension concentrations around 1% or more. The metered dose inhalers containing nedocromil and cromolyn sodium have the highest concentrations (up to 5% drug) on the market because the required doses are the highest. Fisons has countered the aggregate problem by omitting CFC 11 from their formulations and enhancing evaporation kinetics. They use a mixture of the high volatility CFC 12 and 114 as the continuous phase which creates some manufacturing difficulties. The surfactant and drug is blended with propellants at -40°C and the resultant mixture filled through the valve of preassembled containers. While the approach reduces the time taken for aerosol droplets to evaporate, particle aggregation, as described above, remains a problem.

Two other limitations associated with MDI technology are concerned with the surfactants and the injection-molded actuators. Lipophilic surfactants, which are included as suspending agents and, to some extent, valve lubricants in these formulations, slow propellant evaporation by forming a layer at the droplet-air interface.[32] In the actuators, the sophistication of spray jet design is limited for suspension formulations by the ease with which small jets may be blocked with drug and by the precision of injection molding techniques which are used to mass-produce the actuators. It is likely that some large nonrespirable droplets and particles will always be expelled from the spray nozzles of MDIs. Thus, the sensible approach in future developments would be to focus on actuator design in order to retain large nonrespirable aerosol material prior to inhalation.[14] Losing a constant proportion of the metered dose in the device should not be considered a waste when a therapeutic oral dose of drug would be orders of magnitude higher

IV. MODIFIED DELIVERY SYSTEMS

A. RESERVOIRS AND EXTENSION DEVICES

A selection of extension devices and aerosol reservoirs is shown in Figure 4. Although they have been the subject of numerous investigations, only a few studies have sought to design a given device around a particular formulation-valve-actuator combination and some physicians are still skeptical of their value.[33,34] Unlike reservoirs, simple extension devices or spacers do not provide as much opportunity for an aerosol to dwell prior to inhalation. Thus, spacers are usually small devices which are placed between the conventional actuator and the patient and require that aerosol is discharged into them at the same time as inhalation. Spacers are intended to:

1. Provide extra time for propellant droplet evaporation before the aerosol reaches the patient
2. Reduce the droplet velocity and therefore the impaction efficiency of the aerosol at the back of the throat by spacing the actuator further from the mouth
3. Retain some of the extremely large droplets, which are unlikely ever to be respirable, by sedimentation and impaction on the inside walls of the spacer

Reservoirs, on the other hand, are larger and designed to enable actuation prior to inhalation. These enhance the opportunity for evaporation and sedimentation (depending on the aerosol dwell time) but are mainly designed to overcome inhalation difficulties experienced by patients who cannot coordinate actuation and inhalation. In some devices, an audible device usefully informs the patient that they are inhaling too quickly for optimal deposition.[35,36] In others, the intention has also been to optimize patient training (especially small children) so that aerosol therapy becomes possible in the first place (Inhal-Aid for example, Schering/Key Pharmaceuticals, U.S.).

Figure 4 and its legend shows some examples and their main characteristics. While they are bulky and poorly accepted by many patients, they are certainly a good idea. Moren's work with AB Draco (a subdivision of Astra Pharmaceuticals in Sweden) pioneered the field.[37] The diagrams presented in Figure 5A and B summarize some of the validation work on the original cone-shaped device.[14,38] If the values and sites of aerosol deposition are compared for usage of "actuator alone" to "actuator with spacer" it is clear that for a model formulation, lung deposition can be enhanced, while oropharyngeal deposition is reduced by increasing the losses in the device itself. More recent devices have an even more impressive showing in the literature (Figure 5C to 5F).[36,39] Reservoir- and spacer-achieved reductions in oropharyngeal deposition have been advocated to reduce the incidence of oral candidiasis associated with the use of inhaled steroid aerosols. With some of these spacers, however, high oropharyngeal losses continue to occur, indicating that the aerosol segregation function of the total delivery system could be better. It is questionable, indeed, whether the "aid to evaporation" function of these devices is as important as their role in baffling and preventing the emission of nonrespirable droplets and particles. The subject of "baffles" is mentioned later in this chapter alongside formulation effects, where it will be seen that the vast majority of particles and/or droplets which are ultimately to be considered small enough to be "respirable" are actually respirable within a short distance from the spray jet (Figure 2).[40]

B. BREATH-ACTUATED DEVICES

Using an MDI without a reservoir device requires that the patient synchronize valve actuation with the earlier part of inhalation. Some people find this difficult to achieve. The problem can be overcome by the use of an inhalation triggered actuator. Several devices are currently under development[32,41,42] and we can expect to see these launched with increasing levels of sophistication, perhaps even containing electronic components. Figure 6 shows the operating mechanism of Riker Laboratories' automatic inhaler which is presently marketed in Europe. The

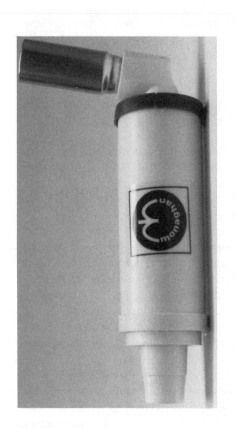

B

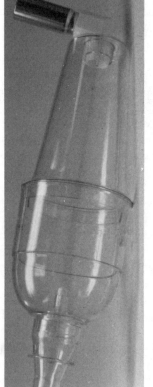

D

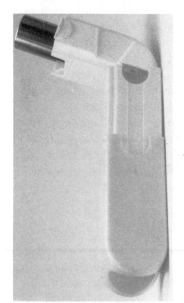

A

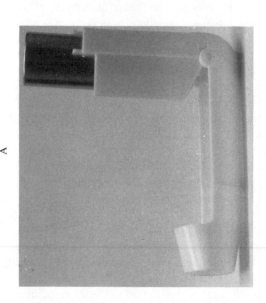

C

FIGURE 4. Spacer and reservoir devices. (A) Astra Pharmaceuticals' Breathhancer or Inhalet; (B) Fisons' open topped extension device; (C) Forest Pharmaceuticals (U.S.) Aerochamber; (D) Astra Pharmaceuticals' Nebuhaler; (E) Key Pharmaceuticals' (U.S.) InspirEase (F) Rorer Pharmaceuticals' (U.S.) Azmacort (MDI marketed with spacer); (G) Valois extension device.

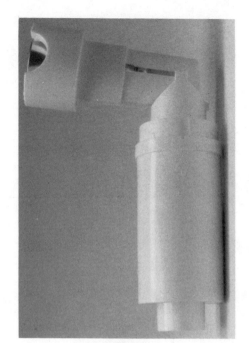

FIGURE 4F.

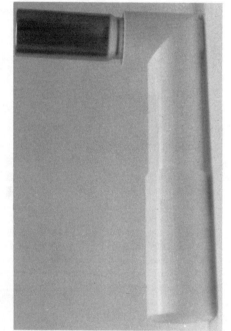

FIGURE 4G.

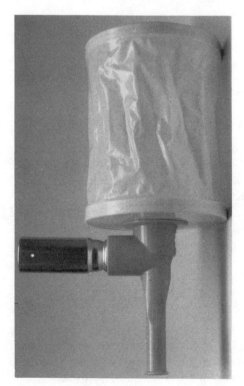

FIGURE 4E.

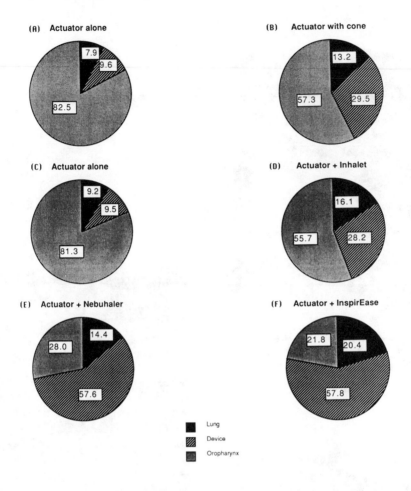

(A) Actuator alone

(B) Actuator with cone

(C) Actuator alone

(D) Actuator + Inhalet

(E) Actuator + Nebuhaler

(F) Actuator + InspirEase

Lung
Device
Oropharynx

FIGURE 5.   Deposition in the lungs oropharynx and device (actuator alone or with spacer/reservoir). A and B show MDI-formulated radiolabeled Teflon particle deposition following administration in the presence and absence of a conical spacer. The remainder show deposition of labeled cromolyn sodium from a model formulation when administration employed the actuator alone or the actuator in addition to the different spacer/reservoir devices.[38,39]

mechanism is primed by closing the mouthpiece cover. To obtain a dose, the patient first opens the cover, then inhales from the mouthpiece. This inhalation effort moves the vane and releases a spring-operated driver. This, in turn, actuates the metering valve and releases drug to the patient's oropharynx. To obtain a second dose, the patient must close the cover to reprime the mechanism. The moment that actuation occurs is accompanied by a "click" which takes a little getting used to. The present device also offers no spacing possibilities. Development of cheap, breath-actuated mechanisms is presently in its infancy. We can await substantial improvements in the future.

V. FORMULATION, MANUFACTURE, AND TESTING MDIs

There is a paucity of literature available on this subject. To some extent this is related to the difficulty and expense of handling volatile propellant blends and the fact that most published work originates from academic institutions with limited funds. The area is becoming increasingly important as some scientists attempt to develop novel formulations to deliver new compounds to various parts of the respiratory tract, while others seek to copy existing MDIs

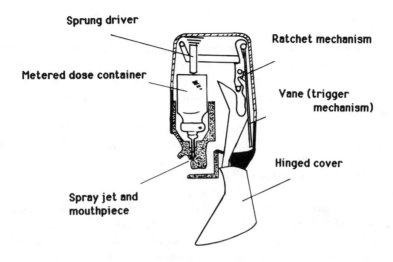

Sprung driver

Ratchet mechanism

Metered dose container

Vane (trigger mechanism)

Hinged cover

Spray jet and mouthpiece

FIGURE 6. Riker's Autohaler. Inspiratory effort triggers the driver mechanism. The device must be closed and reopened in order to gain a second dose.

marketed by companies whose patents are expiring. Several major pharmaceutical manufacturers have accumulated data relating to factors which influence MDI-formulation stability and the subsequent production of "optimized" inhalation aerosol flumes. Much of this work is proprietary and is destined to remain the subjects of internal reports. Nevertheless, some company scientists have pursued the road to publication of the basic principles and further work is available from academe. The following is not intended to be a comprehensive listing, rather they are the key publications which provide these basics. There are various texts which provide some general information on the subjects of formulation and manufacture;[21,42-49] As an example, *The Aerosol Handbook*,[47] which is now in its second edition, is an invaluable reference book. The Chemical Specialties Manufacturer's Association publishes several guides[50,51] which contain much of the essential information concerning propellants and propellant handling. The journal *Aerosol Age* is worth reading on a regular basis and worth catching up on back issues.[52] The larger chemical companies are, of course, a useful source of technical information on propellants, surfactants, and incompatibilities, some of which are as much the property of the cosmetics literature as they are the domain of pharmaceuticals.[53] More specifically, with regard to inhalation, beginners in the field should read the original Riker patent[54] on suspension and solution MDIs which are now more than 28 years old. The work published in 1969 by Polli et al.[55] from Merck Sharp and Dohme is another classic. This group made a series of comparisons between different suspension formulations of dexamethasone. They established some of the effects of suspension and surfactant concentrations, propellant vapor pressure, and spray orifice diameter upon output particle sizes. The latter were determined using cascade impaction, but in such a fashion that propellant evaporation proceeded almost to completion. Polli's group quoted a water content for the formulations investigated of approximately of 0.02% after Karl Fischer titration. The pertinence of this value is highlighted in the appendix to the present chapter where water is shown to wreak havoc within otherwise carefully formulated nonaqueous suspensions. This appendix, prepared by Nicholas Miller of Riker Laboratories, is probably the first to provide a quantitative description of these effects. Dr. Miller's appendix shows explicitly why the physical stability of MDI formulations should be determined at elevated temperature in environments with different humidities. Prior to this, textbook statements on water content[49] such as, "The moisture content of both the suspensoid and the propellant affects the stability of the aerosol system and must be below 300 ppm" were just about all that could be found in the literature. Dr. Miller has begun to place high humidity testing, manufacturing conditions where humidity is strictly controlled, and water diffusion into MDI containers into perspective for aerosol formulators.

The literature which exists is complicated because the aerosol output of any pressurized formulation must also be influenced by the way in which the mechanics of the MDI interact with its contents. Thus, it is difficult to attribute some of the other landmark work to the subject of formulation alone. The work of Rance[25,56] on hairspray formulations detailed the effects that different propellant blends and cosolvents have on aerosol exit velocities only after these formulations had passed through different continuous valves with different orifice diameters and designs. Similarly, the aerosol droplet size data of Pengilly and Keiner[57] by necessity superimposes the valve and spray nozzle effects upon those due to the formulations themselves. Even Gonda's theory for aggregation[30,31] requires that initial droplet sizes are presumed (from a knowledge of spray mechanics) in order to then calculate the probable number of suspended particles which each droplet can contain. In a similar fashion, for specific MDIs, Bell et al.[22] showed that low volatility solution formulations do not evaporate as fast as most suspension systems, resulting in a lower quantity of respirable drug from the former. Conversely, for 0.1% solutions compared to 0.1% suspensions in identical volatile propellant systems and sprayed through identical actuators, we recently found that the solutions provided the greater amount of respirable drug.[23] Although it was known previously that evaporation was incomplete prior to inhalation of MDIs, Moren[58] exploited the observation, and enhanced lung deposition, by increasing the time for evaporation prior to inhalation by extending the actuator mouthpiece. This work has led to a myriad of MDI "add on" accessories in the form of spacers and reservoirs.[34-36,39] When it was originally performed and initiated by Moren,[37] it was combined in a series of articles[6,24,26,27,58-62] which also contain information on the formulation factors which interacted with the different device designs. It is important to observe that some of these interactions between the device and the formulation are specific to the particular formulations, valves, and actuator-spacer combinations being tested.[40]

These references on formulation are not a complete listing. Nevertheless, they do provide the groundwork on which we can found a discussion of formulation and manufacture. With the notable exception of Dr. Miller's appendix to this chapter, most of the literature which details the effects that formulation factors have upon MDI aerosol output uses freshly prepared formulations. Storage may bring about physical changes in formulations. These changes may define resulting aerosol characteristics and thus, it is only after recent preparation that the original formulation can reasonably be expected to describe the multiphase mixture which passes at high velocity through the spray jet. Because it neglects the precise definition of the manufacturing processes leading to MDI production, even this last statement is open to debate. Those who have experience of MDI manufacture will know that a number of process variables can have a profound influence on the aerosol output, even of seemingly identical, freshly prepared products.

Given all these facts as background, it should be apparent that the design, formulation, and manufacture of MDIs is still largely empirical. Thus, in order to be able to function adequately in this area, it is necessary to gain some expertise in formulation, manufacturing processes, device design, and testing. As is the case with any empirical process when a product is the outcome, it is imperative that the testing procedures used to evaluate different product options are clearly defined and the meaning of the data which they provide is understood. Unfortunately, few of the tests which are applied to metered inhalation products are standardized and the interpretation of results remains a matter for debate. Because testing forms the foundation for evaluation of all the other factors we begin by briefly describing available methodology.

A. TESTING MDI OUTPUT

Several techniques are used to characterize output from MDIs, although few provide unequivocal results. Because of the myriad of methods and instruments which are available for use in general aerosol characterization work, no attempt is made here to present a thorough breakdown of each and every possibility. This section on testing has been assembled pragmatically by asking first "what is used most frequently and why?" and second: "What are the problems with these existing techniques and may they be overcome?" With the exception of a small number of compendial methods most instruments and techniques are not standardized between laboratories. The major techniques are defined in this section along with some difficulties associated with their use both from a practical point of view and from that of data interpretation.

1. Determining the Dose

Labeling requirements for MDIs differ between nations. In the U.S., for example, the so-called "dose available to the patient" is the label claim and this is defined as the amount of drug per actuation leaving the actuator as aerosol. In other nations the "metered dose" is used which includes the amount retained in the actuator but not that retained in the valve stem. Whichever definition is used begs the question of how to determine the dose and its reproducibility. If, for example, the actuator (Figure 2) is removed from the device, the container is shaken, allowed to come to rest inverted for sufficient time to prime the valve,[20] and the valve stem compressed against the base of a small beaker containing a collection fluid, an estimate of the dose metered by the valve may be obtained following drug assay in the collection fluid. There are several problems with the determination. First, the valve stem may already contain material from a previous actuation and the exact circumstances of that actuation may define the mass remaining in the valve stem (the contribution of this may be minimized by performing replicate actuations). Second, the amount emitted through the valve may vary depending upon the back pressure due to the depth of the collection fluid and the manner in which the opening of the valve stem is partly occluded by the base of the beaker. Third, aerosolized drug may often escape into the atmosphere by passing in gas bubbles straight through the collection fluid. Finally, the technique is difficult to reproduce between operators because the speed and angle with which the valve stem is depressed into the metering chamber introduce variability in the determination.

Use of a technique in which the MDI and the actuator is submerged in collection fluid suffers from similar problems. While it is possible to minimize the significance of some of these variables, it is hardly surprising that a compendial apparatus is described.[63] This requires actuation of the whole unit into a collection apparatus to which the inhaler is attached while air is drawn by vacuum through the MDI-actuator assembly. The twin stage impinger[64] described later in this section has recently been incorporated in the British compendia, and can function as a particle sizing device and as a means of determining total output simultaneously. Cascade impactors are rarely successful in this regard because of the difficulty in recovering 100% of the drug. Drug captured in the apparatus and the actuator can be determined separately, although there is no guarantee that the respective amounts will be the same following air withdrawal at different rates. Because many actuators contain additional holes for air entry (Figure 2) during the breathing maneuver, aerosolized drug can escape from these ports in amounts which vary depending upon the rate at which air is drawn through the device. To avoid all of these problems, air should be drawn by the collection apparatus through the MDI at a rate which would be used in practice by the patient; further, the means of shaking and actuating the device should be standardized and perhaps automated to avoid operator error. If replicate actuations are needed to obtain sufficient drug in solution for assay, this precludes the estimation of dosing variability. Thus, a sensitive assay is often required early in the development of an MDI to assess the reliability of the metering valve.

2. Aerosol Sampling

A brief section on this subject is important to make the investigator wary of the ways in which he or she performs particle sizing experiments. One of the reasons that cascade impaction is used as the major method of determining aerosol size distributions stems from its capacity to size the whole aerosol output. In short, "sampling" is not required. Because of the need to connect an impactor to an MDI, however, the possibility exists whereby the "connector" can itself classify an aerosol (by impaction or sedimentation; electrostatics are rarely important with MDIs), so that results from the impactor are dependent upon "connector" geometry. It is sensible to choose an "evaporation chamber" as a connector with walls which flare away from the mouthpiece of the MDI[23] and to study the effects of different arrangements upon the results of particle sizing experiments for one or two MDIs. Virtually all other particle sizing techniques involve one form of sampling or another. These always involve experimental problems.[65] If, for example, a microscope slide contains an uneven distribution of small and large particles on its surface, an elaborate sampling scheme to ensure lack of bias in the resultant particle size distribution is required. If, on the other hand, a small aerosol sample is required, then not only must the investigator ensure that the sample is withdrawn isokinetically (where the linear velocity of particles in the sample stream is identical to that in the mainstream[65]), but also that particles within the stream or pool from which the aerosol is withdrawn are distributed homogeneously with repsect to size. The latter is the hardest thing to achieve with MDI output. Small droplets slow down much faster than large ones after leaving the spray jet causing an immediate sampling problem. However, because there are benefits to using a variety of sizing techniques to obtain different types of information, the cautious investigator will study the effect of different sampling techniques upon the results of all determinations.

3. Classification by Impaction

Figure 7A illustrates the principle by which cascade impactors function. So called "imping-ers" (Figure 7B) operate somewhat similarly. Air is drawn through these devices at a constant volume flow rate. Because of decreasing jet sizes, the linear airflow velocity increases as the stages are descended. As a result, smaller and smaller aerosol particles or droplets are made to impact on successive stages. The basics of impactor design were discussed in the previous chapter. Aerosol particles must be endowed with a sufficiently high Stokes' number in order to impact on the surface placed beneath the jet. In the case of impingers, these surfaces are often collection liquids like water. A filter is usually employed beyond the final impaction stage to ensure collection of submicron aerosols which otherwise may escape detection. The major design differences between available impactors relate to the use of multiple or single jets on each stage, slit, or circular orifice (as the jets), removable or integral collection surfaces, and the volumetric air flow rate which is employed for aerosol sampling. Some of these design differences have emerged more for theoretical than practical reasons while some others are due to ease of machining. The most important factors to be considered while selecting a particular impactor are volumetric airflow rate, the maximum stage loading which is possible before significant errors are incurred, and the ease with which the impactor can be dissembled and particulate or drug masses determining on each stage.[66,67] The exact choice will depend upon the job to be accomplished.

Airflow rates define the speed at which the aerosol cloud is drawn through the device and the effective residence time before a given aerosol size range is removed from gaseous suspension. In the "twin stage impinger" shown in Figure 7B, a high flow rate (60 l/min)[64] ensures rapid transit which can be likened to rapid inhalation from a dry powder aerosol generator. Flow is usually slower in cascade impactors but in both types of device, residence times will differ for different sized particles and/or droplets, smaller sizes remaining in suspension longer than their larger counterparts. This fact has clear implications in the case of MDI output being drawn through an impactor while droplets continue to evaporate. The mass median aerodynamic diameter (MMAD) determined by drug assay on each of the stages will underestimate the true MMAD which existed at the aerosol sampling port and the distribution will be skewed toward smaller sizes. It is appropriate at this point also to recognize the fact that MMADs determined by drug assay may be larger than that of the aerosol itself if suspended drug distribution within

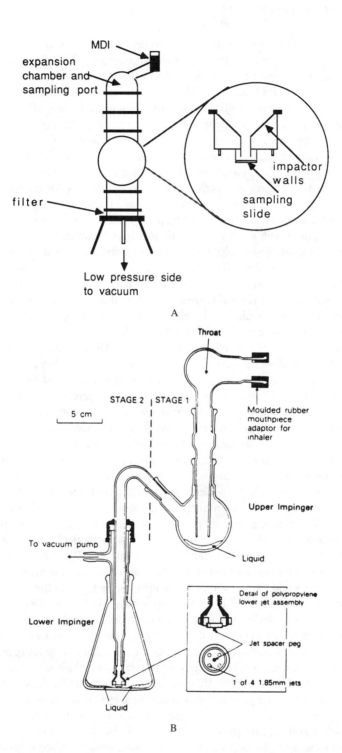

FIGURE 7. A diagram showing (A) a cascade impactor and (B) a twin stage impinger. Both devices operate by segregating airborne droplets and particles according to their inertia. (B reproduced from Hallworth, G. W. and Westmoreland, D. G., *J. Pharm. Pharmacol.*, 39, 966, 1987. With permission.)

the aerosol cloud is skewed toward the larger droplets while the small ones contain mainly surfactant.[68,69] Because the lung itself samples and separates MDI output dynamically (small particles taking longer to deposit than large ones), airflow rates are often chosen to be similar to those which are advised for inhalation (<30 l/min). However, for this rationale to be entirely valid, the time it takes to deposit each size category in the impactor would have to be identical to that in the human lung. This is clearly not the case and, from this point of view, choice of airflow rate in the impactor remains somewhat arbitrary. In summary, the aerosol sizes derived by the methods *in vitro* cannot necessarily be extrapolated to the *in vivo* situation.

Airflow rate in some cascade impactors may be varied and adjusted by flow meter, while in others it is controlled by placement of a critical orifice (below the filter) at the base of the device. Setting up an impactor with a flow meter usually requires adjustment of vacuum at its base with a calibrated flow meter attached to the sampling port. There is a problem with this approach if the sampling mode used with the MDI restricts flow into the impactor. This would result in reduced flow rates through the device due to a pressure drop occurring at the sampling port. As a result, the instrument calibration fails and aerosols appear to be smaller because they penetrate further down the impactor than they would given the correct flow conditions. The critical orifice in the base of many devices, if used correctly, ensures that the flow rate remains constant provided sufficient vacuum is maintained during flow on the low pressure side, while a constant (usually atmospheric) pressure is maintained at the sampling port (Figure 7A). Monitoring flow under these circumstances needs only to be performed as a quality control measure. Once again, however, inaccuracies may result from restricted inflow to the sampling port.

The remaining differences between impactors can be appreciated best by briefly discussing the subject of calibration.[66] To calibrate properly, monodisperse aerosols must be passed through each isolated stage at the chosen volume flow rate. Curves of the form shown by Figure 2 in the previous chapter must be constructed for impaction or collection efficiency as a function of aerodynamic diameter. During this process, information can also be gathered on the maximum mass of a chosen size of aerosol particle which a particular impactor stage can accumulate without the collection efficiency falling off due to stage overload. In the case of more readily cleaned devices with removable glass stages beneath each impactor jet (Figure 7A), losses on the impactor walls should also be determined in order to assess their impact upon resultant size distribution data. The classical way to produce the monodisperse aerosols for calibration purposes is to use a vibrating orifice generator.[70] Even then, theoretical and practical difficulties remain. Fortunately, with most MDI output (the surfactants usually endow particulates with a "sticky" coating), it is not necessary to worry too much about the problem of dry particle rebound from the stage surfaces and subsequent re-entrainment of particles in the airstream.[66,69] Most importantly, the whole process of calibration is very worthwhile. It is rare for the manufacturer's "calibrations" to have been performed in a thorough fashion. This fact is easily discerned by the regular intervals with which the cutoff diameters are quoted for most available devices. In practice, their "calibrations" are usually valid for one, two, or three stages only and large errors may be associated with not knowing the aerosol size range in which a chosen device can be expected to provide reliable results. If, of course, an impactor is only used to provide comparative results between different formulations, then careful calibration is less important.

4. Other Particle Sizing Techniques

In earlier compendia[17,71] the collection of MDI output on a microscope slide held a short distance away from the mouthpiece was advocated as a means of determining the relative percentages of small and large particles and droplets after microscopic examination of the slide. While the method is clearly inadequate (most of the respirable material escapes and drug-containing particles cannot easily be distinguished from other nonvolatile ingredients in the formulation) collection and microscopic examination of the formulation and the aerosol output can often reveal valuable information about the state of aggregation and morphology of particles in a suspension formulation.[72,73] One useful means of reproducibly collecting the dry particle output from an MDI on a microscope slide is to employ an electrostatic precipitator[74] through which the MDI output is drawn after first actuating into an evaporation chamber. Slides from cascade impactors may also be inspected microscopically and electron microscope stubs used in place of the microscope slide when closer detail is required.[73]

While other methods have been used to characterize the output from MDIs,[28,29,56,65,75-80] one major technique which is commercially available employs forward light scattering of a laser source.[57] The most popular device is marketed by Malvern Instruments, Malvern, Worcestershire, U.K. It operates on the principle that large aerosols scatter light at lower angles than small droplets or particles. Information is collected on the intensity of scattered light due to the presence of particles or droplets which are sprayed through the laser beam. In the commercially available device the data are processed by user friendly but rather inaccessible software into a particle size distribution. The systems are popular because of the facility with which they collect and process data.[75] While they have a great deal of potential, there are several practical drawbacks to their use:

1.   Calibration of this instrument using aerosols is difficult. The user must often rely upon calibrations performed with suspensions of known size in liquids with known refractive indices.

2.   Evaporating propellants create vapors which are more dense than air and refract light. This causes apparent particle size distributions to be erroneously large unless some of the low scattering angle data are arbitrarily discarded. Even though "control determinations" can be run with propellant vapor in the laser beam, the situation remains unsatisfactory. With MDI output, the vapor content is variable in different parts of the flume and large droplets which scatter light the least are those which contribute most to the aerosol mass.

3.   The laser beam must not be heavily "obscured" and excessive droplet to droplet scattering must be prevented. This is the case for all forms of light scattering instrumentation where "coincidence errors" must be avoided.[65] The sizing of droplets leaving an MDI results in the fact that the device must be distanced sufficiently from the laser beam to avoid the problem. Thus, apparent droplet sizes can only be determined after substantial evaporation and dispersion of the spray.

4.   The laser beam must be sufficiently "obscured" for the collected data to be reliable. As a result, the device is rarely useful to size dry particles after evaporation unless these are in a fairly concentrated suspension in air. In practice, this may be achieved by arranging some sort of aerosol reservoir without which there are few formulations with sufficient drug and/or surfactant concentrations to enable accurate determinations of dry particle size.

5.   While it may appear that the device could be used easily to assess droplet evaporation rates, this is often not the case. Although different distances (and times) can be used between the actuator and the laser beam, it is difficult to ensure that the same spectrum of droplets is being sized at the two times of determination. This fact is most obvious when the spray is diverging from its origin and thus becomes more dilute, further from the spray jet.

While laser light scattering provides some information on the droplet size distribution emitted by MDIs and other pressurized aerosols, pulsed ruby laser holography[81,82] is the one technique which appears to have the capacity to study and visualize the process of droplet formation within the spray itself. The technique is appealing because of its capacity to "freeze" the motion of microscopic droplets traveling at speeds of approximately 50 m/s. Three-dimensional images of spray droplets can be recreated from the original hologram and used to study the influences of devices and formulations upon spray droplet size distributions. Using holography it may well be possible to study systematically those factors controlling the initial droplet size distribution from MDIs.

Other sizing techniques which can be tempting but require sampling and dilution of the MDI output are rapid data capture laser scanning (available from Brinkman, Inc.), the SPART system (single particle aerodynamic relaxation time analysis[29,76]), and the APS 33 (aerosol particle sizing system, TSI, Inc., St. Paul, MN) which, like the SPART system, sizes particles aerodynamically. All of these systems can be used to provide data on the size of a small number of low concentration evaporated droplets. They all suffer from the need to evaporate the MDI output and subsequently dilute and sample the aerosol stream. The problems inherent in the latter processes cause difficulties with the interpretation of results from these rather sophisticated instruments.

5. Spray Patterns

The shape and size of the aerosol flume produced by an MDI is as much a product of the actuator design as it is of the formulation in the container. While the formulation vapor pressure is of paramount importance, the use of a poorly designed or partly blocked actuator can result in the product losing much of its efficacy. While no compendial method for characterizing the spray pattern from an MDI exists, the technique developed by Benjamin et al.[83] is often employed as a means of characterizing the spray angle from the mouthpiece and/or the spray jet[40] to ensure that no untoward changes have occurred between batches of MDIs in this respect. The technique requires that the MDI is actuated at a fixed distance from a TLC plate and that drug deposition on the plate is then visualized using a suitable technique.[83] High speed photography has also been used to visualize the shape of the spray flume.[84,85] Photographic techniques suffer from the disadvantage that drug distribution within the flume of droplets cannot be determined.

B. MANUFACTURING PROCESSES

Manufacturing techniques and quality assurance procedures are discussed in detail elsewhere.[43,44,47] These will not be repeated except to highlight some of the unique problems associated with MDIs. Thus, it is assumed that the reader is acquainted with the need to control the critical dimensions of valves, containers, gaskets, and actuators as well as controlling the variance of those dimensions within acceptable quality limits.[86] Indeed, all ingredients should be quality controlled prior to use including the propellants, after their delivery and storage at the plant,[63] and the packaging materials from the points of view of chemical constitution, cleanliness, and microbiological contamination. Figure 8 is a schematic showing much of the manufacturing and packaging process for a nonaqueous suspension of drug in propellants. The first major process is usually some form of micronization so that the vast majority of particles have diameters <5 μm. Most comminution techniques are incapable of reducing the size of solid materials to this degree and, because the aerodynamic diameter of a drug particle is given approximately by the product of the square root of its density and true diameter, it is important to use an efficient technique. Several manufacturers try to achieve mass median diameters of approximately 2.5 μm as well as attempting to limit the geometric standard deviation as a measure of the polydispersity of the milled powder. Comminution is commonly accomplished by jet or gas impact milling which is performed in a strictly controlled environment. The manner in which this procedure is performed and the product is handled can often define the success or failure of the subsequent suspension; moisture levels are critical and filtered, pressurized dry nitrogen may be necessary as an inert gas for milling. Ball milling in a low volatility propellant such as CFC 11 and controlled microcrystallization are further options if impact milling is found to be unsuitable. Neither of these techniques is without problems and jet milling is generally the process of choice. The latter functions best with high melting point, brittle, crystalline materials. Jet milling has the advantage that it can be performed with negligible contamination while producing a fluffy, low bulk density product with many fresh active surfaces. Provided the product is not overhandled and not allowed to stand for long periods prior to suspension

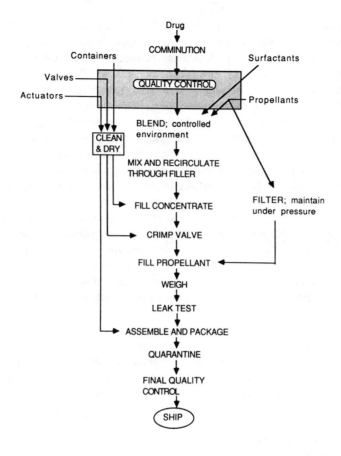

FIGURE 8. A manufacturing scheme for a typical MDI product.

manufacture, it can usually be maintained as a relatively deaggregated powder (the micronized product, as it is collected from the mill tends to have only point-to-point-contact as opposed to aggregates existing which have large crystal faces as their contact surfaces). In this loosely agglomerated form it is much easier to disperse in a suspension concentrate.

Manufacture of a suspension concentrate is the next crucial process. It is essential to achieve maximal dispersion and separate all particles with a layer of the chosen surface active agent. If this is not accomplished the interparticulate attractive forces holding the aggregates together result in the spraying of preformed, nonrespirable clumps of drug. The order and method of mixing, the viscosity of the continuous phase and, most important, the ratio of solid to liquid are all crucial. A typical blend may be surfactant 0.1 to 2%, drug 10 to 20%, and CFC propellant (often CFC 11) to 100%. Choice and control of the manufacturing processes for the suspension can be just as important as the initial formulation work in defining the success or failure of a product. For example, if the drug solubility in the concentrate (which contains a greater surfactant concentration than the final formulation) is greater than that in the final product, changes in the size distribution may occur during the addition of propellant. The mixer which is chosen for concentrate manufacture is usually similar in design to a homogenizer or colloid mill[46,49] in the sense that good mixing and high shear is often required. As a result, contamination from machine bearings should be controlled and it is thus desirable to minimize the mixing and maximize the efficiency with which dispersion is accomplished. Because all mixers impart shear via the liquid phase of the dispersion, the solid content must be kept high for transference of kinetic energy to, and dispersion of, particles in agglomerates. The continuous phase is often chilled to increase viscosity and reduce volatility. The whole operation is usually accomplished in a dry, jacketed pressure vessel which is connected to, or houses, a recirculating mixer. The mixer can then be used to maintain adequate suspension throughout the whole of the filling circuit by continuously circulating it through the concentrate filling unit.

At this stage there are two main options. In some recent products which do not use CFC 11, the whole formulation is prepared in a low temperature pressure vessel and then filled through the valve into evacuated, previously crimped containers. The individual processes of component cleaning, assembly, and crimping must all be optimized to ensure the viability of an uncontaminated, nonleaking, stable product. Although there are advantages to the production of a high volatility formulation, filling suspensions through the valve is a difficult process to optimize. The most popular alternate technique involves the manufacture of a lower volatility concentrate, filling this in a controlled environment into containers, crimping the valves in place, and subsequently adding the high pressure propellants through the valve. This requires that the final dilution step produces a homogeneous, stable dispersion and does not cause aggregation.

Once aggregation has occurred in the diluted suspension it is usually impossible to reverse the process. Sufficient shear can rarely be applied to break down clumps of micronized material. Because surface equilibria in low dielectric media may take considerable time to establish, it is advisable to record the effects of all standing or mixing periods at known temperature upon the adequacy of the final dispersion.

C. FORMULATION

If all forms of metered drug delivery to the respiratory tract were discussed in this section, the chapter would run to several volumes. After a short section on issues of a more general nature, the subject is restricted to a discussion of the formulation of pressurized MDIs containing drugs in suspension.

1. Choosing the Dosage Form

If the screening of a new compound indicates that delivery to the lung has unique advantages over other routes, then a choice must be made fairly quickly between nebulizer, pressurized MDI, or dry powder delivery from a DPG. The pharmacologic screen should be designed to provide information on the minimum dosage required in the respiratory tract for either local or systemic activity to be seen. Even though experimental designs for drug administration to the lung are rarely ideal, with the techniques described in the previous chapter, it is usually possible to arrive at a rough estimate of the minimum effective dose. When high doses (more than about 200 μg) must be deposited (only a fraction of a metered or inhaled dose is actually deposited in the lung), an aqueous formulation administered by nebulizer is usually the dosage form of choice. The other options can both be excluded for toxicologic reasons. Repeated doses from an MDI result in increased systemic levels of propellants[87,88] and increased local doses of surfactants.[89] Large quantities of dry powder can induce irritation and sometimes bronchoconstriction in their own right.

When required doses are small, either an MDI or a dry powder device may be developed. Each of these dosage forms has its own advantages and disadvantages. Moreover, it should be obvious that some compounds may be excluded from one or the other on the basis of the physicochemical nature of the drug. At the outset, however, both systems have similar dosage delivery capabilities. The popularity of DPGs has increased dramatically with the proposed cuts in production of chlorofluorocarbon propellants even though sophisticated DPGs[90] are difficult and expensive to develop. Without trying to detract from some of these successes, the road to a good DPG requires a research group structure which allows routine interaction between powder technologists, process developers, pharmaceutical-aerosol scientists, and engineers. Because this involves significant investment and some restructuring, the development of a more traditional MDI is often seen as the more feasible route. It is probable also that CFC propellants will continue to be used in MDIs as "specialty chemicals" even though their cost will escalate. In short, the pressurized MDI will remain as a relatively inexpensive way of reproducibly metering aerosolized drug doses for inhalation.

The MDI itself may be formulated as either a suspension or solution dosage form. Drug discovery and screening efforts in the last few decades have produced mostly hydrophilic compounds which have had very low solubilities in volatile propellants. Thus, in order to formulate solutions containing adequate drug concentrations, less volatile, polar cosolvents such as ethanol were added. Because of reduced evaporation kinetics, these early solution formulations produced smaller respirable dose fractions than suspension formulations which, in general, could be made more volatile than solutions.[22] With the advent of more polar, volatile propellants such as dimethyl ether, volatile solution formulations with improved respirable fractions may become possible.[23,91-93]

Formulation as it is usually conceived can be subdivided into the three main phases of preformulation, formulation, and stability assessment. These have goals which can be listed separately as:

Phase I — Preformulation: To assess feasibility and the degree of difficulty which is likely to be encountered with drug, formulation, and possible production methods. During this phase the drug must be exposed to a variety of excipients, packaging components, and processing techniques (milling, for example). A validated assay must be developed and used to determine values for such things as solubility in propellants as well as physical and chemical stability under different circumstances. Effects of moisture fall in this category. A decision must be reached on dosage. At the end of this phase, a rational decision on a restricted number of feasible formulations should be possible.

Phase II — Formulation: To screen a variety of formulations in a variety of packages and "optimize" the product. There are numerous packaging and manufacturing variables which require review. The preformulation work should have narrowed the options for the formulation considerably. The effect that the different options have upon dose reproducibility and spray characteristics requires a labor intensive effort using validated techniques. At the end of this phase, you have the formulation-container-valve-actuator combination on which to perform phase III.

Phase III — Stability Assessment: To assess shelf life and formal stability issues for submission to the regulatory authority. This stage usually continues throughout the clinical trials and functions in such a way as to define label claims and requirements for transport, storage, and use.

2. Preformulation and Formulation of Suspensions

Figure 9 illustrates the variables which must be "optimized" or at least fixed in order to produce a marketable suspension aerosol. The complexity of the issues confronting the aerosol formulator is much greater than those facing an individual formulating a conventional dosage form. The former individual needs to consider the impact of each variable upon, not one, but two closely related "formulations". The first of the formulations is held for different time frames at pressure in a metal, glass, or plastic container while the second is formed when the pressurized liquid formulation enters the atmosphere. While it is true to say that a pressurized formulation with poor physical or chemical stability is of little use to anyone, an "optimal" liquid formulation with good physical and chemical stability and reproducible dose metering will not necessarily provide the most respirable aerosol.

Figure 10 shows a possible formulation scheme covering all three development phases from preformulation to stability assessment. The scheme is idealized in some respects in order to rationalize it (in practice a number of short cuts are often demanded due to the rush to get a new drug into the clinic). The initial work should be designed to eliminate time-wasting study of

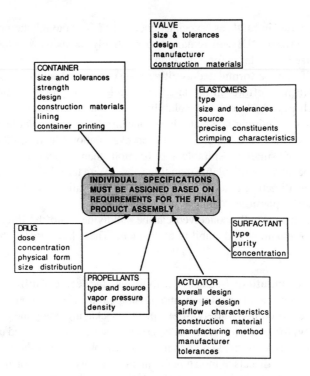

FIGURE 9. Variables which must be fixed and/or optimized in order to
produce a marketable MDI. Specifications for each individual component
must be assigned based upon minimum acceptable quality levels for the
end product.

formulation possibilities which result in chemical or physical incompatibilities and/or instability while the formulation is inside the container. Because many subsequent experimental
determinations depend upon crystal and salt form, the figure assumes that the work begins with
a pure, well-characterized drug. Calorimetry, thermal gravimetry, microscopic examination,
and chemical assay should be performed at the outset and prior to subjecting the drug form to
whichever comminution technique is selected. The options here are usually air impact milling,
ball milling (in an "inert" liquid such as CFC 11) or "controlled" microcrystallization to produce
drug with sizes in the 1 to 5 µm range. Characterization should be repeated after size reduction
in order to assess its impact on the physicochemical properties of the drug.

One of the major goals of the preformulation work is to minimize the solubility of the drug
in the chosen propellants. This is partly achieved by selecting liquified gases with low dielectric
constants as the continuous phase in the suspension. The solubility may be minimized further
by selecting drug (salts, acids, bases, and/or polymorphs) and crystal forms with the smallest
solubilities in propellants. Solvates, especially hydrates, should be excluded if at all possible due
to the doubt associated with the stability of solvent-drug binding in the solid phase. Interestingly,
one marketed steroid product is quoted in the *Physician's Desk Reference*[94] as containing a
clathrate compound with CFC 11 in suspension, showing that solvates involving the continuous
phase of the suspension are both possible and permissible. Ideally, the solubilities of several
characterized drug forms should be determined in pure propellants and several propellant
blends. This can be accomplished by packaging excess solid in aerosol containers with
continuous valves and adding propellant subsequently. Various methods may be devised to
separate the propellant from the solid drug prior to or during actuation, to deliver the liquid
propellant into a collection medium prior to drug assay.[69,73] The weight of propellant delivered
can be found most easily be determining the weight of the container before and after delivery.

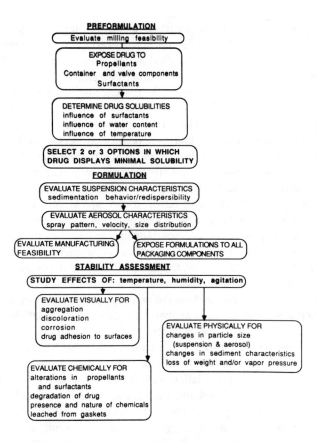

FIGURE 10. Schematic showing steps in the preformulation, formulation, and stability assessment of an MDI.

The rate at which crystal growth can be expected to occur in a suspension should be related to the solubility of the drug in the final formulation.[95,96] Although these solubility determinations are in no way compulsory, they are informative in terms of propellant blend selection and can often be used to predict manufacturing problems. For example, the common practice of preparing a suspension concentrate in CFC 11 can dissolve drug prior to its reprecipitation in different crystal sizes following the addition of CFC 12 and 114.[73,97] Early solubility determinations enable these problems to be flagged before expensive mistakes are made with large batches of material.

It is imperative while performing these experiments to do all packaging in a strictly controlled environment and to control water levels in all ingredients and components. Variable but trace quantities of water can produce large and misleading errors in solubility determinations. Packaging within a glove box may not be absolutely necessary for the final manufacturing process, but early solubility studies should be performed in such a way that trace quantities of solvents such as water are only introduced in a known and controlled fashion. The use of surfactants, of course, can also lead to drug solubility enhancement by solubilization in micelles. The most common surfactants in current use in MDIs are sorbitan trioleate, lecithin, and oleic acid. Only the latter is normally obtained as a pure compound and thus careful control of the true content of these mixed materials is important if reproducible results are required. Other low HLB[98] surfactants are also possible. The preference for nonionic materials stems only from an observation that in general these are less membrane-toxic than cationic or anionic surfactants. Nevertheless, all types have been administered by inhalation and it is extremely difficult to show toxic effects in the doses which are conventionally associated with MDI usage.

The influence of surfactant type, concentration, and temperature on drug solubilities should also be determined (Figure 10). The popular concept of inverted micelles forming in nonaqueous media containing surfactants above their critical micelle concentration, (CMC) should not be assumed without question. Surfactant micellization in aqueous media is believed to be an entropy driven process due, in large part, to the presence of molecular structuring in water (around the hydrophobic portions of surfactant monomers) which can be partly disrupted by the process of micellization.[99] However, the liquid nature of water is due to its tendency to structure or polymerize via hydrogen bonds. Structuring is predictably very much less in low dielectric media with smaller dipole interactions. Indeed, the high vapor pressure of many propellants is a direct measure of the lack of dipole interaction between the propellant molecules. The behavior of low HLB surfactants in low dielectric media is less well documented than that of mid- to high HLB systems in water. The incidence of dimer, trimer, and larger molecular aggregates of surfactant which result in some systems with increasing surfactant concentrations[100] does not necessarily confer micelle structure and solubilizing capacity on the aggregates. In other nonaqueous systems, water is a known promoter of inverted micelle formation.[101] In systems containing micellized or solubilized water, an estimate of drug solubility can result from the sum of three separate phenomena. Drug dissolution in both propellant or solubilized water is possible. Thirdly, drug itself may act as a micelle promoter and sweller[101] in the absence of water to form a surfactant-drug complex of unknown stoichiometry. To conclude on this point, it is necessary to build a substantial database concerning drug solubility in nonaqueous systems if we are to place the subject of MDI suspension formulation on a scientific basis. While this cannot be accomplished overnight, it is to be hoped in the future that an increasing number of papers will be devoted to the use of preformulation predictors of nonaqueous suspension stability.

At some stage during these early solubility determinations, it is advisable to begin to screen a model formulation, packed in plastic coated glass vials, against all prospective packaging components (valve construction polymers, gasket materials, metals, etc.). Gasket swelling, polymer dissolution, corrosion, particle adhesion and aggregation at interfaces, and loss or gain of vapor pressure are all physical properties which may be monitored qualitatively and/or quantitatively. From a chemical viewpoint it is probably worth performing assays on the drug and propellants at this stage. Leachable materials such as plasticizers in gaskets can be a problem from the standpoint of product contamination as well as the likelihood of promoting more rapid propellant loss with lengthened storage times. In some cases it may be worthwhile quantifying nonvolatile residues which cannot be ascribed to drug or surfactant after propellant evaporation. These procedures again act as warning flags to prevent expensive mistakes further down the line. This may preclude further consideration of a gasket or valve material because of the existence of an obvious physical and/or chemical incompatibility. In other cases, it will begin to provide useful control data for comparison to that collected from stability assessment studies performed on one or two major formulation options later (Figure 10). The route toward these major formulation options often requires consideration of manufacturing techniques. For example, filling a volatile suspension formulation through the valve without previously dispensing drug in a low volatility concentrate is a considerable technical challenge. However, aside from the issues of "scale up" for manufacture, several decisions must be made and a series of experiments performed, to enable the selection of the better formulation options.

At this stage we should have some idea of which drug form to suspend and which propellant-surfactant combinations not to choose (the ones in which drug solubility is highest will have the greatest predictable crystal growth and aggregate problems). Assume briefly that we have also decided upon one or two specific propellant blends, a particular drug concentration in suspension, the valve metering volume and the particle size distribution of the drug (these issues are discussed later). If this is the case, optimizing the suspension characteristics of the formulation remains necessary. We can presume for the purposes of MDI formulation that making a viscous or thixotropic gel to keep the particles from colliding to form a nondispersible cake[102] will lead to difficulties in production of a fine spray.[103,104] The dogma on the issue of suspension formulation invokes the DLVO theory[102,105] and states that in a continuous medium (in which solid particles, dissolved surfactant, and propellant molecules are all free to move), we should seek to flocculate (or aggregate) the suspension in a controlled fashion and to stabilize it by secondary minimum flocculation.[30,102,104] In aqueous media this is normally accomplished by carefully titrating interparticulate forces between particles as a function of distance between them.[104] Attractive van der Waal's forces are related to particle size while repulsive forces are usually considered to be steric (due to surfactant tails projecting from the solid surfaces) or electronic (due to counterions and/or surface charge at the solid-liquid interface). Figures 11A and B were generated to show the importance of steric stabilization in nonaqueous systems using the technique described by Schneider et al.[104] Using this method of calculation, the electronic (repulsive) interactions in low dielectric media are much smaller than those values calculated with water as the continuous phase (Figure 11A). Because some charge may well exist at equilibrium on suspended solid particles in a poorly conducting medium,[105] the situation shown in Figure 11A assumes an equal zeta potential[104] in hexane and water. Static surface charge possessed at the time of initial suspension should dissipate slowly in nonconducting media, but surface equilibrium may still take a considerable time to establish. In Figure 11B, the total interaction energy (sum of attractive van der Waal's and repulsive electronic and steric energies) is shown for the same 0.2 μm particles in hexane with different thicknesses of an adsorbed surfactant layer. A comparison of the magnitude of the interaction energies between Figure 11A and B shows the predominance of steric factors in the stabilization of nonaqueous suspension systems. As a generalism it becomes possible to state that steric forces (which presumably are the most dependent upon the molecular characteristics of the chosen surfactant) are the only variable which can reasonably be manipulated in order to achieve secondary minimum flocculation in low dielectric propellants. The theory[104] is complicated by the observation that each individual interaction energy is a different function of particle size.

With propellants, drug concentration, and size distribution held constant, the suspension characteristics must be manipulated by choice of surfactant and its concentration. Reviewing the suspension properties as a function of these variables involves quantification of apparent sedimentation velocities, sedimentation ratios (height of settled sediment/height of original formulation), redispersibility, and the size characteristics of the aerosolized drug after shaking and actuating the trial formulations.[69,73,97,102] It is important when prototype formulations are made to ensure that good deaggregation of the initial micronized drug is achieved in each case; variability in small scale manufacturing technique in this respect (poor mixing leaving clumps of material in suspension) can be interpreted later as effects due to surfactant. Methods of manufacturing small numbers of MDIs with different formulations have been described previously.[23,69,97] Although some mixing shear in the valve is involved, one way of checking to ensure adequate initial powder deaggregation is to collect the product (from the valve) immediately after packaging by actuating under the surface of CFC 11. A microscope slide may be made from this suspension and inspected for aggregates. Assuming that the manufacturing process achieved adequate deaggregation in each case, the sedimentation ratios themselves may still provide little information about the redispersibility or the aerodynamic properties of the product. Figure 12 shows a short series of 1% disodium fluorescein suspension aerosols containing variable quantities of sorbitan trioleate as Span 85 after standing for 20 d at room temperature. The sedimentation ratios are shown in Table 1 alongside the respirable dose fractions (% of dose less than 5.5 μm aerodynamic diameter) obtained from each preparation after sizing by dynamic cascade impaction.[23,97] The suspension with the largest sedimentation ratio is clearly not the best from an aerosol point of view. All preparations were easily redispersible in that one complete revolution of the container was sufficient to produce an apparently homogeneous dispersion and there was no clear difference in the times taken to reach an apparent sedimentation equilibrium. Differences in sedimentation kinetics are usually taken

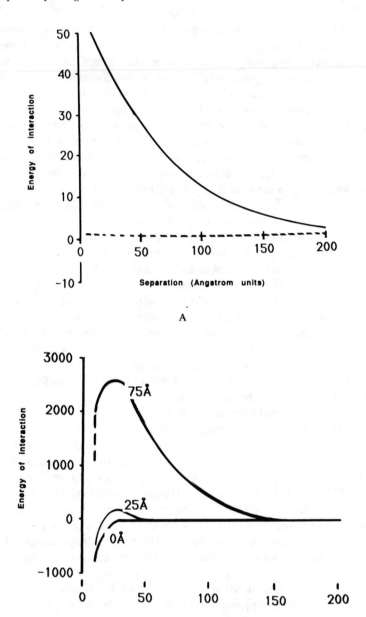

FIGURE 11.   Particle interaction energies calculated according to Reference 104. Dimensionless energies are plotted vs. interparticulate separation for 0.2 μm solid particles in all cases. At zero separation, in the "primary minimum", large negative energy values are typical. Positive energies are repulsive while negative are attractive. (A) Electronic energies of repulsion for particles with identical zeta potential = 25 mV in water (solid line) and hexane (dotted line). Hexane's dielectric constant is 43 times lower than that of water. (B) Total interaction energies in hexane with 0, 25, and 75Å thicknesses of adsorbed surfactant at the particle interface. The total energy is dominated by the term for steric repulsion,[104] despite the existence of a 25-mV zeta potential on the particles.

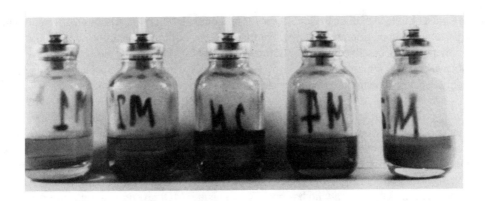

FIGURE 12.   Different sedimentation heights for 1% micronized disodium fluorescein suspensions in chlorofluorocarbon propellants containing sorbitan trioleate as Span 85 in several concentrations (L to R): 1:1, 1:1.2, 1:1.4, 1:1.6, 1:1.8 drug: surfactant.

TABLE 1
Sedimentation Ratios and Percentage of the Dose Showing Aerodynamic Diameters Less than 5 µm for MDIs Containing 1% Micronized Disodium Fluorescein and Different Surfactant Concentrations

Formulation[a]	Sed. ratio[b]	% dose <5.5 µm[c]
1.0	0.40	13.7
1.2	0.70	11.2
1.4	0.50	20.6
1.6	0.50	6.8
1.8	0.85	7.5

[a]   Span 85/disodium fluorescein ratio by weight.
[b]   (sediment height after 20 days at 21°C)/(height of original formulation).
[c]   Percent of disodium fluorescein dose emitted as aerosol with aerodynamic diameters less than 5µm (dynamic sizing).

to indicate differences in the size of "flocs" or aggregates formed as a result of particle collisions. Hiestand[102] has observed the difficulty, even with aqueous dispersions, of discerning the precise nature of flocculation and whether the aggregates are broken apart during agitation. Gonda[30] believes that the forces holding flocs together in MDIs are small and can be broken during the processes of actuation and aerosolization. While I am in general agreement with these presumptions, the subject is far from clear. The most important tests in this regard are to discern (1) whether the drug material is adequately deaggregated during manufacture, (2) whether redispersibility is easy and allows doses to be metered reproducibly, and (3) which surfactant concentration-drug combination gives the greatest respirable fraction.

The values for sedimentation ratio in propellant blends can vary dramatically between formulations. The values shown in Table 1 are relatively high. In a suspension with 1% solid material by volume, closest packing would produce a sedimentation ratio a little over 0.01. With no apparent redispersibility problems, our values for the sedimentation ratio with the bronchodilator drug, terbutaline sulfate, stabilized in 1% suspension by lecithin were much smaller than those shown in Table 1 and about 0.05.[73] Terbutaline sulfate has a density <1.4 g/cm^3 and floats to the surface in a CFC 11/12/114 blend with a ratio by weight of 1:2:1, respectively. The density of this blend is approximately 1.4 g/cm^{3,} while disodium fluorescein has a density[106,107] of 1.46 to 1.49 g/cm^3 and therefore sinks in the same blend (Figure 12). If the form of these relatively stable suspensions has anything to do with secondary minimum flocculation, any unifying theory must be able to explain these differences in sedimentation ratio. Although differences in interparticulate separation are possible, the major explanation is probably to be found in the experimentally inaccessible particle coordination number.[102] This can be viewed as the average number of particles which any other particle within a floc contacts via a surfactant bridge and is highly dependent on the interfacial tension between the solid and continuous phase. Figures like that shown in Figure 11B only help to visualize the distance between *two single particles* which a particular surfactant layer may promote from an unstable to a metastable state, where an energy barrier must be overcome in order to proceed from a secondary minimum to the stable primary minimum shown in Figure 11B.

Deciding on a particular propellant blend involves a series of compromises. From a marketing standpoint, the bad press which the CFC propellants are presently receiving would no doubt give the salesperson who has no CFCs in his/her MDI an edge over the competition. Because our discussion is restricted to the formulation of suspension systems, however, it is difficult to suggest good substitutes to these pharmacologically and chemically inert propellants. The proposed chlorofluorohydrocarbons (CFHC) are purposefully more reactive chemically to reduce their lifetimes in the atmosphere. While this does not preclude them from MDI usage, they are not the agents of choice in a pharmaceutical preparation over the CFCs. Flammability can also pose problems.[108] While the CFHCs are likely to possess greater chemical and pharmacologic reactivities, any anesthetic properties which may be expected are likely to be minor when the doses are taken into account (25 μl of a typical propellant produces about 6 cm^3 of gas at room temperature[109]). From a suspension formulator's point of view, the smaller the dielectric constant of the propellant chosen, the lower the drug solubility is likely to be. This is why CFC 11 is usually quoted as a "better solvent" than CFC 12 and 114.[44] It is also why CFC 12 is so much more volatile than CFC 11; the intermolecular attractive forces of the latter are much greater and its escaping tendencies much smaller than those of CFC 12. From a pharmaceutical point of view, the move toward CFHCs is less rational than a move toward FCs[110] or totally fluorinated derivatives. These should have minimal reactivity with the ozone layer whose destruction is believed to be due to the reactivity of the chlorosubstituents in the CFCs.[11] Market forces are the reason for the seemingly irrational trend; CFHCs and CFCs are about 100 times cheaper to produce than FCs and the market for either is negligibly associated with MDI manufacture. To preserve and improve a successful dosage form in the face of the CFC-ozone issue, the pharmaceutical industry can take one or two routes. A campaign could usefully be mounted to educate physicians and the public concerning the trivial contribution of CFCs in MDIs to overall usage of these chemicals. Even in the U.S., the public still seems to suffer from the delusion that aerosols are the major cause of the CFC pollution problem. Considering that these propellants have been banned in the U.S. in all except a small number of medicinal aerosols for application to mucous membranes since 1978, it is hardly surprising that the U.S. aerosol industry has been through some lean times recently. Alternatively, the pharmaceutical industry itself could produce CFCs and other propellants for use specifically in these dosage forms. If the lung can also be used as a route of systemic drug administration for low dose peptides and proteins[111], the investment would be well worthwhile.

There are two other issues concerned with selection of an appropriate propellant blend. Neither of these are discussed in detail here because information is readily available elsewhere.[43,44,47,51] Vapor pressure and density vary with temperature and the selected propellant blend. These properties are usually predictable from ideal solution theory (Raoult's and Henry's laws[43]) because of the inert nature of the CFCs. The propellant manufacturer literature is an enormous and reliable source of information on different blends and their properties and is well worth studying with a simple text on physical properties in hand.[43] Unlike the hydrocarbons, the density of the major CFCs and their blends is approximately the same as that associated with many pharmaceutical solids.[112] Therefore, settling velocities of micronized powders can be minimized fairly readily and some MDI preparations, if left in a nonisothermal environment,

TABLE 2
Densities and Vapor Pressures of the Major Blends of CFC Propellants Used Currently in Suspension MDIs

Blend[a]	Example[b]	V.P.[c]	Density[d]
25.0/50.0/25.0	Brethaire (Geigy)	42.1	1.44
28.0/72.0/0.0	Ventolin (Glaxo)	52.2	1.37
0.0/60.0/40.0	Intal (Fisons)	52.9	1.38

[a] Parts ratio by weight. CFC11/CFC12/CFC114.
[b] A single example of each is provided. Brethaire is an Astra product, marketed under license in the U.S. by Geigy.
[c] Pounds per square inch (psi) gauge; 21°C. Absolute pressure is 14.7 psi (1 atm = 14.7 psi = 101.3 knm^{-2}) more.
[d] Calculated, assuming ideality, g cm^{-3}.

show little tendency to settle at all. The density of any blend will decrease at elevated temperatures and this can lead to several problems. Because propellants are usually metered by volume into containers, fill weights often change during manufacture. Check weighing is an important quality assurance step. More importantly, with increased temperatures, consideration must be given not only to changing pressures of the gas phase within the container, but also to changing volume of the liquid phase. At some temperature, dependent upon the percentage of the container volume which the liquid phase originally occupied, the container will be completely filled with liquid and the pressure will rise precipitately; the pressure will cease to be dictated by the vapor-liquid equilibrium and the container will burst.

The choice of propellant blend can be thought of most simply as one which ensures a good compromise among (1) an optimum density for minimal settling at normal ambient temperatures, (2) an optimum vapor pressure for spray formation, yet one which is safe to transport, (3) ease vs. difficulty in handling (safe scale-up and manufacture), (4) the display of minimal drug solubility, and (5) a lack of chemical incompatibilities. While the number of options is infinite, it is necessary to start somewhere and the blends which are on the market were not arrived at by accident! Although other options also have their merits, Table 2 shows three blends of CFCs marketed in different MDIs alongside their vapor pressures and densities. While density has obvious influences on the metered dose through suspension concentration and metering volume, vapor pressure variations have the most profound effects on the nature of the aerosol produced during actuation.[55-57,83,103,113] The subject will be discussed as it relates to the production of respirable aerosol with aerodynamic diameters <5 µm and gradually complicated by the introduction of additional variables: metering volume, suspension concentration, drug particle size, and surfactant concentration.

The liquid in an MDI suspension occupies 95 to 100% of the sprayed formulation. Not surprisingly, therefore, the nature of this liquid or propellant and the speed with which it is propelled by its own vapor tend to dictate the droplet sizes formed at the spray nozzle of the actuator. Despite the fact that low surface tension liquids are known to produce smaller droplets upon spraying than their high tension counterparts, the fact is difficult to exploit. Low dielectric materials have low surface tensions[114] to begin with and surfactants are not believed to orient at the liquid-gas interface quickly enough to affect the droplet size distribution upon spraying.[103] Furthermore, suspension concentrations which are normally used in MDIs are unlikely to be high enough to significantly influence bulk spray characteristics. While there may be differences in spray characteristics due to changes in the drug and/or surfactant concentrations in some droplet size ranges, the previous statements are supported by the data shown in Table 3. Here, a series of suspensions containing disodium fluorescein and sorbitan trioleate in different

TABLE 3

Percent Dose Emitted as Aerosol and Percent Retained in the Actuator for Identically Packaged MDIs with Substantially Different Formulations[40]

Formulation[a]	Actuator (%)[b]	Aerosol (%)[c]
0.1	29.4 (1.4)	70.6
0.5	31.0 (1.4)	69.0
1.0	32.4 (1.3)	67.6
2.0	32.8 (1.4)	67.2

Note: Actuator (Valois IN2) retention remained effectively constant despite the wide variation in formulations tested.

[a] Percent weight/volume disodium fluorescein (DF) in suspension in CFC propellants. Surfactant (Span 85) was present in a ratio of 1:4:1 surfactant:DF in all cases.
[b] Percent of dose of DF retained by the actuator. Value in parenthesis is S.D.
[c] Percent emitted as aerosol. Particle size of the aerosol flume varied with formulation.

concentrations were packaged identically and are shown to have almost identical actuator retention due to impaction of large droplets (the spray diverges as it leaves the jet and collides with the internal walls of the mouthpiece shown in Figure 2). Because the droplet spray characteristics are almost identical for the large droplets in these distributions, fractional drug deposition on the walls due to impaction is independent of suspension and surfactant concentration and represents a constant proportion of the metered dose in each case.

Figure 13, taken from Rance,[25] shows aerosol flume velocity as a function of distance from the jet for a spray jet with a diameter of about 0.4 mm and several different propellant vapor pressures. Volume median diameters for droplets about 10 cm distant from this jet would be expected to be in the range of 15 to 20 μm[69] for the higher vapor pressure formulation, while those at the jet itself should be nearer to 35 μm.[27] Although it is possible to use nozzles with smaller jets and smaller droplet size distributions may result, it is important to note that this is not always true and because patients do not always keep their inhalers clean, jet blockage can result if very small diameters are used. Literature reports which indicate that smaller droplets result from higher vapor pressure systems[35,78] often do not emphasize that the effects are due in large part to higher rates of droplet vaporization. While higher driving pressures are known to produce somewhat smaller droplets *at the jet,* an increase of about 1 atm in vapor pressure (Table 2) probably does little in this regard[103] until we make allowances for the fact that the continuous phase of the suspension begins boiling the moment it reaches the inside of the valve stem (Figure 2). Under these circumstances, and until the liquid cools substantially due to evaporation, suspended particles in large droplets probably act as vapor nuclei or "boiling granules" causing droplets to explode and become rapidly smaller. Whether this hypothesis is true and what the size limit for such a phenomenon may be requires research and visualization of the actual spray phenomenon. Studies may be possible with the aid of high resolution pulsed laser holography.[81,82] While smaller spray jets effectively limit the rate of flow and lengthen spray duration for a particular propellant, doubling the driving pressure while holding the actuator constant does the opposite.

Although the trend more recently has been to formulate higher pressure systems,[26] the approach is not without its problems. Taking values for velocity at 10 cm from the spray jet from the upper curve of Figure 13 and calculating[115] √(Stokes' number) for 15 to 20 μm droplets with densities = 1.4 g/cm[3] traveling in a 5-cm diameter airstream, one produces values in the range 0.68 to 0.9. Comparison of these values to those required for impaction 10 cm from the jet (approximately the distance to the back of the throat), using Figure 2 in the previous chapter, reveals that the majority of these droplets will impact in the case of the higher vapor pressure formulations used in MDIs. Raising the exit velocity by increasing the vapor pressure will increase the probability that smaller droplets will also impact in the oropharynx (Equation 2,

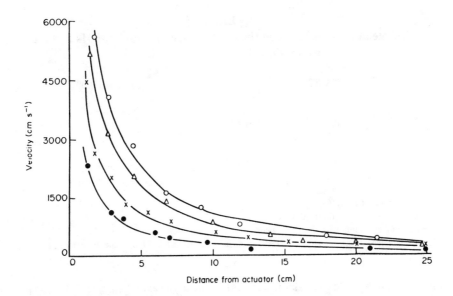

FIGURE 13.   Variation of the velocity of sprays with distance from the spray jet for differently pressurized aerosols. Key: O, Δ, X, • are 359, 290, 221, and 152 kNm⁻², respectively. (From Rance, R. W., *J. Soc. Cosmet. Chem.*, 25, 545, 1974. With permission.)

Chapter 6). Thus, while higher pressures may create smaller droplets and spacers may be used, an optimum vapor pressure may exist for each system. There is obviously a need to find out exactly what the most crucial factors are and to determine the impact of drug and surfactant concentration upon those factors. To decide between different vapor pressure systems it may be possible to use throat deposition models[116,117] at appropriate volume flow rates. Because of the existence of different oropharyngeal geometries occurring with different inhalation flows,[118] from the point of view of the laboratory worker, it would be nice to see one or two of these models validated *in vivo* for different inspiratory flows.

Selecting a metering volume involves the estimation of the required respirable dose. This is normally determined based upon pharmacologic results obtained from an inhaled nebulized solution, given estimates of deposition as described in Chapter 6. If, for example, a 10% deposition is presumed for the MDI, then the metered dose must be 10 times larger than the required respirable dose. A knowledge of the propellant density and proposed drug concentration is then all that is really necessary to fix the metering volume, unless a purpose built unit is designed and validated. Because a limited range of volumes are usually offered by valve manufacturers, the concentration of drug is usually manipulated to fit the available sizes. For toxicologic reasons and due to the work performed by Moren[26] there is a tendency to choose the smaller metering volumes (and higher suspension concentrations) where there is a lower requirement for propellant evaporation prior to the production of dry micronized particles as the aerosol. Unfortunately, this approach involves a compromise due to the spraying of aggregates of increased sizes at increased suspension concentrations. The subject is treated in depth by Gonda.[30,31] As the metering volume is reduced, the drug concentration must be increased to hold the dose constant. Because a fixed volume of a particular propellant will spray through a jet into an approximately constant number of droplets, the required inclusion of a larger number of micronized particles necessitates the formation of aerodynamically larger clusters or aggregates of drug leading to a less respirable system. Because Gonda's theory deals only with monodisperse (with respect to particle size) drug particles in mono- or polydisperse droplets, it is difficult to apply to a situation where the particles are actually polydispersed. The data in Table 4 are reproduced[30] to show the way in which different volumetric suspension concentrations, C, and

TABLE 4

Numerical Relationships Between the Drug Concentration in MDIs and the Size Distribution of the Aerosol Product[30]

C%V/V[a]	D/d[b]	n[c]	MMAD/d[d]
0.1	5.0	1.06	1.0
0.1	10.0	1.58	1.07
1.0	5.0	1.75	1.12
1.0	10.0	10.0	1.98
2.0	10.0	20.0	2.46
3.0	10.0	30.0	2.81

[a]   Volumetric concentration (%).
[b]   Droplet, D, to particle , d, diameter ratio.
[c]   Average number of drug particles per cluster.
[d]   Mass median aerodynamic diameter of evaporated aerosol product divided by the diameter of the primary particle, d.

different droplet to particle diameter ratios, D/d, relate to the average number of drug particles per cluster, n, and the ratio of MMAD for cluster to that of the original drug particle. Although this table assumes that monodisperse particles are sprayed in monodisperse droplets, the results are generally also true[31] for the case when monodisperse particles are sprayed in polydisperse droplets (when these are log-normally distributed with respect to size). The primary difference in the latter case is that the polydispersity of the droplets endows a similar or equivalent geometric standard deviation on the final dry aerosol product. This statement is true despite the original powder in suspension possessing monodispersity. At high values of C (Table 4; C = 2 or 3%) the MMAD is raised more than 2-fold by aggregates of 20 or 30 particles existing per cluster. The smaller increases in MMAD for lower values of C are, of course, much more permissible when the droplet size, D, is halved relative to the primary particle diameter (Table 4; D/d = 5). The importance of this D/d ratio to the subject of cluster formation further begs the question of what drug size to select. Although the tendency may be to comminute to as small a size as possible,[55] there must be limits to the usefulness of this approach. The subject of cluster formation clouds the issue because of the tendency to subdivide a constant dose between a fixed number of droplets following actuation. It should be clear from this discussion that even to optimize a formulation in terms of drug concentration, particle size, and metering volume is not straightforward. The need for expanded theory backed up by experiment is evident.

To increase the respirable dose we must maximize the number of smaller satellite droplets which contain respirable drug clusters. The current practice of formulation optimization, however, has changed little since the presentation of the early but excellent work by Polli et al.[55] in 1969. The basis of the work involved the comparison of aerosol size distributions (after the bulk of droplet evaporation had occurred) from different formulations for the whole of the dose emitted by the MDI. Size information after evaporation is important not only because smaller aerosols should contain greater respirable dose fractions, but also because the importance of cluster formation[30,31] can only be detected given size information for the complete aerosolized dose. Nevertheless, this experimental approach[55] fails to consider droplet inertia and impaction efficiency. Also, sizing the aerosol under dynamic conditions[23,64] where complete evaporation is not allowed due to the use of a smaller evaporation chamber and/or more rapid flow rates prevents the contamination of data for the *respirable dose fraction close to the actuator* by large masses of drug from much larger droplets. These large droplets and the drug which they contain are only respirable after a substantial velocity reduction and evaporation opportunity. Sizing MDI output by impaction in these different ways (during and after evaporation has occurred) is a valuable means of collecting additional information.

A typical aerosol flume following actuation of an MDI extends about 40 cm from the spray jet and is roughly conical in shape. Droplet evaporation commences at the time of initial spray formation. The spray consists of a broad range of droplet diameters and thus, even ignoring the process of evaporation, the small respirable droplets tend to stop much sooner than their larger counterparts. Considering the calculations which are presented graphically in Figure 14, it is obvious that the smaller satellite droplets[15] with smaller stopping distances[115] will be concentrated in the flume closer to the spray jet than the larger primary droplets, even though their velocity at the spray jet was identical. In recent work we inserted a series of baffles into the actuators of some model MDIs with calculated vapor pressures of 41.4 psig.[40] Spray formation appeared to be effectively complete for these systems at about 1 cm from the opening of the jet to the atmosphere. The work on the baffles themselves showed that the ratio of (respirable)/(nonrespirable) aerosol output could be maximized by optimal placement of a spherical baffle close to the spray jet. While the individual results were a function of formulation and MDI design, the conclusions in that work would have been masked if sufficient opportunity had been allowed for large droplets to evaporate and thus contribute to the apparent respirable fraction in the aerosol flume. Similarly, laser light scattering also has its place because it can provide comparative information on spray droplet sizes at different distances from the actuator.[57]

As a summary of this section on formulation, it is unwise to rely on one or two experimental methods to perform the job of formulation and device optimization. Numerous techniques provide valuable information and in some cases different operating procedures (e.g., impaction at different flow rates, light scattering at different points in the flume and times after actuation) can be used to enhance the information content of the data in a way dependent upon the experimental goals. Data interpretation from all experimental techniques is at least as important as its collection and requires an adequate understanding of basic aerosol science.[115] Some of the material emitted from the spray jet is small enough to be respirable at the outset. Some drug is issued in droplets which are so big that complete evaporation may take several seconds to occur, and some solid aggregates which are most likely emitted in larger droplets will never be respirable with or without this evaporation. It is the job of the pharmaceutical aerosol scientist to find a means of studying all of these drug categories, maximizing and ensuring reproducibility of the respirable material, and eliminating the nonrespirable drug from the aerosol.

3. Stability Assessment

There are two aspects of this subject which need to be considered here. The first involves the selection of conditions under which the stability of the chosen formulation(s) is to be evaluated, while the second concerns the selection of testing procedures. It is not the function of this chapter to describe compendial methods or to list the demands of regulatory agencies like the U.S. Food and Drug Administration. Furthermore, it will be apparent to some of the industrial users of this text that many test procedures must be evolved during the preformulation and formulation stages of the work, and as a result, these will be product and formulation specific. Nevertheless, because stability testing will define a shelflife and many of the label requirements for the product, it is pertinent to discuss protocol design and some of the more general aspects of stability testing at this juncture.

Table 5 is a list of independent and dependent variables which are commonly studied within a stability testing protocol for a suspension MDI. As far as protocol design is concerned, transport and personal carriage induced vibration or agitation can be a cause of reduced shelflife. Large external pressure (and temperature) reductions occur in the storage holds of airplanes and can cause leaks and explosions. While label disclaimers are one approach to this problem, it is wiser to produce a product which will stand up to air travel in checked baggage in the first instance. Other predictable variations in temperature, pressure, and relative humidity should also be covered. While the influence of low pressure and temperature should be studied for short periods, most of the protocol is usually concerned with ambient and elevated conditions of

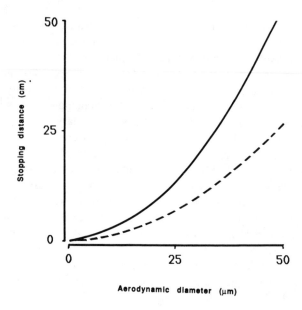

FIGURE 14.   Stopping distances in still air vs. aerodynamic diameter for droplets traveling at an initial velocity of 50 m/s (solid line) or
25 m/s (dotted line).

temperature and relative humidity under static and cycling conditions. As one example, a static
test of stability at 40°C and 75% relative humidity is used by several manufacturers. Dramatic
failures like exploding containers or severely leaking valve seals should have been sorted out
much earlier by making adjustments in packaging components and manufacturing variables. It
is common practice to include overage in the formulation to extend shelflife. This practice
requires tighter control of the manufacturing function than would otherwise be required to
produce units complying with compendial dose-uniformity tests. Current good manufacturing
practice and quality control procedures which emanate from some of the larger manufacturers
of MDIs ensure that products are manufactured far more stringently than compendial tests would
imply.

The most obvious dependent variables in Table 5 are particle size distribution, total output
from the unit, and reproducibility. Spray patterns (including spray duration and spray velocity),
valve function, and the color, taste, and odor of residues are important "customer accessed"
variables which can influence the marketability of an otherwise acceptable product. Weights and
vapor pressures of all units should be recorded systematically because all MDIs leak and lose
the most volatile propellants preferentially. It is also wise to chill and open a representative
number of each test batch to inspect for obvious crystal growth, container and valve interactions,
product agglomeration, and/or creeping up the walls of the container prior to performing
analyses to identify nonformulation components in the residues. Chemical assay and control of
all purchased or synthesized ingredients is a presumed function of a quality control department
prior to manufacture of the MDIs. Assays for drug and ingredients are then repeated during
stability assessment on samples obtained for total output determination. The occasional
presence of unknown contaminant peaks on HPLC determinations sometimes requires identification, quantification, and limits to be imposed upon degradation products and materials which
can be leached from gasket materials. Minute doses of contaminating materials are usually of
minimal consequence toxicologically. Nevertheless, because the patient must inhale the aerosol
as it is created by the complete MDI, regulatory authorities insist that the toxicologic evaluation
is performed upon the final product and not upon a prototype. In practice, the stability assessment

TABLE 5
Some Dependent and Independent Variables for Consideration in the Design of MDI Stability Trials

Independent	Dependent
Temperature	Particle size
Relative humidity	Total output
Agitation	Dosage reproducibility
Environmental pressure	Valve function
	Spray pattern
	Nature and distribution of chemicals in nonvolatile residues
	Leakage; weight and vapor pressure change
	Odor and taste
	Nature of residue remaining inside the container; agglomerates and corrosion products

extends throughout the various phases of clinical trials and may take several years to complete. It is during this phase that acceptable quality limits (AQLs) must be set and adhered to. Frequently these AQLs become more stringent as the time which a product has spent on the market becomes greater.

This chapter has described the formulation, generation, and delivery aspects of drugs from MDIs. The emphasis has been placed on pressurized suspension systems which are most popular in the U.S., even though DPGs are currently undergoing a renaissance in Europe. There are numerous possibilities for further exploitation of drug delivery by inhalation though our understanding of this route is presently in its infancy. The chapter was intended to demystify the subject by presenting it simply and logically, while identifying and highlighting areas of ignorance which, as they are researched, will enhance our ability to exploit this route in the future.

REFERENCES

1. **Powell, M. L., Chung, M., Weisberger, M. S., Gural R., Radwanski, E., Symchowicz, S., and Patrick, J. E.,** Multiple dose albuterol kinetics, *J. Clin. Pharmacol.,* 26, 643, 1986.
2. **Jonkman, J. H. G., Freie, H. M. P., van der Boon, W. J. V., and Grasmeijer, G.,** Single dose absorption profiles and bioavailability of two different salbutamol tablets, *Arzneim. Forsch.,* 36, (II), 1133, 1986.
3. **Brittain, R. T., Jack, D., and Ritchie, A. C.,** Recent β-adrenoceptor stimulants, *Adv. Drug Res.,* 5, 197, 1970.
4. **Walker, S. R., Evans, M. E., Richards, A. J., and Paterson, J. W.,** The clinical pharmacology of oral and inhaled salbutamol, *Clin. Pharmacol. Ther.,* 13, 861, 1972.
5. **Weisberger, M., Patrick, J. E., and Powell, M. L.,** Quantitative analysis of albuterol in human plasma by combined gas chromatography and chemical ionization mass spectrometry, *Biomed. Mass.,* 10, 556, 1983.
6. **Moren, F.,** Pressurized aerosols for oral inhalation, *Int. J. Pharm.,* 8, 1, 1981.
7. **Bronsky, E., et al.,** Comparison of inhaled albuterol powder and aerosol in asthma, *J. Allergy Clin. Immunol.,* 79, 741, 1987.
8. **Persson, G., Gruvstad, E., and Wiren, J. E.,** Therapeutic effect of Turbuhaler in comparison with metered dose inhaler in adults, in *A New Concept in Inhalation Therapy,* Newman, S. P., Moren, F., and Crompton, G. K., Eds., Medicom, Bussum/London, 1981, 136.
9. **Rogers, A.,** Counselling on inhaler therapy, *Pharm. J.,* 239, 652, 1987.
10. **Self, T. H. and Fuentes, R. J.,** Metered dose inhalers and extender devices, *U.S. Pharmacist,* May 1985, 36.

11. **Cicerone, R. J., Stolarski, R. S., and Walters, S.,** Stratospheric ozone destruction by man-made chlorofluoromethanes, *Science,* 185, 1165, 1974.
12. **Pover, G. M., Browning, A. K., Mullinger, B. M., Butler, A. G., and Dash, C. H.,** A new dry powder inhaler, *Practioner,* 226, 565, 1982.
13. **Newman, S. P.,** Production of radioaerosols, in *Aerosols and the Lung: Clinical and Experimental Aspects,* Clark, S. W. and Pavia, D., Eds., Butterworths, London, 1984, 71.
14. **Byron, P. R.,** Some future perspectives for unit dose inhalation aerosols, *Drug Dev. Ind. Pharm.,* 12, 993, 1986.
15. **Byron, P. R.,** Pulmonary targeting with aerosols, *Pharm. Tech.,* 11, 42, 1987.
16. **Vidgren, M. T., Karkkainen, A., Paronen, T. P., and Karjalainen, P.,** Respiratory tract deposition of 99mTc-labelled drug particles administered via a dry powder inhaler, *Int. J. Pharm.,* 39, 101, 1987.
17. **Byron, P. R., Davis, S. S., Bubb, M. D., and Cooper, P.,** Pharmaceutical implications of particle growth at high relative humidity, *Pest. Sci.,* 8, 521, 1977.
18. **Moss, G. F., Jones, K. M., Ritchie, J. T., and Cox, J. S. G.,** Plasma levels and urinary excretion of disodium cromoglycate after inhalation by human volunteers, *Toxicol. Appl. Pharmacol.,* 20, 147, 1971.
19. **Vidgren, M., Karkkainen, A., Karjalainen, P., Paronen, P., and Nuutinen, J.,** Effect of powder inhaler design on drug deposition in the respiratory tract, *Int. J. Pharm.,* 42, 211, 1988.
20. **Fiese, E. F., Gorman, W. G., Dolinski, D., Harwood, R. J., Hunke, W. A., Miller, N. C., Mintzer, H., and Harper, N. J.,** Test method for evaluation of loss of prime in metered-dose aerosols, *J. Pharm. Sci.,* 77, 90, 1988.
21. **Porush, I.,** Pharmaceutical products, in *Aerosols: Science and Technology,* Shepherd, H. R., Ed., Interscience, New York, 1961, 387.
22. **Bell, J. H., Brown, K., and Glasby, J.,** Variation in delivery of isoprenaline from various pressurized inhalers, *J. Pharm. Pharmacol.,* 25(Suppl.) 32, 1973.
23. **Dalby, R. N. and Byron, P. R.,** Comparison of output particle size distributions from pressurized aerosols formulated as solutions or suspensions, *Pharm. Res.,* 5, 36, 1988.
24. **Newman, S. P., Pavia, D., Moren, F., Sheahan, N. F., and Clarke, S. W.,** Deposition of pressurized aerosols in the respiratory tract, *Thorax,* 36, 52, 1981.
25. **Rance, R. W.,** Studies of the factors controlling the action of hair sprays. III. The influence of particle velocity and diameter on the capture of particles by arrays of hair fibres, *J. Soc. Cosmet. Chem.,* 25, 545, 1974.
26. **Moren, F.,** Drug deposition of pressurized inhalation aerosols. II. Influence of vapour pressure and metered volume, *Int. J. Pharm.,* 1, 213, 1978.
27. **Moren, F and Andersson, J.,** Fraction of dose exhaled after administration of pressurized inhalation aerosols, *Int. J. Pharm.,* 6, 295, 1980.
28. **Kim, C. S., Trujillo, D., and Sackner, M. A.,** Size aspects of metered dose inhaler aerosols, *Am. Rev. Resp. Dis.,* 132, 137, 1985.
29. **Hiller, C., Mazumder, M., Wilson, D., and Bone, R.,** Aerodynamic size distribution of metered dose bronchodilator aerosols, *Am. Rev. Resp. Dis.,* 118, 311, 1978.
30. **Gonda, I.,** Development of a systematic theory of suspension inhalation aerosols. I. A framework to study the effects of aggregation on the aerodynamic behaviour of drug particles, *Int. J. Pharm.,* 27, 99, 1985.
31. **Chan, H. K. and Gonda, I.,** Development of a systematic theory of suspension inhalation aerosols. II. Aggregates of monodisperse particles nebulized in polydisperse droplets, *Int. J. Pharm.,* 41, 147, 1988.
32. **Kirk, W.,** Aerosols for inhalation therapy, *Pharm. Int.,* 7, 150, 1986.
33. **Lewis, R. A., Cushley, M. J., Fleming, J. S., and Tattersfield, A. E,** Is a nebulizer less efficient than a metered dose inhaler and do pear shaped extension devices work?, *Am. Rev. Resp. Dis.,* 25, 94, 1982.
34. **Konig, P.,** Spacer devices used with metered dose inhalers: breakthrough or gimmick?, *Chest,* 88, 276, 1985.
35. **Sackner, M. A. and Kim, C. S.,** Auxillary MDI delivery systems, *Chest,* 88(Suppl.), 161S, 1985.
36. **Newman, S. P., Woodman, G., Clarke, S. W., and Sackner, M. A.,** Effect of InspirEase on the deposition of metered dose aerosols in the human respiratory tract, *Chest,* 89, 551, 1986.
37. **Moren, F.,** Studies on Pressurized Aerosols for Oral Inhalation, Ph.D. thesis, University of Uppsala, Sweden, 1980.
38. **Newman, S. P.,** *Deposition and Effects of Inhalation Aerosols,* AB Draco, Lund, Sweden, 1983.
39. **Vidgren, M. T., Paronen, T. P., Karkkainen, A., and Karjalainen, P.,** Effect of extension devices on the drug deposition from inhalation aerosols, *Int. J. Pharm.,* 39, 107, 1987.
40. **Byron, P. R., Dalby, R. N., and Hickey, A. J.,** Optimized inhalation aerosols. I. The effects of spherical baffle size and position upon the output of several pressurized nonaqueous suspension formulations, *Pharm. Res.,* 6, 1989.
41. **Hart, J.,** personal communication.
42. **Gorman, W. G. and Hall, G. D.,** Inhalation aerosols, in *Current Concepts in the Pharmaceutical Sciences: Dosage form Design and Bioavailability,* Swarbrick, J., Ed., Lea & Febiger, Philadelphia, 1973, 97.
43. **Sciarra, J. J. and Stoller, L.,** *The Science and Technology of Aerosol Packaging,* John Wiley & Sons, New York, 1974.
44. **Sanders, P. A.,** *Handbook of Aerosol Technology,* Van Nostrand Reinhold, New York, 1979.

45. **Shepherd, H. R., Ed.,** *Aerosols: Science and Technology,* Interscience, New York, 1961.
46. **Sciarra, J. J.,** Aerosols, in *Remington's Pharmaceutical Sciences,* 16th ed., Osol, A., Ed., Mack Publishing, Easton, PA, 1980, 1614.
47. **Johnsen, M. A.,** *The Aerosol Handbook,* 2nd ed., Wayne Dorland Publishing, Mendham, NJ, 1982.
48. **Kanig, J. L.,** Pharmaceutical aerosols, *J. Pharm. Sci.,* 61, 513, 1963.
49. **Sciarra, J. J. and Cutie, A. J.,** Pharmaceutical aerosols in *Theory and Practice of Industrial Pharmacy,* 3rd ed., Lachman, L., Lieberman, H. A., and Kanig, J. L., Eds., Lea & Febiger, Philadelphia, 1986, 270.
50. *The Aerosol Guide,* 7th ed., Chemical Specialties Manufacturer's Association, Washington, D.C., 1981.
51. *Hydrocarbon, Dimethyl Ether and Other Propellants: Considerations for Effective Handling in the Aerosol Plant and Laboratory,* Chemical Specialties Manufacturer's Association, Washington, D.C., 1981.
52. **CSMA Aerosol Division,** Aerosol division identifies critical issues affecting the industry, *Aerosol Age,* January, 12, 1988.
53. **Blakeway, J.,** Comparative study of alternative propellants to the chlorofluorocarbons in aerosols, *Soap Perfum. Cosmet.,* 53, 19, 1980.
54. **Riker Laboratories, Inc.,** U.K. Patent, 837465, Her Majesty's Stationery Office, London, 1960.
55. **Polli, G. P., Grim, W. M., Bacher, F. A., and Yunker, M. H.,** Influence of formulation on aerosol particle size, *J. Pharm. Sci.,* 58, 484, 1969.
56. **Rance, R. W.,** Particle size distribution measurement of hair sprays using an image splitting particle size analyser, *J. Soc. Cosmet. Chem.,* 23, 197, 1972.
57. **Pengilly, R. W. and Keiner, J. A.,** The influence of some formulation variables and valve/actuator designs on the particle size distributions of aerosol sprays, *J. Soc. Cosmet. Chem.,* 28, 641, 1977.
58. **Moren, F.,** Drug deposition of pressurized inhalation aerosols. I. Influence of actuator tube design, *Int. J. Pharm.,* 1, 205, 1978.
59. **Gortz, R. and Moren, F.,** Pressure drop across inhalation aerosol actuators. Influence of position and area for air passage, *Int. J. Pharm.,* 3, 101, 1979.
60. **Newman, S. P., Moren, F., Pavia, D., Little, F., and Clarke, S. W.,** Deposition of pressurized aerosols inhaled through extension devices, *Am. Rev. Resp. Dis.,* 124, 317, 1981.
61. **Newman, S. P., Moren, F., Pavia, D., Corrado, O., and Clarke, S. W.,** The effect of changes in metered volume and propellant vapour pressure on the deposition of pressurized inhalation aerosols, *Int. J. Pharm.,* 11, 337, 1982.
63. <601> Aerosols, in *The United States Pharmacopeia,* 21st ed., U.S. Pharmacopeial Convention, Rockville, MD, 1985.
64. **Hallworth, G. W. and Westmoreland, D. G.,** The twin impinger: a simple device for assessing the delivery of drugs from metered dose pressurized aerosol inhalers, *J. Pharm. Pharmacol.,* 39, 966, 1987.
65. **Allen. T.,** *Particle Size Measurement,* 2nd ed., Chapman & Hall, London, 1975, 1.
66. **Gonda, I., Kayes, J. B., Groom, C. V., and Fildes, F. J. T.,** Characterization of hygroscopic inhalation aerosols, in *Particle Size Analysis,* Stanley-Wood, N. G. and Allen, T., Eds., Wiley Heyden, Ltd., London, 1981, 31.
67. **Groom, C. V., Gonda, I., and Fildes, F. J. T.,** Prediction of equilibrium aerodynamic diameters for inhalation aerosols, in *2nd Int. Conf. on Pharmacy Technology,* Vol. 5, AGPI, Paris, 1980, 124.
68. **Malton, C. A., Hallworth, G. W., and Padfield, J. M.,** The association and particle size distribution of drug and surfactant discharged from a metered dose inhalation aerosol, *J. Pharm. Pharmacol.,* 34(Suppl.), 65p, 1982.
69. **Dalby, R. N.,** Reducing the Particle Size and Decreasing the Release Rate of Drugs Delivered by Metered Dose Inhalers to the Respiratory Tract, Ph.D. thesis, University of Kentucky, Lexington, 1988.
70. **Berglund, R. N. and Liu, B. Y. H.,** Generation of monodisperse aerosol standards, *Environ. Sci. Tech.,* 7, 147, 1973.
71. Ergotamine Aerosol Inhalation, *British Pharmaceutical Codex,* Pharmaceutical Press, London, 1973, 645.
72. **Dalby, R. N. and Byron, P. R.,** Relationship between particle morphology and drug release properties after hydration of aerosols containing liposome forming ingredients, *Pharm. Res.,* 5(Suppl.), S-94, 1988.
73. **Dalby, R. N. and Byron, P. R.,** Sustained release terbutaline sulfate aerosols, in *Interphex USA Proceedings,* Cahners Exposition Group, Des Plaines, IL, 1988, 23.
74. **Byron, P. R. and Hickey, A. J.,** Spinning disk generation and drying of monodisperse solid aerosols with output concentrations sufficient for single breath inhalation studies, *J. Pharm. Sci.,* 76, 60, 1987.
75. **Ho, K. K. L., Kellaway, I. W., and Tredree, R. L.,** The determination of aerosol output during size analysis by laser diffraction, *J. Pharm. Pharmacol.,* 39(Suppl.), 77p, 1987.
76. **Hiller, F. C., Mazumder, M. K., Wilson, J. D., and Bone, R. C.,** Effect of low and high relative humidity on metered dose bronchodilator solution and powder aerosols, *J. Pharm. Sci.,* 69, 334, 1980.
77. **Hallworth, G. W. and Hamilton, R. R.,** Size analysis of metered suspension pressurized aerosols with the Quantimet 720, *J. Pharm. Pharmacol.,* 28, 890, 1976.
78. **Porush, I., Thiel, C., and Young, J. G.,** Pressurized pharmaceutical aerosols for inhalation therapy, *J. Am. Pharm. Assoc.,* 49, 70, 1960.
79. **Moren, F. and Jacobsson, S.,** *In vitro* dose sampling from pressurized inhalation aerosols: investigation of procedures in BPC and NF, *Int. J. Pharm.,* 3, 335, 1979.

80. **Davies, P. J., Amin, K. K., and Mott, G. A.,** Particle size of inhalation aerosol systems. II. Uniformity of delivery of some commercial inhalation aerosols, *Drug Dev. Ind. Pharm.,* 6, 653, 1980.
81. **Thompson, B. J., Ward, J. H., and Zinky, W. R.,** Application of hologram techniques for particle size analysis, *Appl. Optics,* 6, 519, 1967.
82. **Hathaway, D.,** Particle size measurement of an aerosol deodorant using laser holographic microscopy, *Aerosol Age,* September, 28, 1973.
83. **Benjamin, E. J., Kroeten, J. J., and Shek, E.,** Characterization of spray patterns of inhalation aerosols using thin-layer chromatography, *J. Pharm. Sci.,* 72, 380, 1983.
84. **Miszuk, S., Gupta, B. M., Chen, F. C., Clawans, C., and Knapp, J. Z.,** Video characterization of flume pattern of inhalation aerosols, *J. Pharm. Sci.,* 69, 713, 1980.
85. **Dhand, R., Malik, S. K., Balakrishnan, M., and Verma, S. R.,** High speed photographic analysis of aerosols produced by metered dose inhalers, *J. Pharm. Pharmacol.,* 40, 429, 1988.
86. **Bellersen, M.,** A statistical approach to quality control, *Aerosol Age,* December, 32, 1986.
87. **Amin, Y. M., Thompson, E. B., and Chiou, W. L.,** Fluorocarbon aerosol propellants. XII. Correlation of blood level of trichloromonofluoromethane to cardiovascular and respiratory responses in anesthetized dogs, *J. Pharm. Sci.,* 68, 160, 1979.
88. **Aviado, D. M.,** Toxicity of aerosol propellants in the respiratory and circulatory systems, *Toxicology,* 3, 311, 1975.
89. **Niven, R. W. and Byron, P. R.,** Effect of surfactants on the penetration of fluorescein across the pulmonary barrier of the isolated perfused rat lung, *Pharm. Res.,* 5(Suppl.), S-111, 1988.
90. **Wetterlin, K.,** Turbuhaler: a new powder inhaler for administration of drugs to the airways, *Pharm. Res.,* 5, 506, 1988.
91. **Bohnenn, L. J. M.,** Update and review of dimethyl ether propellant-1986, *Aerosol Age,* September, 30, 1986.
92. **Bohnenn, L. J. M.,** Recent European developments in DME technology. I., *Aerosol Age,* September, 26, 1988.
93. **Bohnenn, L. J. M.,** Recent European developments in DME technology. II., *Aerosol Age.,* November, 40, 1988.
94. Beclovent™ Oral Inhaler, *Physician's Desk Register,* 42nd ed., Medical Economics, Oradell, NJ, 1988, 1003.
95. **Randolph, A. D. and Larson, M. A.,** *Theory of Particulate Processes,* Academic Press, New York, 1971, 16.
96. **Rodriguez-Hornedo, N. and Carstensen, J. T.,** Crystallization kinetics of oxalic acid dihydrate: nonisothermal desupersaturation of solutions, *J. Pharm. Sci.,* 75, 552, 1986.
97. **Hickey, A. J., Dalby, R. N., and Byron, P. R.,** Effects of surfactants on aerosol powders in suspension. Implications for airborn particle size, *Int. J. Pharm.,* 42, 267, 1988.
98. **Martin, A., Swarbrick, J., and Cammarata, A.,** *Physical Pharmacy,* 3rd ed., Lea & Febiger, Philadelphia, 1983, 445.
99. **Ong, J. T. H. and Manoukian, E.,** Micellar solubilization of timobesone acetate in aqueous and aqueous propylene glycol solutions of nonionic surfactants, *Pharm. Res.,* 5, 704, 1988.
100. **Tikhonov, V. P., Lebedev, R. A., and Fuks, G. I.,** Study of micelle formation of surfactants in nonpolar liquids by means of infrared spectroscopy, *Kolloidnyi. Zhurnal.,* 44, 57, 1982.
101. **Fowkes, F. M.,** The interactions of polar molecules, micelles, and polymers in nonaqueous media, in *Solvent Properties of Surfactant Solutions,* Shinoda, K., Ed., Marcel Dekker, New York, 1967, 65.
102. **Heistand, E. N.,** Theory of coarse suspension formulation, *J. Pharm. Sci.,* 53, 1, 1964.
103. **Dombrowski, N. and Munday, B.,** Spray drying, in *Biochemical and Bioengineering Sciences,* Blakebrough, N., Ed., Academic Press, London, 1968, 209.
104. **Schneider, W., Stavchansky, S., and Martin, A.,** Pharmaceutical suspensions and the DLVO theory, *Am. J. Pharm. Ed.,* 42, 280, 1978.
105. **Parkins, D. A.,** The Electrophoretic Mobility of Non-Aqueous Dispersions, Ph.D. thesis, University of Bath, Bath, U.K., 1986.
106. **Groom, C. V.,** Effects of Relative Humidity on Inhalation Aerosols, Ph.D. thesis, University of Aston, Birmingham, U.K., 1981.
107. **Hering, S. V., Freidlander, S. K., Collins, J. J., and Richards, L. W.,** Design and evaluation of a new low pressure impactor, *Environ. Sci. Tech.,* 13, 184, 1979.
108. **Johnsen, M. A.,** Aerosol gas house construction, *Aerosol Age,* January, 30, 1988.
109. **Byron, P. R. and Niven, R. W.,** A novel method for drug administration to the airways of the isolated perfused rat lung, *J. Pharm. Sci.,* 77, 693, 1988.
110. **Thiel, C.,** personal communication.
111. **Niven, R. W., Byron, P. R., and Rypacek, F.,** Transfer of a potential drug carrier, poly (2-hydroxyethyl) aspartamide, across the airways of the isolated rat lung, *Pharm. Res.,* 5(Suppl.), S-111, 1988.
112. **Swintosky, J. V., Reigelman, S., Higuchi, T., and Busse, L. W.,** Specific surface area and average particle size of some drugs determined by the BET method, *J. Am. Pharm. Assoc.,* 38, 210, 1949.
113. **Wiener, M. V.,** How to formulate aerosols to obtain the desired spray pattern, *J. Soc. Cosmet. Chem.,* 9, 289, 1958.
114. **Weast, R., C., Ed.,** *Handbook of Chemistry and Physics,* 59th ed., CRC Press, Boca Raton, FL, 1979, F43.

115. **Reist, P. C.,** *Introduction to Aerosol Science,* Macmillan, New York, 1984, 11.
116. **Hallworth, G. W. and Andrews, U. G.,** Size analysis of suspension inhalation aerosols by inertial separation methods, *J. Pharm. Pharmacol.,* 28, 898, 1976.
117. **Martin, G. P., Bell, A. E., and Marriott, C.,** An *in vitro* method for assessing particle deposition from metered pressurized aerosols and dry powder inhalers, *Int. J. Pharm.,* 44, 57, 1988.
118. **Chan, T. L., Schreck, R. M., and Lippman, M.,** Effects of laryngeal jet on particle deposition in the human tracheal and upper bronchial airways, *J. Aerosol Sci.,* 11, 447, 1980.

Chapter 8

CLINICAL TESTING OF AEROSOL DRUGS

Tahir Ahmed

TABLE OF CONTENTS

I. INTRODUCTION

Delivery of aerosolized drugs in the tracheobronchial tree is increasingly becoming an important part of modern respiratory pharmacology. Although aerosol therapy is regarded as a relatively modern practice, inhalation of primitive remedies for respiratory and nonrespiratory ailments has been described in ancient Greek, Roman, Chinese, Indian, Hebrew, and Arabic cultures. Although a large number of the current drugs have been used as crude extracts for centuries,[1] respiratory pharmacology is undergoing the most innovative and successful approaches of the Western pharmaceutical industry. During the last 25 years, new drug development has had a profound effect on the treatment and understanding of respiratory diseases.

The U.S. Food and Drug Administration (FDA) in 1938 set up rigorous standards that any new drug had to pass before it was approved for marketing. This was the result of legislation that had been introduced with the intent of protecting the public from hazardous or ineffective drugs. Pharmaceutical companies are now required to submit a new drug application containing

TABLE 1
Goals Of Aerosol Drugs

Bronchodilatation
Prevent bronchospasm
Inhibit bronchial hyperreactivity
Suppress airway inflammation
Increase mucociliary clearance
Experimental uses

detailed information about the drug for the FDA to review, including controlled trials to demonstrate the safety and effectiveness of new drugs.[2,3] Less rigorous standards and far less bureaucratic regulatory rules in Europe and U.K. have resulted in rapid development and marketing of innovative drugs for respiratory pharmacology, such as cromolyn sodium, salbutamol, and beclomethasone. Rigorous FDA standards have also delayed the entry of established foreign drugs into the U.S. market. The development of a new drug requires a complex and cooperative effort that involves basic chemists, pharmacologists, animal experiments, and clinical investigators. In the case of aerosol drugs, additional information is provided by an aerosol physicist to determine the appropriate particle size, physical characteristics of aerosol, delivery, and deposition of the drug in the airway. Thus, clinical studies for determining the safety and efficacy of an aerosol drug are even more complicated than an oral or parenterally administered drug.

II. GOALS OF AEROSOL DRUGS

For centuries aerosol drug delivery has been used primarily for pulmonary disorders and has included bronchodilator and mucokinetic agents. The lung has an extensive absorptive surface area and alveolo-capillary membrane network which make it easy for rapid absorption into the systemic circulation. However, at present few drugs are administered as an aerosol for systemic effects. Thus, aerosol drugs can be divided into two groups: (1) agents that act on the lung and (2) agents with systemic effects.[4]

The main group of drugs given for their pulmonary action are those used for the treatment of asthma and other chronic obstructive pulmonary diseases. The major goal of aerosol drugs in asthma and other related disorders is alleviation and prevention of bronchospasm. However, continued research into the pathophysiology of these disorders is revealing new therapeutic insight. In addition to treating bronchospasm, increasing stress is being placed on preventing the bronchospasm and other related pathophysiological abnormalities of asthma. Thus, the goals of aerosol drug delivery in asthma and obstructive airway disease are bronchodilation, prevention of bronchospasm, inhibition of bronchial hyperreactivity, suppression of airway inflammation, increase of mucociliary clearance, and experimental use (Table 1). Although currently used aerosol drugs were initially tested and approved for a specific indication (e.g., bronchodilation), many of these drugs are able to achieve more than one goal. However, as newer and more specific agents are being discovered (e.g., mediator antagonists), more specific and cumbersome studies would be required to establish their clinical efficacy.

The use of the aerosol mode for systemic administration of drugs is quite limited at present, and mainly includes anesthetic gases and vapors. Many hormones can be delivered via the lungs for systemic absorption, however, at present this is considered experimental. The lungs could also be a target organ for complications of systemic diseases. Involvement of the lungs with *Pneumocystis carinii* and other opportunistic infections in patients with acquired immune deficiency syndrome (AIDS) is a case in point for possible experimental use of prophylactic antibiotics and other antiviral agents as aerosols.

TABLE 2
Sympathomimetic Bronchodilators

Drug	B_1-action	B_2-action	Onset	Duration of action (h)
Epinephrine	++++	+++	Rapid	Short (2—3)
Isoproterenol	++++	++++	Rapid	Short (2—3)
Rimetrol	(+)	++++	Rapid	Short (2—3)
Isoetharine	+(+)	+++	Rapid	Medium (3—4)
Metaproterenol	++	+++	Rapid	Long (4—5)
Albuterol	+(+)	++++	Rapid	Long (4—5)
Terbutaline	++	+++	Intermediate	Long (4—5)
Fenoterol	+(+)	++++	Intermediate	Long (5—6)

III. TESTING OF AEROSOLIZED BRONCHODILATOR AGENTS

Bronchodilator drugs can be classified into three main groups: β-adrenergic agonists, phosphodiesterase inhibitors (theophylline), and anticholinergic agents. Since theophylline derivatives are relatively ineffective when given as an aerosol,[5] the present discussion is limited to β-adrenergic agonists and anticholinergic agents.

A. β-ADRENERGIC AGONISTS

Ephedrine is the oldest adrenoreceptor stimulant and has been used by the Chinese for over 5000 years. In 1910, Bargar and Dale[6] described the activity of several adrenaline-like amines with sympathomimetic activity. Konzett[7] in 1940 observed that isoprenaline was a very effective bronchodilator when given by aerosol. Since then, isoprenaline has become an important agent for research, and serves as an important therapeutic and reference agent for clinical drug trials. Since the discovery of α- and β-adrenergic receptors,[8] β receptor subtypes[9] (β_1- and β_2-receptors) and subsequent demonstration that β_2-receptor activation is necessary for bronchodilatation, the search for selective β_2-receptor agonists has been intensified. This has led to the development of highly selective β_2-agonists, replacing epinephrine and isoprenaline as the main aerosol bronchodilator agents.

1. Selective β_2-Agonists

The first relatively selective β_2-agonist, metaproterenol, was introduced in Europe in 1961. Since then, a variety of selective β_2-agonists has been investigated and marketed worldwide. Table 2 lists the commonly used β_2-agonist aerosols. Dose-response curves in patients with asthma show that nonselective and selective β_2-agonists attain the same maximal bronchodilating effect when given intravenously (i.v.) (Figure 1).[10] The bronchodilator and cardiac effects of isoprenaline run parallel, suggesting that β_1- and β_2-receptors are equally stimulated. However, with a very high dose of isoprenaline giving maximal bronchodilatation, the heart rate continues to increase. In contrast the selective β_2-agonist, salbutamol, achieves the same maximal bronchodilatation but initially is not associated with tachycardia, a sign of selective β_2-receptor stimulation. Even at the highest dose, the percent increase in heart rate was lower than the percent bronchodilatation. There could be limitations in evaluating selectivity *in vitro* and transferring the results to *in vivo*. One limitation is that drugs can be full or partial agonists. *In vitro* metaproterenol and fenoterol appear to be full β_1-agonists, but with lower potency than isoproterenol, whereas albuterol and terbutaline are partial β_1-agonists.[11] This suggests that there could be dose-dependent differences in their cardiac effects (β_1-agonist); whether this is of any clinical significance can only be determined by *in vivo* clinical studies. In spite of differences in β_1-agonist activity, similar clinical β_2 selectivity has been established for albuterol, fenoterol, and terbutaline, and from a clinical point of view there is no major difference in their therapeutic efficacy or selectivity.[12]

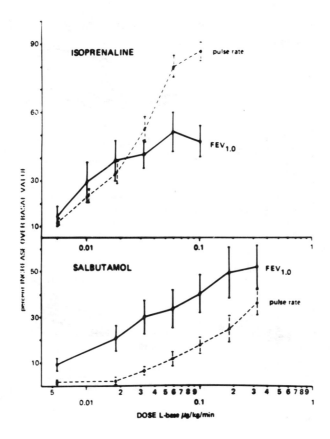

FIGURE 1. Mean dose-response curves for i.v. isoprenaline and salbutamol (albuterol) in patients with asthma. For similar increases in forced expired volume in 1 s (FEV₁), isoprenaline had a greater increase in pulse rate. Each dose was infused during 6 min with 30-min intervals. (From Svedmyr, N. and Thiringer, G., *Postgrad. Med. J.*, 47(Suppl.), 44, 1971. With permission.)

2. Aerosol vs. Parenteral Administration

The administration of a drug by inhalation has many advantages since the drug is delivered directly to the airways.[13] Potential benefits include rapid onset of action, high efficacy, lower dose for optimal effect, and reduced incidence of side effects. This was clearly pointed out by the studies of Thiringer and Svedmyr,[14,15] who compared the bronchodilating effects and side effects of inhaled forms to oral or i.v. forms of β_2-agonists. Intravenous terbutaline which exceeded the therapeutic doses did not produce maximal bronchodilation but increased the heart rate by 25% and doubled the Tremor ratio.[14] Inhaled terbutaline not only produced greater bronchodilator response, but an equivalent level of bronchodilatation was obtained without any significant effect on heart rate, blood pressure, or tremors, indicating a local effect with an increased therapeutic range and a lessened risk of side effects (Figure 2).[14] Similar observations were made when inhaled salbutamol was compared to oral forms.[15] Inhaled salbutamol produced significantly less tremor for a comparable degree of bronchodilatation.

3. Powder vs. Aerosol

The preferred formulation of β_2-agonist for inhalation has been either a solution for use with a nebulizer or with a metered dose inhaler (MDI) with freon propellant. However, greater concern over fluorocarbon propellants has triggered the search for alternative forms of administration. Although aerosolized albuterol has been available since 1969, a dry powder formulation of albuterol was introduced in the U.K. in 1971. The powder formulation has been

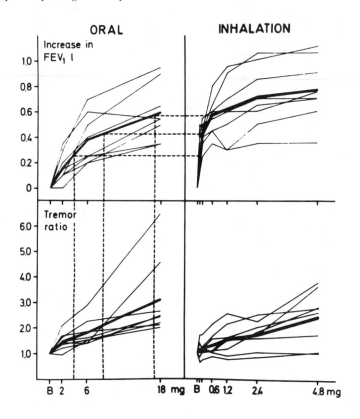

FIGURE 2.   Effects on 1-s FEV_1 and tremor ratio of increasing doses of inhaled
and oral salbutamol. For identical increases in FEV_1 inhaled salbutamol caused
less tremors. (From Larsson, S., et al., *J. Allergy Clin. Immunol.*, 59, 93, 1977.
With permission.)

particularly useful in patients who are unable to properly use pressurized aerosols with MDI or
who prefer an alternative delivery system. A capsule containing albuterol powder is inserted into
a flow-activated device (Rotahaler™, Glaxo, Inc.), that helps the patient avoid the difficulty of
synchronizing release of medication with the start of inspiration. Preliminary studies with a
small study population suggested that efficacy of dry powder albuterol was comparable with
aerosol formulation.[16,17] A recent multicenter study involving a study population of 231 subjects
demonstrated that albuterol powder produced similar improvements in pulmonary function to
those observed with two puffs (metered dose = 180 μg) of albuterol.[18] There was also no
significant difference between the two formulations in terms of clinical efficacy, symptoms
scores, cardiovascular effects, adverse effects, or patient preferences.

4. Assessment of Bronchodilator Response

   When drugs are administered systemically, the concentration present in the plasma often has
a known relationship to the pharmacologic effects achieved. The kinetics of plasma concentration, therefore, can be used to determine optimal dosages and dosing frequencies. However,
when drugs are administered as an aerosol to the lung, the desired therapeutic effect depends
upon local tissue concentration, which is very difficult to determine and has no immediate
relationship to plasma concentration. Methods of measuring responses to a bronchodilator
usually require pulmonary function tests before and at various time intervals after bronchodilator administration or initiation of a trial of bronchodilator therapy. A number of factors
influence the measured response to a bronchodilator (Table 3), and thus may confound the

TABLE 3
Factors Influencing Bronchodilator Response

Intrinsic responsiveness of airway smooth muscle
Severity of baseline obstruction
The class of bronchodilator agent being evaluated
Dose of bronchodilator
Mode of aerosol generation and technique of inhalation
Timing of test in relation to peak action of drug
Possible residual effect of a previously administered not "washed out drug"
Tests used for measuring the response

interpretation:[19] (1) intrinsic responsiveness of airway smooth muscle, (2) severity of baseline obstruction, (3) the class of bronchodilator agent being evaluated, (4) dose of bronchodilator, (5) mode of aerosol generation and technique of inhalation, (6) timing of test in relation to peak action of drug, (7) possible residual effect of a previously administered not "washed out drug", and (8) tests used for measuring the response.

a. Methods

A variety of pulmonary function tests has been used to evaluate a bronchodilator response. These include:

1. Measurements of forced expired volumes (FEV) and flow rates from the forced expiratory spirogram (forced vital capacity, FVC; FEV in the first second, FEV_1; and FEV_1/FVC ratio)
2. Maximal expiratory flow-volume curve (MEFV) obtained from a timed spirogram and various indices of maximal flow rates (peak expiratory flow rates, PEFR; maximal midexpiratory flow rates, MMFR; and maximal expiratory flow rates at different percentages of vital capacity [$\dot{V}max_{25}$, $\dot{V}max_{50}$, $\dot{V}max_{75}$])
3. Partial expiratory flow-volume curve (since MEFV can cause either transient bronchoconstriction or bronchodilatation, partial expiratory flow-volume curve can be used to avoid the possible airway effects of deep inspiration prior to forced expiration)
4. Plethysmographic measurements of airway resistance (Raw) and lung volumes (functional residual capacity, FRC); since airway resistance depends upon the lung volume, generally data are described as airway conductance (Gaw = 1/Raw) and corrected for lung volume and designated as specific airway conductance (SGaw = Gaw/FRC).

b. Expression of Data

The simplest and most commonly used test to evaluate a bronchodilator response is FEV_1. The methods of expressing the bronchodilator response in quantitative terms can influence the interpretation of the "statistical" as well as "clinical" significance of the response. These include percent improvement of baseline, absolute improvement, and percent of maximal achievable improvement. Percent improvement of baseline is the most common method of expressing the bronchodilator results. Use of each of these methods can lead to problems in interpretation of data and degree of bronchodilatation would depend upon the prebronchodilator FEV_1 (Figure 3).[19] When lung function is near normal, relatively little absolute improvement is possible. As obstruction increases, more reversible bronchospasm is present and improvement is greater. However, with more severe obstruction acute bronchodilator response decreases, probably due to less readily reversible bronchial pathological conditions, including secretions, inflammation, and edema. As shown in Figure 3, the small bronchodilator response noted when obstruction is severe (low baseline FEV_1) is indicated by shallow slopes of all the curves on the left side of the figure. On the other extreme, when obstruction is mild and there is relatively little room for

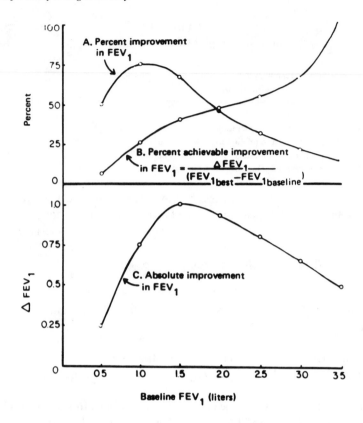

FIGURE 3.   Three ways of representing the bronchodilator responses in a hypotheti-
cal patient studied on seven different occasions at seven different baseline values
(FEV$_1$ ranging from 0.5 to 3.5 l) with seven different arbitrary responses. (From
Jenne, J. W. and Tashkin, D. P., in *Provocative Challenge Procedures*, Vol. 2,
Spector, S. L., Ed., 1983. With permission.)

improvement, full achievement of the small degree of possible improvement is reflected by a
high level of percent achievable improvement (curve B), but only an intermediate level of
absolute improvement (curve C) and a strikingly low level of percent improvement. The percent
improvement (curve A), in this situation appears as a misleading way of representing a
bronchodilator response since it is most dependent on baseline lung function. However, as is
apparent from inspection of all three curves, none of the methods of expressing a bronchodilator
response obviate the confounding effect of the level of baseline lung function on the response.
Consequently, in comparative studies of bronchodilator drugs, including different agents or
different dosages of the same agent, it is important that each subject have fairly comparable
baseline lung function at each testing session. As a general principle, subjects should not be
tested unless the prebronchodilator FEV$_1$ values fall within a predetermined range, usually
within 10 to 20% of each other.

c. What is a Significant Response?

Significance of a bronchodilator response can be defined in terms of clinical response or
statistical response. In an individual subject, a number of factors can influence the expected
bronchodilator response, including variability of tests and baseline FEV$_1$ on different days.
When examining responses to a bronchodilator in a group of subjects, statistical tests can be
applied to ascertain whether there has been a significant change compared to a placebo.
However, statistically significant responses to a bronchodilator do not necessarily correlate with

the clinical response. A bronchodilator response may be statistically significant and yet not be important clinically and vice versa. For example, a 15 to 20% improvement in FEV_1 in a COPD patient may be statistically significant, but its clinical relevance can be argued. For this reason, other indices of effectiveness, such as symptoms score and exercise tolerance, should also be evaluated.

5. Pharmacodynamics of Aerosol β-Agonists
a. Onset of Action

The onset of bronchodilator action of catecholamine β-agonists such as isoproterenol and isoetharine is rapid, with maximal effect being achieved within 5 min of inhalation. In contrast, the noncatecholamines such as albuterol, fenoterol, and terbutaline produce about 80% of their effects within 5 min, but require 15 to 60 min to reach maximal effect.[12,20] There are no apparent major differences in onset of action of different noncatecholamine bronchodilators. An agent with a more rapid onset of action may be desirable in some specific clinical situations. Furthermore, performing pulmonary functions in the clinical laboratory 5 min postinhalation may underestimate the magnitude of bronchodilator action of some noncatecholamine agents.

b. Intensity and Duration of Action

Studies of intensity and duration of action of a bronchodilator aerosol are of major clinical importance. Choice of a selective β_2-agonist, dosage, and dosing interval for clinical treatment are based upon these studies. This is especially true when around-the-clock efficacy is needed, such as for the treatment of a prolonged exacerbation of symptoms of asthma, or for preventive maintenance therapy of chronic asthma. The dosing frequency in such clinical situations should be such that each successive dose is administered before the effects of a prior dose have become insufficient to control symptoms.[21]

The therapeutic action of a particular β-agonist aerosol will depend upon the length of time over which optimal concentrations of drug remain at the receptor site. This, in turn, will depend not only on the amount of drug deposited in the airway, but also on the rate at which the drug is removed. Thus, the mean duration of action of an inhaled β_2-agonist is a function of three independent factors: (1) the dosage of inhaled drug, (2) the potency of the drug, and (3) the rate of elimination of the drug (Figure 4).[21] The higher the dosage of a specific β_2-agonist delivered, the longer the overall duration of action of that drug. A more potent drug will produce a greater initial effect and, therefore, will have a longer duration of action. A lower rate of elimination of the drug from the vicinity of β_2-receptor will result in a greater duration of action.

Studies of drug-induced bronchodilator responses have been very useful in providing information about the intensity and duration of action of inhaled β-agonists. These studies have clearly shown that the duration of action of catecholamine agents is much shorter than noncatecholamine β-agonists.[22] The effects of metaproterenol (150 μg) and albuterol (200 μg) were sustained for greater than 3 h, whereas the effects of isoproterenol (1000 μg) were not significantly different from placebo after 2 h (Figure 5). Because of their shorter duration of action, drugs such as isoproterenol have almost become obsolete as therapeutic agents.

In general, the differences in the intensity and duration of bronchodilator action of selective noncatecholamine β_2-agonists are subtle and not of any clinical significance. These differences may be partly related to the limitations of tests used, the manner in which data were expressed, or the differences in peak effect or rate of decline of the bronchodilator effect. Several published studies have compared equal numbers of MDI puffs of terbutaline (250 μg/puff) and albuterol (100 μg/puff). Depending upon the study cited, it is possible to reach entirely different conclusions. For example, it has been suggested that puff for puff, terbutaline has: (1) virtually the same initial effect, rate of decline, and duration of action as albuterol;[23] (2) has the same initial effect, but a slower rate of decline of effect, and, therefore, a longer duration of action than albuterol;[24] or (3) has a lesser initial peak effect, a slower rate of decline, and thus, a duration of

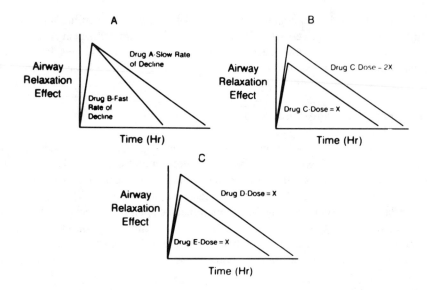

FIGURE 4. Hypothetical examples of factors affecting duration of action of inhaled β_2-agonists. (A) Rate at which effects diminished with time. Slow vs. fast rate of decline. (B) Dosage. Smaller vs. larger dose. (C) Relative potency. (Reprinted from Jenne, J. W. and Ahrens, R. C., in *Drug Therapy for Asthma,* Jenne and Murphy, Eds., Marcel Dekker, New York, 1987. With permission.)

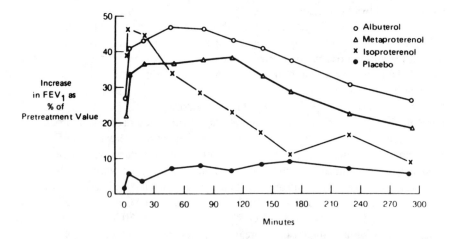

FIGURE 5. Percentage increase in FEV_1 after metered dose inhalation of albuterol (200 µg; ○), metaproterenol sulfate (1500 µg; Δ), isoproterenol sulfate (1000 µg; X), and placebo (●). Effects of metaproterenol and albuterol were significantly longer than isoproterenol. (From Choo-Kang et al., *Br. Med. J.,* 2, 287, 1969. With permission.)

action which is similar to albuterol.[25] The reasons for these conflicting results are not completely clear. Variability in the baseline pulmonary functions, technique of aerosol administration and consequently the differences in the airway deposition dose may be some of factors responsible for these differences.

c. Prevention of Induced Bronchospasm

An alternative approach for estimating the duration of action of inhaled bronchodilators is to measure the ability of these drugs to inhibit bronchospasm induced by various stimuli. Many studies have shown that the bronchodilatation induced by oral and inhaled β_2-agonists does not correlate with the ability of these agents to inhibit bronchospasm induced by either pharmacologic effect or exercise.[26-29] Ahrens et al.[26] have demonstrated that whereas the bronchodilator effects of inhaled metaproterenol last over 4 h, the bronchoconstrictive effects of methacholine are prevented for only 2 h. It has also been demonstrated that inhaled metaproterenol completely inhibits exercise-induced bronchospasm immediately after administration, while it was ineffective when exercise challenge was performed 3 to 4 h later in spite of persistence of significant bronchodilatation.[29] Similar observations were made when metaproterenol was compared to albuterol with histamine as the provocative agent.[28] A temporal correlation between the disappearance of protective effects of β_2-agonist against histamine-induced bronchoconstriction and increase in asthma symptom score was also observed.[28] These data suggested that use of bronchial provocation tests could be a useful tool for determining the duration of action of β_2-agonists and assessment of appropriate dosing frequencies with these agents. Using this technique, several recent studies have compared the relative potency and duration of action of various inhaled selective β_2-agonists available in MDI forms, including metaproterenol, albuterol, terbutaline, fenoterol, and bitolterol.[25-28,30] Jenne and Ahrens[21] have suggested the estimation of half-lives of disappearance from the vicinity of airway β_2-receptors. This technique also required estimation of airway reactivity. Although somewhat cumbersome and not uniformly accepted, they did estimate the half-life of disappearance for metaproterenol as 1.0 h, 1.4 h for albuterol, and 2.3 h for terbutaline.[21]

d. Dosage and Potency

While analyzing studies that compare the different selective β_2-agonists, attention should be given not only to technique and expression of data, but also to relative dosages and potency of each drug. For example, it has been shown that two puffs of metaproterenol appear to have a shorter duration of action than two puffs of albuterol, simply because this dosage of metaproterenol produces a less intense initial effect than albuterol.[28] On the other hand, two puffs of terbutaline appear to be less potent than two puffs of albuterol, but because of slower rate of decline, the duration of action of terbutaline is similar to that of albuterol. A comparison between two puffs of albuterol and three puffs of bitolterol suggests that at these dosages the drugs have similar initial potency, but because of a slower rate of decline, bitolterol has a longer duration of action.[30] Similarly, the effectiveness of fenoterol (400 μg) on airway reactivity has been reported to be 5 to 6 h;[27] such data are difficult to interpret as direct comparison with other selective β_2-agonists was not performed. Two puffs of fenoterol appear to be more potent than two puffs of albuterol, which may account for its longer duration of action. A major limitation of the studies assessing the duration of bronchodilator action of selective β_2-agonists is that many newer drugs are compared to isoproterenol rather than to other selective β_2-agonists. It would be much more appropriate to compare newer agents to other selective β_2-agonists (perhaps more than one), so that comparisons are performed under identical conditions.

6. β-Adrenergic Tolerance and Tachyphylaxis

Prolonged use of β-adrenergic agonists has been suggested to result in tolerance or tachyphylaxis.[31-35] However, others have been unable to demonstrate this phenomenon.[36] Although data remain somewhat controversial, it is very likely that chronic β-agonist therapy, if not discontinued for a sufficient period, may underestimate the bronchodilator response to a β-agonist. This diminished bronchodilator response to a newer or same β-agonist may be especially pronounced in terms of duration of action, rather than peak response. Repsher et al.,[35] in fact, observed that β-agonist tolerance was best detected by area under the response curve (ARC), which is mainly dependent upon the duration of action. These investigators studied 58 asthmatics, using albuterol by MDI on a regular basis. The bronchodilator response to albuterol

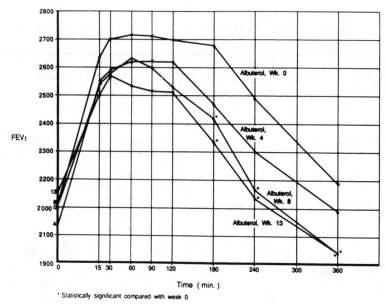

* Statistically significant compared with week 0

FIGURE 6. Absolute values of mean FEV_1 after inhalation of albuterol aerosol at study weeks 0, 4, 8, and 13. There is a significant difference in duration of bronchodilation between week 0 and weeks 8 and 13, due to tachyphylaxis. (From Repsher et al., *Chest,* 85, 34, 1984. With permission.)

was studied on weeks 0, 4, 8, and 13. Although there was no significant difference in peak bronchodilator response, as measured by FEV_1, the duration of bronchodilator effect was significantly less at weeks 8 and 13 (Figure 6). It has also been demonstrated that β-agonist tachyphylaxis can persist for about 2 weeks after discontinuation of therapy.[31] Many earlier studies have neglected to withdraw patients from their usual β-agonist therapy for a sufficient period (2 weeks) before commencing the study, thus potentially suppressing the bronchodilator action of a new β-agonist. This is of particular importance when testing β-agonists with a crossover design. In this case, it is imperative that the protocol design should include a washout period of at least 2 weeks prior to each crossover phase. While designing such studies, it is important to note that results and interpretation of data in terms of tachyphylaxis may be influenced by certain factors which are not constant and controversial:[31]

1. Occurrence of tachyphylaxis is more pronounced in normals than asthmatics.
2. Degree and duration of tachyphylaxis may vary with duration of exposure.
3. Concurrent therapy must remain constant or discontinued if possible. Corticosteroids may reduce development of tachyphylaxis, which is an important consideration when comparing different studies.
4. In crossover design studies, a concurrent placebo group must be included with equal washout periods.
5. Data analysis should include both peak effect as well as duration of action.
6. Baseline pulmonary function should be comparable on different study days: "Rising" or "falling" baseline pulmonary functions during the study period should not be ignored, as they may signify development or improvement of tachyphylaxis, and thus, may affect the results.

The clinical demonstration of down-regulation of β-adrenoreceptor function has been correlated with cellular function as well as with radioligand studies.[37-39] Szentivany, initially

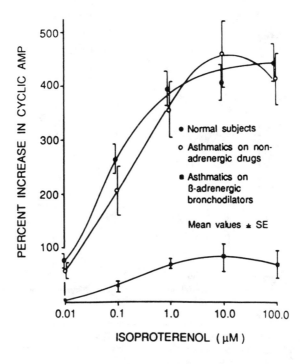

FIGURE 7. Percentage increase in lymphocyte AMP after a 15-min incubation at 37°C with isoproterenol. Lymphocytes were taken from normal subjects and two groups of asthmatic patients. (From Conolly, M. E. and Greenacre, J. K., *J. Clin. Invest.*, 58, 1307, 1987. With permission.)

suggested that suppressed β-receptor function was the primary defect in asthma.[37] The alternative hypothesis put forward by Conolly et al.[38] was that the reduced β-adrenergic function was a result of prolonged exposure to β-agonist bronchodilators (thus, a down-regulation of β-receptors). These investigators found a marked depression of cyclic AMP (cAMP) response to isoproterenol in lymphocytes of asthmatics using β-adrenergic drugs, but not in asthmatics who were being treated with nonadrenergic drugs (Figure 7). Radioligand studies on lymphocyte cell membranes from asthmatic subjects have shown a 40% loss in β-receptor density after 3 to 5 weeks of oral terbutaline therapy.[39] It was also observed that a single injection of methylprednisolone restored the receptor density when tested 16 h later (Figure 8).[39] These data underscore the importance of steroids in influencing the results of β-agonist bronchodilators.

B. ANTICHOLINERGIC AGENTS

Anticholinergic agents such as atropine and stramonium were a mainstay of bronchodilator therapy in the 19th and earlier part of the 20th century. However, with the discovery of epinephrine and other β-agonists, they almost disappeared from clinical use. In the past 20 years interest in anticholinergic bronchodilators has been revived. This is due in part to an understanding of the role of the parasympathetic system in the control of airway tone and in part to the development by the pharmaceutical industry of synthetic compounds devoid of the undesirable side effects of atropine.

The bronchodilator effects of anticholinergic agents in both normal subjects and patients with obstructive airway disease have been studied by many investigators and reviewed in some recent publications.[40-45] Compared to β-agonists, the onset of action of anticholinergic agents is somewhat slower and reaches a peak between 30 min to 2 h and persists for a longer period

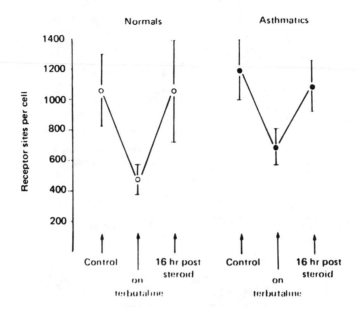

FIGURE 8. [^{3}H] DHA binding sites in 4 normal subjects and 4 asthmatic subjects before terbutaline, at the end of 3–5 weeks on 5 mg 3 times daily, and 16 h after 2 mg/kg i.v. methylprednisolone. (From Hui, K., et al., *Clin. Pharmacol. Ther.*, 32, 566, 1982. With permission.)

TABLE 4
Anticholinergic Agents

Agent	Chemical type	Duration (h)
Atropine sulfate	Tertiary ammonium	3—4
Atropine methonitrate	Quaternary ammonium	5—6
Ipratropium bromide	Quaternary ammonium	5—6
Oxitropium	Quaternary ammonium	6
Glycopyrrolate bromide	Quaternary ammonium	6—8
Thiazinamium chloride	Quaternary ammonium	6

because of a slow decline in action. However, the duration of action is dependent upon the inhaled dose, the agent being used, and the study population, i.e., normals, asthmatics, or chronic bronchitics. The different anticholinergic agents used for nebulization include atropine (sulfate or methonitrate), ipratropium bromide, oxitropium, glycopyrrolate, and thiazinamium (Table 4). Although atropine solution has been used for nebulization, ipratropium bromide is the only approved drug available as MDI in the U.S. under the brand name of Atrovent.

1. Atropine

Atropine has a very narrow therapeutic index because it is well absorbed from mucus membranes and readily crosses the blood-brain barrier. Nevertheless, Klock et al.[44] found aerosolized atropine to be an effective bronchodilator over a 3-week study period, at a dose of 1 mg 4 times a day, in patients with chronic bronchitis. However, the majority of patients complained of symptoms related to urinary hesitancy, blurring of vision, and dry mouth. Subsequent studies have shown the optimal nebulized dose of atropine sulfate is 25 μg/kg in adult patients with chronic bronchitis,[45,46] and somewhat lower for atropine methonitrate.[46] Even at this lower dosage, long-term administration of atropine does produce side effects in adult patients. Children, however, are able to tolerate higher doses of nebulized atropine, and optimal effects are achieved at 50 μg/kg.[47] Atropine and glycopyrrolate can produce lower oropharyngeal sphincter pressure, and atropine sulfate at a dose of 50 μg/kg in adult asthmatics has been shown to cause gastric stasis.[48] In addition, nebulized atropine has been shown to cause hallucinations, flushings, and tachycardia. Although nebulized atropine is used randomly, at present its use has not been approved by the FDA.

2. Ipratropium Bromide

Ipratropium bromide is a quaternary methyl isopropyl derivative of atropine. The pharmacologic spectrum of systemically administered ipratropium bromide is similar to atropine with respect to inhibition of salivary and gastric secretion, tachycardia, mydriasis, and urinary retention. However, the aerosolized ipratropium bromide is devoid of many of these side effects because it does not cross the blood-brain barrier and has poor gastric mucosal absorption.[51]

Inhaled ipratropium bromide has been shown to possess significant bronchodilatory effects in normals and patients with asthma.[49-52] In normal subjects inhalation of ipratropium has been shown to increase FEV_1 by about 10%, decrease airway resistance by about 50%, and increase SGaw by about 100% at the time of peak effect.[42,52] Like atropine, it produced greater bronchodilatation in the larger central airways than smaller peripheral airways.

Several small-scale, short-term studies in patients with chronic bronchitis and emphysema (COPD) have shown that anticholinergic agents produce bronchodilatation equivalent or superior to that produced by β-adrenergic agonists.[40-44] Single inhalation of 10, 20, and 40 μg of iprotropium bromide produced a significant increase in FEV_1 for 3 to 4 h, while 80 μg was effective for 5 h. Furthermore, the initial studies also demonstrated that ipratropium bromide was superior to isoproterenol, salbutamol, or fenoterol, both in terms of peak efficacy and duration of effect.[40] These studies also noted an absence of any tolerance to ipratropium. In a recent multicenter study involving 261 COPD patients, 40 μg ipratropium bromide was compared to 1.5 mg metaproterenol in a randomized, double blind, 90-d, parallel group trial.[53] Subjects were studied on 3 test days, i.e., days 1, 45, and 90. Mean peak responses (FEV_1 and FVC) as well as mean area under the time-response curve were higher for ipratropium bromide than for metaproterenol, while side effects were lower with ipratropium bromide. The onset of action of ipratropium bromide occurred within 15 min, the action peaked within 1 to 2 h, and the mean duration of action was 3 to 5 h.[53]

In contrast, the role of ipratropium bromide for the treatment of asthma is controversial and the drug is currently not approved by the FDA for its treatment. Over 300 studies have been conducted in patients with asthma, and the majority of these studies were conducted in stable asthmatics. Comparative bronchodilator responses to ipratropium bromide vs. placebo, isoproterenol, salbutamol, terbutaline, metaproterenol, and fenoterol have been reported. These studies were reviewed by Schlueter[49] and showed that ipratropium bromide had almost the same peak effect as isoproterenol, salbutamol, and terbutaline, but was only 75% as effective as metaproterenol or fenoterol. The peak effect of ipratropium bromide is achieved in about 60 min, which is less rapid than that of β-agonists. However, in most of these studies ipratropium bromide was not superior to β-agonists. It has also been suggested that ipratropium bromide has better efficacy in patients with intrinsic asthma, those with a smoking history, and those with a history of psychogenic asthma, underscoring the importance of cholinergic pathways in these subgroups. Recently, ipratropium bromide (40 μg 4 times a day) was compared to metaproterenol (1500 μg 4 times a day) in a double-blind, randomized, parallel, multicenter 90-d study in 144 patients with asthma.[54] Seventy-one patients received ipratropium bromide and 73 received metaproterenol. Both drugs were equally effective bronchodilators, as demonstrated by comparison of the areas under the curves for the two drugs. However, ipratropium bromide had different bronchodilator kinetics than metaproterenol, as it had a slower onset of action and a more prolonged duration of action.[54] The only significant side effects noted with ipratropium bromide were cough (9.9%) and exacerbations of symptoms (7.4%).

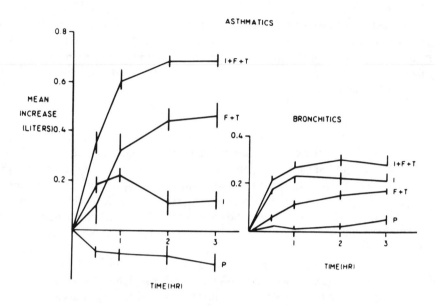

FIGURE 9. FEV$_1$ responses of patients with asthma and chronic bronchitis to agents indicated: I, ipratropium 40 μg aerosol; F, fenoterol 5 mg orally; T, oxtriphylline 400 mg orally, P, placebo. (From Lefcoe, N. M., et al., *Chest,* 82, 300, 1982. With permission.)

3. Adjuvant Therapy

Several studies have examined the role of ipratropium bromide as an adjuvant bronchodilator in the treatment of COPD and asthma, and the subject was reviewed recently.[42,50] In general, addition of adrenergic bronchodilators to ipratropium bromide in patients with chronic bronchitis and emphysema resulted in slightly greater bronchodilatation than ipratropium bromide alone.[42,50] However, the slightly additional bronchodilatation observed is perhaps not of any clinical importance. This was best demonstrated by the study of Lefcoe et al.,[55] who did not find a significantly greater increase in FEV$_1$ with a combination of ipratropium bromide, fenoterol, and oxtriphylline (Figure 9) compared to ipratropium bromide alone. In contrast, patients with asthma demonstrated a significantly greater bronchodilator response to combination therapy than with ipratropium bromide.[55] This has been borne out by other studies.[42,50] It has also been suggested that treatment with cromolyn and steroids may enhance the responsiveness to anticholinergic agents. In Europe, where ipratropium bromide has been in clinical use for 1 decade, fixed combinations of fenoterol and ipratropium bromide have been introduced, either 50 plus 20 μg (Berodual) or 100 plus 40 μg (Duovent), respectively. The aim of combination therapy is to provide rapid bronchodilatation with β$_2$-agonists, and prolonged bronchodilatation with anticholinergic agents.[56] There is limited information available on the use of ipratropium bromide in acute exacerbations of asthma and COPD. Both in children and adult patients with status asthmaticus, addition of ipratropium bromide to a β-agonist resulted in greater bronchodilatation than with a β-agonist alone.[57] However, the results are difficult to interpret because of concomitant therapy with steroids and xanthines.

4. Site of Action

Some of the differences between the COPD and asthmatic patients may have been related to differences in predominant site of obstruction, relative role of cholinergic mechanism, density of muscarinic receptors in large vs. small airways, and finally, the predominant site of action of ipratropium bromide (i.e., large vs. small airways) in relation to muscarinic receptor density. In normal lungs, muscarinic receptor density is higher in large airways,[58] which is consistent with the concept that the predominant site of action of muscarinic agonists and antagonists is in the large airways.[59] Although it is not known at present, it is possible that muscarinic receptor density may be altered differently in the two diseases, which may contribute to differences in bronchodilator response to ipratropium bromide between patients with asthma and COPD. Finally, the most commonly used parameter (i.e., FEV_1) may not be the most appropriate test to study the bronchodilator response to anticholinergic agents such as ipratropium bromide. FEV_1 is a measure of both large and small airway functions, whereas SGaw predominantly estimates large airway function. It is, therefore, possible that FEV_1 may underestimate the bronchodilator response to anticholinergic agents. The available data are limited and conflicting. Douglas et al.[60] studied the effect of ipratropium on normal airway function and concluded that it produced bronchodilatation in both large and small airways. In contrast, Pistelli and associates[61] reported that the major effect is on large airways. Several studies in patients with asthma confirmed this finding,[62,63] whereas other investigators concluded that both large and small airways are affected.[49]

5. Other Anticholinergic Agents

A number of newer anticholinergic agents are at different stages of clinical testing. These include oxitropium, glycopyrrolate, and thiazinamium. Glycopyrrolate was recently studied as MDI. Inhaled doses of 240, 480, and 960 µg produced dose-related bronchodilatation. Maximum bronchodilatation was achieved in 2 to 3 h and with higher doses lasted up to 12 h.[64] An attempt is being made to develop compounds with selective action on muscarinic-receptor subtypes, which may have a higher therapeutic index.

IV. TESTING OF AEROSOLIZED BRONCHOPROTECTIVE AGENTS

The clinical evaluation of bronchodilator antiasthmatic drugs (BAAD) is a relatively straightforward procedure, since the administration of these compounds is followed by an acute and easily measurable increase in bronchial potency. The testing of nonbronchodilator antiasthmatic drugs (NBAAD) for bronchoprotection is somewhat complicated and difficult to quantify. The major goals of bronchoprotective agents are to prevent bronchospasm, airway hyperreactivity, and airway inflammation.

A. PREVENTION OF BRONCHOSPASM

The rationale for the use of NBAAD to prevent bronchospasm suggests that bronchial provocation studies should play an important role in their assessment. The bronchial provocation studies are of undeniable value in exploring the pharmacological profile of a new compound, optimal dose, and duration of action. However, as predictors of clinical efficacy, the value of these tests is controversial. The tests of bronchial reactivity are of two main types, specific and nonspecific. The specific bronchial provocation testing primarily consists of an inhalation challenge with the specific antigen to which the subject has demonstrated cutaneous allergy. The nonspecific bronchoconstrictor agents would produce bronchoconstriction in every asthmatic subject and these agents include histamine, methacholine, and osmotic challenge. In addition, exercise-induced bronchoconstriction (EIB) has also been used as a model of bronchoprovocation. NBAAD are generally tested against one or more of these stimuli.

The procedure of bronchial provocation generally involves measuring pulmonary functions (FEV_1 or SGaw) before and after each increasing concentration of antigen, histamine, or methacholine until FEV_1 has decreased by 20% or SGaw has decreased 35% from the baseline.[65] From the dose-response curve the cumulative dose of agonist which caused a 20% decrease in FEV_1 (PD_{20}) or a 35% decrease in SGaw (PD_{35}) is calculated as an indicator of airway reactivity. To test for bronchoprotection, the above procedure is repeated following pretreatment with NBAAD. Bronchoprotection is demonstrated by a shift in the dose-response curve to the right along with a marked increase in PD_{20} or PD_{35}. For EIB, pulmonary functions are obtained before

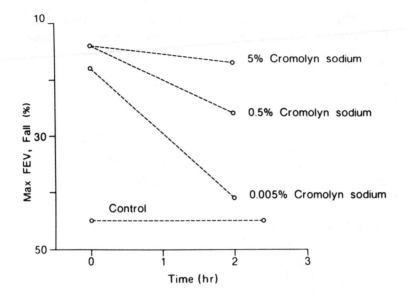

FIGURE 10.   Maximum FEV$_1$ reduction after antigen alone (control line) and after antigen
following pretreatment with varying concentrations of cromolyn sodium inhaled either 5 min
or 2 h before antigen challenge. (From Cox, J. S. G. and Altounyan, R. E. C., *Respiration*,
27(Suppl.), 292, 1970. With permission.)

and after a sustained submaximal exercise, and bronchoconstriction is estimated as percent
decrease in FEV$_1$ or SGaw. Bronchoprotective effects of a drug would be demonstrated by a
lesser decrease in FEV$_1$ or SGaw. Since EIB is dependent upon respiratory heat loss, it is
imperative that minute ventilation, temperature, and humidity be kept constant on placebo and
drug days.

1. Cromolyn Sodium: A Gold Standard?

Disodium cromoglycate (DSCG) has become the gold standard of NBAAD drug therapy
possibly due to unavailability of anything better. The drug became available in the U.K. in 1968
and in the U.S. in 1973.[66] Until recently, cromolyn sodium had been available as a powder to be
used with a "spinhaler", which had limited its use. Recently, it also became available as an
MDI.[67] Although its exact mode of action is still not clearly known, it is well accepted that its
primary mode of action is stabilization of mast-cell membrane and prevention of release of
chemical mediators.[68] Recent data have suggested that besides acting on mast cells, cromolyn
sodium may have a direct suppressive effect on other cells, such as neutrophils and alveolar
macrophages.[69] It is generally believed that cromolyn sodium does not possess significant
bronchodilating activity. Cromolyn sodium is an effective NBAAD agent, and in human
subjects it has been shown to inhibit both allergic and nonallergic bronchoconstriction produced
by stimuli including exercise, cold air, SO$_2$, and distilled water.[70] The history of the clinical
development of cromolyn sodium has become a model for clinical testing of newer NBAAD
agents. Cromolyn sodium was developed through the use of *in vivo* antigen challenge in
asthmatic volunteers. Altounyan, who himself was an asthmatic, demonstrated that inhalation
of 20 mg cromolyn sodium "before" antigen challenge markedly inhibited the antigen-induced
decrease in FEV$_1$.[66,68] The drug became progressively less effective when inhaled 1, 6, and 45
min "after"antigen challenge. Inhalation of various concentrations of cromolyn sodium 10 min
before antigen challenge showed that the protective effect is present over a wide range of dosages
of 0.005 to 5% (Figure 10). However, the degree of protection lessens when the time between

drug inhalation and antigen challenge is lengthened to 2 h or more. Multiple studies have been carried out since the original work of Altounyan, and have demonstrated the relative efficacy of cromolyn sodium in protecting against acute antigen-induced bronchoconstriction.[70] The efficacy rate was about 37% complete and 49% partial protection in the first 140 subjects challenged.[71] Cromolyn sodium has also been shown to inhibit bronchoconstriction mediated by nonimmunologic stimuli, including SO_2, exercise, cold air, and a variety of industrial agents including toluidine disocyanate and Western red cedar.[70]

Inhalation challenge with antigen results in an immediate or early asthmatic reaction (EAR) in patients with allergic asthma. Some asthmatics will exhibit a second bronchoconstrictor response 4 to 12 h after the first, which is known as delayed or late asthmatic reaction (LAR).[72] Whereas the EAR can be rapidly reversed by β_2-agonists, the LAR responds poorly to these agents, is prolonged, and more severe. LAR are of clinical importance, as these reactions are associated with prolonged increases in nonspecific bronchial hyperresponsiveness as well as frequency of asthma attacks. Drugs that will inhibit LAR should be regarded as particularly valuable for prophylaxis of asthma.

Cromolyn sodium given prior to a variety of different types of challenges has been shown to block both the EAR and LAR in human asthmatics as well as in animal models of asthma.[70] In a recent study, Cockcroft and Murdock[73] compared the effects of inhaled salbutamol (200 µg), cromolyn sodium (10 mg), and beclomethasone (200 µg) on antigen-induced EAR and LAR as well as the antigen-induced increases in bronchial hyperresponsiveness to histamine. They found that EAR was inhibited by a single dose treatment with inhaled salbutamol and cromolyn sodium, but not with inhaled beclomethasone, whereas the LAR was inhibited by pretreatment with cromolyn sodium and beclomethasone and not salbutamol (Figure 11). It was also observed that drugs (DSCG and beclomethasone) which inhibited the late phase also attenuated the postallergen increase in bronchial reactivity to histamine, while salbutamol which only attenuated the EAR (and not LAR) was ineffective. This comparative study confirmed early findings on the effects of different drugs on EAR and LAR.[70,72] Implications from these studies toward clinical testing of NBAAD are of pharmaceutical and clinical importance. Testing of NBAAD by showing inhibition of EAR is, perhaps, inadequate and must include studies of LAR as well as prevention of bronchial hyperreactivity which follows LAR.

In certain asthmatic groups, (e.g., intrinsic), identification of specific allergen is not possible, which offers a great difficulty in direct testing of NBAAD drugs in such patients. Long-term studies in such patients have demonstrated that cromolyn sodium may also be effective in intrinsic asthma. There are many published studies which support the clinical efficacy of cromolyn sodium in both extrinsic and intrinsic asthmatics.[67,74] The formulations of cromolyn sodium used in these studies have included powder, solution, and MDI. Many of the earlier studies in the U.K. had limitations because of the absence of control groups and concomitant use of isoproterenol, which makes interpretation of the data somewhat difficult. Despite these problems, the majority of the results were favorable with success rates ranging from 60 to 89% in different studies, as evaluated by symptoms score, decreased use of β_2-agonists, and improved pulmonary functions. Recent, well-controlled studies have confirmed these earlier observations in both adults and children, with comparable efficacy of powder, solution, or MDI formulation of cromolyn sodium.[67,70,74]

2. Inhaled Steroids

A variety of inhaled steroids is currently used for the prevention of asthma, including beclomethasone dipropionate, triamcinolone acetonide, flunisolide, budesonide, and betamethasone valerate. Budesonide and betamethasone valerate are not available for clinical use in the U.S. Although the mechanism of action of steroids is not known, their value in acute severe asthma (systemic steroids) or for prophylaxis (oral or inhaled) is well established.[75] Testing of inhaled steroids for bronchoprotection is mainly dependent upon clinical studies. Such studies

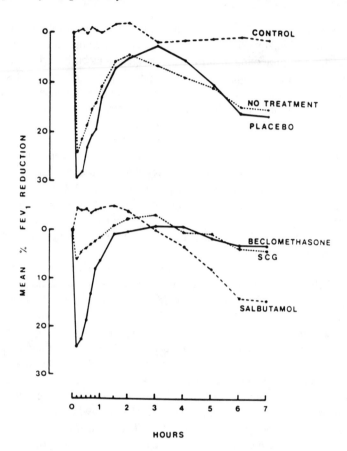

FIGURE 11.   Modification of antigen-induced early and late phase bronchoconstriction by drug pretreatments. FEV_1 (percent fall) on the control and 5 allergen
days is shown before and at hourly intervals after the antigen challenge. The top
panel includes responses on day 1 control inhalation (dashed line) and to allergen
on day 2 (solid line) and day 6 (dotted line), no treatment and placebo pretreatment, respectively. The bottom panel demonstrates allergen response on days 3
to 5 with pretreatments of beclomethasone dipropionate, 200 μg (solid line),
salbutamol, 200 μg (dashed line), and cromolyn sodium, 10 mg (dotted line).
(From Cockcroft, D. W. and Murdock, K. Y., *J. Allergy Clin. Immunol.*, 79, 734,
1987. With permission.)

have demonstrated that patients vary not only in their initial responsiveness to a clinical trial of
inhaled steroids, but also in their long-term dose requirement. Certain patient groups and disease
characteristics have been found to correlate significantly with the degree of responsiveness to
inhaled steroids; however, such predictors cannot be applied to individual patients.[75] It has also
been observed that many patient groups who do not respond to regular doses of 400 μg/d of
beclomethasone, may respond with higher initial doses.[76,77] Higher dose trials seem to give more
accurately predictable results than low dose trials. These clinical studies have also suggested that
in addition to symptoms score and decreased use of oral steroids and bronchodilators,
normalization of pulmonary function tests is an important parameter to follow. Recent studies
have also demonstrated that higher dose inhaled steroids or use of concentrated formulations
may help wean steroid-dependent patients from oral therapy.[77]

Bronchial provocation studies have been less helpful in the clinical testing of inhaled steroids.
This may have been partly related to the design of experimental protocols. Earlier studies
demonstrated that both systemic as well as inhaled steroids had no effect on EAR, yet blocked

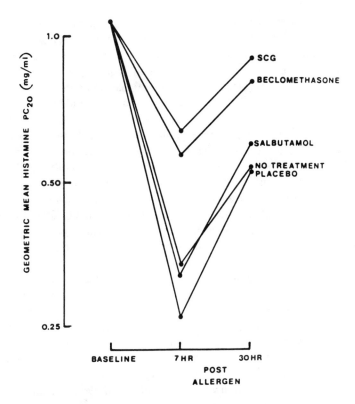

FIGURE 12.   Modification of antigen-induced increase in nonspecific airway hyperresponsiveness by drug pretreatments. Geometric mean PC_{20} is shown for the baseline and at 7 and 30 h after the 5 allergen challenges with pretreatment (control, placebo, cromolyn sodium, salbutamol, and beclomethasone dipropionate). (From Cockcroft, D. W. and Murdock, K. Y., *J. Allergy Clin. Immunol.*, 79, 734, 1987. With permission.)

the LAR.[78,79] Recent studies have confirmed these earlier investigations. Cockcroft and Murdock[73] have shown that inhaled beclomethasone, administered just prior to antigen challenge, had no effect on EAR, but prevented the LAR as well as nonspecific bronchial hyperreactivity to histamine, which followed the LAR (Figures 11 and 12). LAR and bronchial hyperreactivity are more closely related to airway inflammation than EAR, thus underscoring their importance in testing NBAAD agents.

The failure of steroids (both inhaled and systemic) to prevent EAR may have been related to a shorter time interval between the drug administration and antigen challenge. This is borne out by studies conducted in allergic sheep, which demonstrated that systemic administration of methylprednisolone 4 h prior to antigen challenge attenuated the EAR, whereas administration of drug just prior to the antigen challenge was ineffective.[80] Both modes of administration, however, prevented the LAR. Recent studies in asthmatic patients with inhaled steroids support these observations. One study demonstrated that 800 μg daily of beclomethasone for 7 d, prevented the EAR in 50% and LAR in 80% of the subjects.[81] Thus, evaluation of newer inhaled steroids should include studies with both short- and long-term administration of these drugs and perhaps be correlated with clinical studies.

3. Anticholinergic Agents

Anticholinergic agents have been studied in terms of their ability to protect against a wide variety of induced bronchoconstriction. However, the significance of these studies is limited by at least four problems: (1) site of action of agonist vs. the site of action of anticholinergic agent, (2) tests used to determine the response, (3) role of parasympathetic reflex, and (4) change of resting air flow resistance by anticholinergic agents. Keeping these factors in mind, it has been demonstrated that anticholinergic agents (ipratropium bromide) are much more effective against specific muscarinic agonists (e.g., methacholine) than nonmuscarinic bronchoconstrictors.[82] Cockcroft et al.[83] studied the effects of ipratropium bromide against methacholine, histamine, and allergen-induced bronchoconstriction. Ipratropium bromide (80 μg) offered 97% protection against methacholine-induced bronchospasm even when the provocating dose was increased by 400%, while histamine and allergen-induced bronchoconstriction were protected by 57 and 30%, respectively. In another study, Ruffin and colleagues[84] observed that whereas fenoterol (800 μg) significantly reduced the antigen-induced EAR by 76%, ipratropium bromide (80 μg) caused an insignificant reduction of 21%. These data are generally consistent with studies of Howarth et al.,[85] who failed to show any protection of EAR with ipratropium bromide, while albuterol effectively attenuated the EAR. In contrast, some of the earlier studies showed partial protection against antigen-induced bronchoconstriction.[86,87] However, these differences may be related to the changes in resting airway tone produced by anticholinergic agents; furthermore, protection was partial and observed in some subjects only. Anticholinergic agents are unlikely to offer any protection against LAR, and this has been confirmed in animal and human studies.[72] The data are also conflicting on the protective effects of anticholinergic agents against exercise, cold air, and SO_2-induced bronchoconstriction.[82] Some carefully conducted studies showed that ipratropium bromide did not change the magnitude of the bronchoconstrictor response to exercise, and the apparent improvement was entirely due to the bronchodilator effect of the drug.[88] Others, however, believe that there is a subgroup of asthmatics who show partial protection with ipratropium bromide, especially those with large airway EIB.[82]

4. Newer Bronchoprotective Agents

As newer concepts of the pathophysiology of asthma are being evolved, extensive research is being conducted by the pharmaceutical industry for developing newer bronchoprotective agents. Most of the studies so far have been conducted in the animal models of experimental asthma, including sheep, guinea pigs, rats, and monkeys. In these animal studies, effects of investigational drugs on antigen-induced early and late phase bronchoconstriction and bronchial hyperreactivity have been evaluated. These studies are based on the hypothesis that prevention of late phase bronchoconstriction and bronchial hyperreactivity plays a major role in the symptomatic control and exacerbation of asthma. Abraham has demonstrated that inhaled and systemically administered leukotriene antagonists (e.g., FPL-55712, FPL- 57231, LY-171883, WY-48252), attenuated antigen-induced LAR and bronchial hyperresponsiveness in sheep, without affecting the EAR. Similar observations have been made with inhibitors of 5-lipoxygenase enzyme (L-651392).[89] These animal studies underscore the importance of arachidonic acid and related metabolites in the pathophysiology of asthma. Similarly, antagonists of platelet-activating factor (PAF) (WEB-2086, BN52063, BN52021, CV-3988) are being evaluated for prevention of EAR and LAR as well as bronchial hyperreactivity.[90] PAF has been demonstrated to cause prolonged bronchial hyperreactivity in human subjects, and preliminary studies in human subjects have demonstrated partial attenuation of EAR.[91]

Calcium antagonists are currently being investigated as possible bronchoprotective agents. Oral calcium antagonists (verapamil and nifedipine) have been of limited value in human subjects and generally have no significant bronchodilating activity. Both nifedipine and verapamil in oral form prevent the exercise-induced asthma and partly attenuate the histamine and methacholine-induced bronchoconstriction. Oral nifedipine is generally more effective than oral verapamil against acute antigen-induced bronchoconstriction, however, its efficacy may be limited by systemic side effects. Inhaled calcium antagonists may be more effective and free of systemic side effects, as demonstrated by greater efficacy of inhaled verapamil. A new calcium antagonist, gallopamil, is being investigated as an aerosol, and in preliminary studies in sheep and humans was shown to inhibit histamine, carbachol, and antigen-induced bronchoconstriction in sheep and humans. Although the currently available calcium antagonists are of limited value in the treatment of asthma, it is hoped that newer, potent agents, when administered as aerosol, may be of potential clinical use.[92]

The animal studies are quite useful in studying the pathophysiology of asthma and evaluating newer NBAAD agents. Whether such studies could be duplicated in human asthmatics or if these drugs would be of any clinical value remains to be demonstrated. If these studies ultimately appear to be of no or of doubtful clinical importance, then the work of Dr. Altounyan, who performed earlier studies of cromolyn sodium upon himself,[66] would be of major practical importance. It may strongly suggest that once the toxicity, safety, and efficacy studies of NBAAD agents have been conducted, these drugs should be directly tested in human asthmatics.

B. AIRWAY HYPERREACTIVITY

Nonspecific airway hyperreactivity (AHR) is now recognized as one of the most characteristic features of asthma. The degree of bronchial hyperresponsiveness as measured by PD_{20} to histamine or methacholine correlates with the severity of asthma, with airway responses to allergen, and with treatment requirements to control symptoms.[72,93] Thus, reduction of bronchial hyperreactivity by pharmacological means may become central to chronic asthma therapy.

Evaluation of nonspecific bronchial hyperresponsiveness generally involves estimation of bronchoconstrictor response to an agonist such as histamine or methacholine. This requires performing a dose-response curve with increasing concentrations of agonist, and determining the PC_{20} of agonist. Asthmatic subjects have low PC_{20}, compared to normal nonallergic subjects. However, low PC_{20} is not synonymous with asthma, as many patients with chronic bronchitis or hay fever may also have low PC_{20}. A transient increase in AHR, as demonstrated by further lowering of PC_{20}, has also been demonstrated by pollutant exposures, upper respiratory tract infection, hypoxia, as well as after acute antigen challenge.[93]

The increase in AHR after antigen challenge is of clinical and pharmacological importance. Although AHR has been observed after EAR, prolonged increase in AHR is observed after LAR, which has also been related to exacerbations of asthmatic symptoms.[72] It has also been demonstrated that drugs that prevent LAR are also likely to prevent the increase in AHR, and thus by increasing the threshold to bronchoconstriction may be of potential value in the prophylaxis of perennial and seasonal allergic asthma.[72,73] Altounyan[94] reported an inhibitory effect of inhaled cromolyn sodium on increased AHR during the pollen season. Others have confirmed his observations in well-controlled studies.[95] Similarly, reversal of seasonal increase in AHR in allergic subjects by corticosteroids has also been demonstrated.[96] Cockcroft and Murdock[73] recently studied the comparative effects of inhaled salbutamol, cromolyn sodium, and beclomethasone on antigen-induced EAR, LAR, and AHR to histamine. The prevention of increased AHR by these drugs after antigen exposure was closely related to their inhibitory effects on LAR. Thus, cromolyn sodium inhibited the antigen-induced EAR, LAR, and AHR, whereas salbutamol which only attenuated the EAR was ineffective in preventing the increased AHR to histamine (Figure 12). In contrast, beclomethasone, which had no effect on EAR, attenuated the LAR and AHR. It is important to realize that drugs such as cromolyn sodium and beclomethasone generally do not affect the basal airway responsiveness to histamine or methacholine, but prevent the increase in response following antigen exposure, thus increasing the threshold to bronchoconstriction. It has also been suggested that prolonged therapy with cromolyn sodium may also reduce the basal bronchial reactivity to histamine;[97] however, this remains controversial.

Newer drugs under development must be evaluated for their effect on AHR. It has been demonstrated in experiments with allergic sheep that leukotriene antagonists (FPL-55712, FPL-

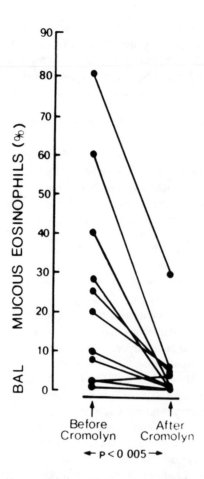

FIGURE 13. Reduction in mucous eosinophils obtained in bronchoalveolar lavage before and after 3 months of cromolyn sodium
therapy. (From Diaz, P., et al., *J. Allergy Clin.
Immunol.*, 74, 41, 1984. With permission.)

57231, LY-171883) not only inhibit antigen-induced LAR, but also diminish AHR.[89] Similarly, pretreatment with FPL-57231 and cromolyn sodium prevented the hypoxia-induced enhancement of nonspecific bronchial reactivity.[98] The effects of other investigational drugs (PAF-antagonists) on AHR are also being investigated.

The role of drugs which prevent an increase in AHR without attenuating EAR or LAR is less well known. For example, the cyclooxygenase inhibitor, indomethacin, has been shown to prevent the increase in AHR following exposure to ozone[99] and antigen[100] without affecting the EAR or LAR. On the other hand, indomethacin has been shown to unmask the late response in sheep with EAR only.[101] Similarly, aspirin has been suggested to exacerbate the symptoms of asthma in asthmatic subjects with aspirin hypersensitivity.[102] Thus, clinical significance of drugs which affect AHR without affecting LAR remains to be demonstrated.

C. AIRWAY INFLAMMATION

Airway inflammation is closely related to LAR and AHR. Many of the drugs which attenuate the LAR and AHR may also affect the airway inflammation. However, the direct clinical testing of the anti-inflammatory effects of these drugs is not possible, as it requires performing bronchial mucosal biopsies or lung lavage. In one study, Diaz and associates[103] studied the effects of inhaled cromolyn sodium on the accumulation of inflammatory cells in the lung lavage fluid of asthmatic subjects. These subjects underwent BAL before and after a 28-d course of either cromolyn sodium or placebo. The percentage of eosinophils in bronchial mucus and BAL fluid was significantly less after cromolyn sodium than after placebo (Figure 13). When the cromolyn sodium-treated patients were divided into responders and nonresponders on the basis of daily symptoms scores, the responders had significantly fewer bronchial eosinophils. However, it is not known whether it represented a direct anti-inflammatory action or an effect secondary to inhibition of chemical mediators released from mast cells.

Antigen-induced EAR in asthmatic subjects is associated with an increase in plasma levels of histamine and serum neutrophil chemotactic activity. It has been shown that drugs such as cromolyn sodium and β_2-agonists which attenuate the EAR, prevent the increase of histamine and neutrophil chemotactic factor (NCF) in blood.[85] In contrast, ipratropium bromide is without effect on EAR as well as mediator release. However, inhibition of mediator release during EAR cannot be taken as an evidence of the anti-inflammatory effect of the drug, as β_2-agonists are devoid of any antiinflammatory effect.

Activation of blood neutrophils *in vitro* was observed during EAR and EIB.[104] This was demonstrated by an increased expression of cell-surface membrane receptors for complement as well as an increased cytotoxic activity of these cells. Cromolyn sodium pretreatment prevented these responses. *In vitro* experiments suggested that cromolyn sodium has significant direct effects on the activation of neutrophils.[69] Thus, it is possible that effects of cromolyn sodium in asthma and other related conditions may be associated with its capacity to directly inhibit leukocyte activation. This may also explain its efficacy in inhibiting LAR and AHR, both of which are closely related to inflammatory response.

V. MUCOCILIARY TRANSPORT

The main purpose of inhaled pharmacological agents used for the treatment of asthma or other obstructive airway diseases is prevention and treatment of bronchospasm. However, many of these drugs affect mucociliary transport, which may or may not be clinically beneficial. Mucociliary transport is decreased in patients with asthma and other obstructive airway diseases such as chronic bronchitis, bronchiectasis, and cystic fibrosis.[105]

β-Adrenergic agonists generally increase mucociliary transport, whether administered as an aerosol or systemically. This has been observed with isoproterenol, epinephrine, and selective β_2-agonists including fenoterol, salbutamol, carbuterol, and terbutaline.[106] β_2-Agonists also prevent the acute antigen-induced decrease in mucociliary transport associated with bronchospasm.[107] It is important to note that freon per se has no effect on mucociliary transport.

Anticholinergic bronchodilator agents such as atropine have been shown to depress mucociliary transport.[105] In contrast to atropine, ipratropium bromide does not slow mucociliary transport in animals or human subjects with or without bronchial asthma.[108]

NBAAD agents have no effect on mucociliary transport, but may prevent mucociliary dysfunction associated with antigen-induced bronchoconstriction. Mezey et al.[109] observed that pretreatment with inhaled cromolyn sodium prevented the antigen-induced mucociliary dysfunction. Subsequent studies demonstrated that inhaled FPL-55712, a leukotriene antagonist, also prevented the antigen-induced decrease in mucociliary transport (Figure 14).[110] No information is currently available in human asthmatics on whether inhaled PAF antagonists or inhaled steroids would prevent antigen-induced mucociliary dysfunction. Inhaled beclomethasone, had no deleterious effect on mucociliary transport in sheep and subjects with chronic bronchitis.[111]

Although mucolytic agents change the rheological properties of respiratory secretions *in vitro*, their effects on mucous secretions and mucociliary transport *in vivo* is not clear. Generally, inhaled agents such as bromhexine and glycerol guaiacolate had no effect on mucociliary

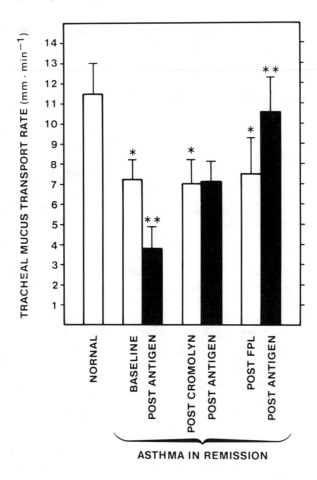

FIGURE 14. Tracheal mucous velocity in normals and subjects with asthma. In the asthmatic subjects tracheal mucous transport is shown before (open bars) and after antigen challenge (solid bars) without and following pretreatment with cromolyn sodium and FPL-55712 (leukotriene antagonist).

transport in normal subjects, although slight improvement has been noticed in subjects with chronic bronchitis.[105] On the other hand, oral 5-carboxymethylcysteine does not appear to stimulate mucociliary transport in patients with COPD.[112] The demonstration of a beneficial effect of mucolytic agents and expectorants in patients with COPD has been based on subjective symptoms without direct *in vivo* evidence on mucociliary transport. Thus, further studies are needed to assess any beneficial effect of these drugs.

VI. EXPERIMENTAL USES

The vast surface area of alveocapillary membrane with its close proximity to blood flow, provides an opportune location for deposition and possible absorption of drugs both for pulmonary and extrapulmonary conditions. Table 5 lists various situations (other than asthma and COPD) in which aerosolized drugs could potentially be of therapeutic use.

A. HEPARIN
Heparin is administered as a subcutaneous injection for prophylaxis of thromboembolism.

TABLE 5
Experimental Uses Of Aerosol Drugs

Pharmacologic agent	Clinical entity
Heparin	Thromboembolism
Cromolyn/vasodilators	Pulmonary hypertension
Calcium antagonist	Asthma
Pentamidine	Pneumocystis (AIDS)
Antibiotics	Cystic fibrosis
Ribavirin	RSV, Influenza; HIV; Lassa fever
α_1-Antitrypsin	α_1-Antitrypsin deficiency
Surfactant	Respiratory distress syndrome
Intranasal	
Desmopressin (DDAVP)	Diabetes insipidus
Pituitary snuff	Panhypopituitarism
Growth hormone	Growth hormone deficiency
Insulin	Diabetes mellitus

Inhalation of heparin has been tried experimentally in dogs, mice, rats, and human volunteers to produce hypocoagulability.[113] In all species a single administration of a large quantity of aerosolized heparin resulted in a prolonged state of moderate hypocoagulability (3 d in dogs, 14 d in man) due to production of a sustained low concentration of heparin in plasma. The lengthening of clotting time and duration of this response increased with higher dosage (effective dosage was about 1300 U/kg). In animals, examination of the lungs, body fluids, and tissues showed that heparin is cleared rapidly from lungs after inhalation. It was postulated that heparin enters a cellular body compartment (probably macrophages) from which it is slowly released into plasma. No toxic effects from inhaled heparin were observed. In another study of 86 patients with thromboembolism, heparin was nebulized 100 mg 4 times daily for 5 d, followed by 100 mg twice daily for 5 months, thus nebulizing an effective maintenance dose of 20 mg/kg/week. Thus, aerosolized heparin has clinical potential for patients needing long-term anticoagulant therapy for prophylaxis of thromboembolism.

B. PULMONARY VASODILATORS

Pulmonary hypertension may be primary or secondary (from intrinsic lung disease and hypoxia). Treatment of pulmonary hypertension may include administration of oxygen and/or pulmonary vasodilators. Since no selective pulmonary vasodilators are available at present, oral pulmonary vasodilators (calcium antagonists, for instance) are generally of limited value because of side effects resulting from systemic hypotension. In conscious sheep, it has been postulated that hypoxic pulmonary hypertension may be caused by chemical mediators released from mast cells, as demonstrated by prevention of hypoxic pulmonary hypertension by i.v. cromolyn sodium.[114] Subsequent studies have also demonstrated the efficacy of aerosolized cromolyn sodium in preventing hypoxic pulmonary hypertension.[115] However, since cromolyn sodium is not a pulmonary vasodilator, it does not reverse the established pulmonary hypertension. It may be possible to administer pulmonary vasodilator drugs as an aerosol for absorption and local action in the pulmonary vascular bed, thus reducing the systemic side effects. No such studies have been performed in human subjects.

C. PENTAMIDINE

More than 60% of patients with AIDS develop *Pneumocystis carinii* pneumonia (PCP). Conventional therapy with either parenteral pentamidine or trimethoprim-sulfamethoxazole is associated with a 50% incidence of significant toxicity. However, systemic toxicity could be significantly lowered, if these drugs could be effectively nebulized into the lungs. Studies in normal rodents have shown that inhaled pentamidine results in higher pulmonary and lower kidney and liver concentrations than parenteral pentamidine.[116] Immunosuppressed rats with PCP infection can be successfully treated with aerosolized pentamidine.[117] In a pilot study, Conte et al.[118] treated 13 patients with inhaled pentamidine (4 mg/kg/d). Nine patients responded satisfactorily and three had early relapse. It has been suggested that relapse can be prevented by increasing the duration of treatment or dose of pentamidine. Since pentamidine was delivered directly into the lungs, the drug concentration in the lavage fluid was 10-fold higher than that in the i.v. group.[118,119] Furthermore, very little inhaled pentamidine was absorbed into the systemic circulation and two thirds of plasma samples had no detectable pentamidine. It has also been shown that pentamidine delivery can be markedly enhanced by administration in liposomes.[120] Aerosolized pentamidine had no deleterious effects on pulmonary function, while some patients reported pentamidine-related cough, bronchospasm, and temperature elevation.[118]

D. ANTIBIOTICS

Antibiotic aerosol therapy was first used in 1945 when various antibiotics were inhaled either as nebulized solutions or dry powder to treat respiratory infections.[121] Although this practice waned in popularity, it has recently been revived, particularly for treatment and prophylaxis of pseudomonas infections in some patients with cystic fibrosis.[122] Studies in patients with chronic bronchitis, pneumonia, bronchiectasis, and lung abscess have not led to any general support for the use of nebulized antibiotics in the management of these diseases. As mentioned above, aerosol pentamidine therapy is being evaluated for treatment of PCP infection in patients with AIDS.[118,119] Antibiotics used for cystic fibrosis patients have included polymyxin, gentamicin, and carbenicillin. The major problem with all nebulized antimicrobial agents is that they can cause airway irritation and bronchospasm. The efficacy of aerosol antibiotic treatment also depends upon the site of deposition of the drug in the airways, and thus, indirectly on the choice of nebulizer equipment.[123] It may be difficult to get the antibiotic aerosol to the desired site as secretions in the proximal airways may prevent peripheral deposition.

E. ANTIVIRAL AGENTS

Respiratory syncytial virus (RVS) infection in infants and young children and influenza infection in adults remain the most important respiratory pathogen viruses in this country. Immunity to these viruses is of short duration, and until recently, no effective treatment or prophylaxis were available. Ribavirin, a new experimental antiviral agent, is a synthetic nucleoside that possesses antiviral properties *in vitro* against a variety of both RNA and DNA viruses and has shown clinical efficacy against influenza and RSV infections.[124-127] The course of both influenza A and B infections in adults has been shown to be ameliorated by ribavirin therapy, especially when this agent is administered by small particle aerosol.[124,125] Ribavirin aerosol has also been evaluated in young adults with experimental RSV infection.[126] Volunteers treated with ribavirin aerosol appeared to have diminished systemic symptoms, fever, and viral shedding, as compared with a placebo-treated group. In 1983, Hall et al.[127] evaluated ribavirin for the treatment of infants hospitalized with RSV infection of the lower respiratory tract. Ribavirin or placebo aerosol was administered to 33 infants in a double-blind manner as a continuous aerosol for 3 to 6 d. Seventeen infants who received ribavirin had significantly greater improvement in their overall score for severity of illness, clinical signs of bronchial infection, and arterial oxygenation, as well as diminished viral shedding. More recently, ribavirin aerosol was administered to elderly COPD patients at high risk for influenza.[128] No significant side effects on pulmonary function were observed after 96 h of therapy. Whether this drug would be of prophylactic value in preventing viral-induced exacerbations of COPD remains to be demonstrated. The FDA approved the aerosolized ribavirin for lower respiratory tract infection due to RSV virus in infants and children in 1987.

F. α₁-ANTITRYPSIN

In patients with emphysema due to α_1-antitrypsin deficiency, replacement therapy with α_1-antitrypsin has been investigated. So far the trials have been with weekly parenteral replacement. Such parenteral replacement therapy has been demonstrated to elevate the α_1-antitrypsin to adequate levels.[129] In addition, assessment of lower respiratory tract antielastase activity by bronchoalveolar lavage demonstrated that parenteral replacement of α_1-antitrypsin resulted in establishment of effective antielastase activity within the alveoli. Currently, trials with aerosolized α_1-antitrypsin are being conducted at the National Institutes of Health.

G. SURFACTANT

Surfactant deficiency due to immaturity is characteristic of the respiratory distress syndrome in premature infants. Surfactant replacement is effective in prevention and amelioration of the respiratory distress syndrome of the newborn. Robillard and associates[130] felt that the aerosol may have alleviated the respiratory distress somewhat. Chu et al.[131] noted a change in lung compliance but no changes in clinical status after surfactant aerosol exposure. Subsequent studies in animals and in human infants born with surfactant deficiency have established an important new way to reduce morbidity and mortality in premature infants by replacing one component of pulmonary surfactant, i.e., dipalmitoyl phosphatidylcholine.[132] The essential differences between the earlier unsuccessful studies and more recent studies that have met with unequivocal success relate to the mode of administration and the nature of the surfactant delivered. The best results are achieved when 60 to 120 mg of surfactant, derived from bovine lungs or human amniotic fluid, are introduced into the lung through an endotracheal tube as a bolus of 3 to 5 ml.[133,134] Efforts are underway to synthesize the ideal artificial surfactant. Because of the failure of the pioneering work of Chu et al., interest in the aerosolized mode of administration has not been revived. However, aerosol technology has become very sophisticated and it may be worthwhile reinvestigating this mode of administration.

H. INTRANASAL AEROSOLS (SPRAYS)

The nasal mucosa has an extensive blood supply and is easily accessible. Intranasal deposition of drugs could be used for absorption into the circulation and in achieving systemic effects. This mode of administration of drugs for systemic effects is being investigated for experimental or clinical use in the following conditions: (1) desmopressin for diabetes insipidus, (2) pituitary snuff for panhypopituitarism, (3) growth hormone for growth hormone deficiency, and (4) insulin for diabetes mellitus. In addition, nasal sprays are clinically used for treating primary allergic or nonallergic disorders of the nose. These agents include cromolyn sodium (Nasalcrom) and beclomethasone (Beconase or Vancenase) for allergic rhinitis and other nonspecific nasal decongestants containing α-agonists.

I. LIPOSOMES

Liposomes are lipid vesicles composed of a bilayer membrane enclosing an aqueous space. Because of their unique properties, they have been studied extensively as drug carriers. Hydrophilic agents can be encapsulated in the internal aqueous spaces and lipophilic substances can be incorporated into the lipid bilayer. Liposomes are composed of naturally occurring, biodegradable lipids and appear largely nontoxic *in vivo*, even after systemic administration in high doses. Drug delivery in liposomes can significantly alter retention, metabolism, absorption into circulation, and intracellular fate of encapsulated agents. It was recently demonstrated that uptake of pentamidine in the lung was selectively enhanced by delivery in liposomes.[135] It is possible that aerosol drug delivery in liposomes may enhance drug efficacy by greater intrapulmonary retention. In addition, because of poor absorption into circulation, systemic side effects may be lessened. This would be ideal for β-agonist aerosols and may greatly increase their therapeutic index and duration of action.

TABLE 6
Side Effects of
Inhaled Drugs

Cardiac
Respiratory
Neurologic
Endocrine
Oropharyngeal
Candidiasis
Dysphonia
Cough
Ocular

VII. SIDE EFFECTS OF AEROSOL DRUGS

Inhaled drugs may exhibit adverse reactions which are either "general" — related to the use of aerosols, or "specific" — related to pharmacologic actions of drug (Table 6).

A. ARE AEROSOL SPRAYS HAZARDOUS?

The three essential components of an aerosol spray are the propellant, the solvent, and the active ingredient; each component may be hazardous. The most common propellants are fluorochlorohydrocarbons, bearing the tradename freon. Originally, fluorocarbons were considered nontoxic, a view that is no longer tenable. In acute animal experiments the major toxic effect is on the heart, and depending upon the experimental conditions depression of myocardial contractility, conduction, and irritability has been observed.[136] Cardiac arrhythmias are more likely to occur in the presence of hypoxemia. It is also possible that fluorocarbons may sensitize the myocardium for the arrhythmogenic effects of β-agonists. Peak arterial plasma concentrations of fluorocarbons that follow use of MDI in human subjects for the treatment of asthma are quite small, occur within 20 s, and then rapidly decrease.[137] These levels are 12 to 25% of those associated with arrhythmias in dogs.

Recent studies in dogs and human subjects revealed variable effects of freon on cardiac output.[138,139] In dogs, 20 puffs of freon caused a 16% increase in cardiac output.[138] In human subjects with reversible airway obstruction, two puffs of freon had no significant effects on pulmonary blood flow, whereas eight puffs increased pulmonary blood flow, which was not significantly different from that with isoproterenol.[139] The increased mortality from asthma in England and Wales in the 1960s, followed the introduction of MDIs. The cause of increased mortality remained unexplained and may have been partly related to excessive use of concentrated forms of isoproterenol, in the presence of freon and hypoxemia. Thus, it is possible that excessive use of MDI in an asthmatic patient with severe hypoxemia may produce cardiac toxicity and arrhythmias.

B. CARDIOVASCULAR

The cardiovascular effects of nonselective β_2-agonists (for example, isoproterenol) are well known.[138-140] Selective β_2-agonists, although less likely, do produce cardiac effects in the form of tachyarrhythmias. These effects are more likely to occur with excessive use in patients with severe asthma attacks and underlying coronary artery disease. Electrocardiographic abnormalities of T-wave and ST-depression have been observed in 4% of patients.[140] In contrast, ipratropium bromide, even at higher doses, has no significant cardiovascular effects.[139]

C. PULMONARY

The pulmonary effects of inhaled drugs are uncommon and consist of cough and bronchospasm. Bronchoconstriction has been reported with all inhaled agents including selective and nonselective β-agonists, however, the incidence remains low. In some instances, it may be related to the preservative. For example, ipratropium bromide nebulizer solution containing benzalkonium chloride can cause paradoxical bronchoconstriction, but not the preservative-free solution.[141] Although freon is generally considered devoid of any airway effects, in one study it decreased SGaw in some subjects.[139]

Rare cough is not an uncommon observation; however, irritating cough occurs infrequently. With ipratropium bromide, the incidence is 9.9%[54] and β-agonists produce cough less frequently. Both inhaled cromolyn sodium (powder or solution) and inhaled steroids have been reported to produce cough.[75,142] If the episode of cough is severe, it may produce bronchospasm. In one study, cough and wheezing from inhaled beclomethasone resulted in discontinuation of the drug in 24% of the patients.[142] It has also been reported recently that compared to beclomethasone, inhaled triamcinolone has a much lower incidence of cough and wheezing.[142]

D. OROPHARYNGEAL

The oropharyngeal complications of candidiasis and dysphonia are related to the use of inhaled steroids. Although positive throat cultures of candida are quite frequent, clinical thrush is reported in about 4 to 13% of cases treated with beclomethasone or triamcinolone.[75] It has been suggested that use of spacer devices may lower the incidence of candidiasis. Different degrees of dysphonia have been reported in 5 to 50% of cases, and can occur in the presence or absence of candidiasis. These symptoms tend to get better with temporary lowering of the steroid dose and rarely necessitate withdrawal of drug.

E. ENDOCRINE

Long-term use of oral steroids produces suppression of hypothalamic-pituitary-adrenal (HPA) axis. Initial studies with inhaled beclomethasone reported no suppression of HPA-axis at a dose of 400 µg/d. However, recent studies with 1600 µg/d, have shown a significant suppressive effect.[75] Children are more susceptible to HPA-axis suppression than adults and even doses of 400 to 800 µg/d have demonstrated some suppression of HPA-axis. It has been suggested that HPA-axis suppression in children or adults is more likely to occur with inhaled doses of greater than 14 µg/kg/d.[75,143]

F. NERVOUS SYSTEM

Inhaled drugs generally have no chronic effects on the central nervous system. Nervousness, anxiety, and tremors have been reported with the use of β-agonists.[140]

G. OCULAR

Ocular side effects are infrequent with most inhaled agents. Intraocular pressure in patients with glaucoma and chronic obstructive airway disease does not change with the use of ipratropium or salbutamol.[144] However, when these drugs were used in combination intraocular pressure rose in patients with narrow-angle glaucoma, but not in patients with open angle glaucoma. Anticholinergic agents can also produce mydriasis because of the local effect related to the use of spray.

VIII. GUIDELINES FOR CLINICAL TESTING

The U.S. Food and Drug Administration, with the assistance of its Scientific Advisory Committee and other outside consultants, including those from academia and the Pharmaceutical Manufacturers Association, have developed guidelines for the clinical evaluation of new drugs. These guidelines present acceptable, current approaches to the study of investigational drugs in man, and pertain to phases I through III of the investigation. These guidelines present generally accepted principles for the study of specific classes of drugs and for reaching valid conclusions concerning safety and effectiveness of new drugs.

The guidelines are not mandatory requirements by the FDA for clinical trials with investigational drugs or to obtain approval of a new drug for marketing. Under the FDA regulations (21CFR 10.90), all clinical guidelines constitute advisory opinions on an acceptable approach to meeting regulatory requirements, and research begun in good faith under such guidelines will be accepted by the Agency for review purposes unless this guideline has been formally rescinded for valid health reasons. It is also clear that studies conducted under these guidelines will not necessarily result in the approval of an application or that the studies suggested will produce the total clinical information required for approval of a particular drug.

In 1978, the FDA published guidelines for the clinical evaluation of "bronchodilator" antiasthmatic drugs,[145] while guidelines for "nonbronchodilator" antiasthmatic drugs were published in 1986.[146] These guidelines are for all drugs included in BAAD and NBAAD categories; however, no special attention was paid to aerosol drugs. In April and May, 1988, another meeting was held under the auspices of the FDA to update the guidelines for bronchodilator drugs, which included some discussion on aerosol drugs. The final updated guidelines, after undergoing regular bureaucratic process, will be available for publication at a later date. However, one can obtain the preliminary minutes of the meeting by writing to:

Food and Drug Administration
Freedom of Information Staff, HF1-35
5600 Fishers Lane
Rockville, MD 20857

A. GENERAL CONSIDERATIONS

Clinical evaluations of a particular drug must include well-designed studies from phase I to phase III and postmarketing surveillance of phase IV (Table 7). For aerosol drugs, special attention must be paid to actuated dose, as well as comparable aerosol delivery systems (Table 8).

The "efficacy/risk" ratio is a critical parameter in determining acceptability of a particular drug. In addition to comparison with a placebo, careful comparison of the new drug with an acknowledged reference drug is needed for adequate appraisal and labeling of the drug. However, for some new drugs with a novel mode of action, no useful comparison may be available.

Efficacy should be considered in relation to realistic, clinical circumstances and interactions with other drugs should be studied. Likewise, risks and toxicity should be studied with attention to relevant clinical circumstances, e.g., the drug might induce cardiac arrhythmias in hypoxic individuals but not in normoxic ones. A careful search for potential toxicity should be undertaken using appropriate methods, particularly in the areas of cardiovascular effects, metabolic effects, and neurologic effects.

The determination of safety and efficacy of bronchodilator and nonbronchodilator antiasthmatic drugs should be based upon objective data obtained with pulmonary functions and bronchoprovocation tests, respectively, as well as subjective data with symptoms score and evidence of the reduction of the requirements for other concomitant drugs. Finally, for aerosol drugs, study of the role of the carrier material (vehicle) to be administered with the drug should also be performed.

1. Phase I

Phase I follows completion of initial *in vitro* and *in vivo* animal studies which have demonstrated desired activity, potency, and safety. It consists of studying pharmacokinetics and

TABLE 7
Clinical Evaluation Of A New Drug

Phase I
  Radioisotopic investigations
  Drug assay in biological fluids
  Single dose pharmacokinetics
    Rate of absorption
    Protein binding
    Distribution parameters
    Route of elimination
    Extent of absorption
  Multiple single-dose studies
  Number of subjects

Phase II
  Single dose studies
  Multiple dose studies
  Potency, efficacy, safety,
    drug interaction

Phase III
  Extended phase II
  Other patient groups
  Other population groups

Phase IV
  Postmarketing surveillance (logistics)
  Safety, toxicity, loss of effect

TABLE 8
Factors Influencing the
Response to Inhaled Drugs

Standardization
  Actuated dose
  Dose delivered to oropharynx
  Dose delivered to conducting airways

Assessment
  Patient coordination
  Patient compliance
  Severe side effects with abuse
  Systemic toxicity, e.g., steroids

Comparable delivery system

Estimation of response

metabolic effects of drug, safety, and determination of a preliminary dose-range for further study. The initial study may be a limited, single-dose pilot study, for example, to demonstrate bronchodilator activity in patients with reversible airway obstruction, or prevention of antigen-induced bronchospasm. If these results are promising, studies of dose-response and dose-toxicity relationships in several animal species should be undertaken.

Pharmacokinetics and metabolism of the drug should be performed in normal subjects and patients with mild disease. This should be followed by single-dose, short-term studies to determine a safe, therapeutic dose of the drug. Studies should be placebo-controlled, double-blind, and compared with a reference aerosol drug. These studies should provide preliminary information about onset and duration of action and dose-response information in terms of efficacy and adverse reactions.

2. Phase II

The objective of phase II studies are to evaluate potency, efficacy, safety, tachyphylaxis, cumulative drug effect, and drug interaction with other agents. Phase II studies should provide detailed information on onset and duration of action and dose-response characteristics regarding efficacy and adverse reactions. These studies should be performed in a homogeneous patient population, e.g., with demonstrable, reversible airway obstruction, while testing a bronchodilator agent.

Studies should be conducted over a 3-month period with parallel or crossover design (6 weeks ×2), in a double-blind fashion and should utilize at least one reference agent. There should be a sufficient washout period of 2 to 4 weeks prior to investigation, and drugs with a mechanism of action similar to the test drug should be withheld. If crossover design is considered, a second washout period of 2 weeks is necessary, since there could be substantial carryover effect and/ or tachyphylaxis. Because of this and intrasubject variability, parallel design studies may be preferable.

3. Phase III

The objective of phase III studies is to further define the safety and effectiveness of the drug, including its usefulness in certain subgroups of patients. The design of phase III studies, generally, is similar to that of phase II; however, emphasis is placed on studying "larger groups" of subjects, as well as longer term side effects and tachyphylaxis. Phase III subjects should be subclassified into well-defined disease groups so that the spectrum of clinical usefulness of the drug can be evaluated and information included in the labeling. For example, patients with obstructive airway disease due to chronic bronchitis and emphysema should be distinguished from those with asthma. Likewise, patient subgroups with extrinsic asthma, intrinsic asthma, exercise-induced asthma, and asthma associated with aspirin sensitivity should be clearly separated. These large-scale studies should be of at least 3 months' duration, double-blind, and should use (except for novel agents) a reference drug. Studies with concomitant drugs should also be conducted.

4. Phase IV

Because phases II and III studies are of shorter duration (i.e., 3 to 4 months), it is desirable to perform long-term observational studies for safety in the postmarketing period.

B. SPECIAL CONSIDERATIONS
1. Aerosol Dose

Studies should be well controlled in terms of particle size of aerosol, inhalation technique, delivered and deposited dose, and aerosol delivery system.

2. Bronchodilator Agents

Clinical assessment of aerosol bronchodilator agents is generally a straightforward procedure, as inhalation of agents is followed by a measurable change in indices of bronchodilatation. However, special attention should be paid to side effects. Study design should be either parallel or crossover design. Generally, parallel studies are preferable, and crossover design should be followed by an adequate washout period to avoid carryover effect. In addition, data should be carefully analyzed for tachyphylaxis and drug interaction.

While comparing two or more aerosol bronchodilator agents in a single-dose study, special attention should be focused on factors which may influence the bronchodilator response (Table

TABLE 9
Designing a Single-Dose Bronchodilator Study
(Comparing 2 or More Bronchodilators)

Dosages should be equipotent (same FEV_1)
Dosages should be submaximal
Comparable baseline lung function
Placebo-controlled, random order, and double blind
Withhold other bronchodilators if possible (β-agonists,
  theophylline, steroids)
Comparable patient groups
Diurnal variation (same time of the day)

TABLE 10
Design Errors

Use of single-blind design
No placebo or positive control
Poor control of factors that cause variation of clinical response
Crossover study does not include a long enough washout period
Poorly regulated concomitant treatment
Inadequate sample size
Inappropriate data analysis
NBAAD
  No study of late response

9), including comparable drug potency, baseline pulmonary functions, patient groups, concomitant drug therapy, and aerosol delivery system.

3. Nonbronchodilator Agents

Clinical testing of nonbronchodilator agents is somewhat complicated and requires well-designed "objective" bronchoprovocation studies as well as clinical "subjective" studies to demonstrate efficacy as bronchoprotective agents. Subjective clinical studies of symptoms scores and decreased use of concomitant agents are difficult to quantitate as they are overlayed on the spontaneous variability of asthma.

The task force of the American Association of Allergy and Immunology in cooperation with the National Institute of Allergy and Infectious Disease, the FDA, academia, and the pharmaceutical industry held a workshop in June 1985 at the NIH and made recommendations for guidelines for the evaluation of NBAAD agents, which were published in 1986. Eight workshops were held including: (1) overview of past lessons, (2) special pharmacologic considerations for the NBAAD agent, (3) study design, (4) role of bronchoprovocation, (5) assessment of efficacy, (6) compliance factors, (7) special pediatric problems, and (8) data analysis. In spite of the fact that two major NBAAD agents are used as aerosol drugs (i.e., cromolyn sodium, steroids), very little attention was paid to special consideration for this mode of administration. As mentioned in Table 8, in addition to nebulized dose, airway deposited dose and a comparable delivery system would be very important for the testing of NBAAD agents.

4. Design Errors

Possible design errors for bronchodilator and nonbronchodilator drug testing have been listed in Table 10. These errors include the use of single-blind studies, absence of placebo control, lack of washout period for crossover designs, poorly regulated concomitant treatment, inadequate sample size, and inappropriate data analysis. In addition, for an NBAAD agent, the absence of studies evaluating its effect on late response and bronchial hyperreactivity may be a potential

TABLE 11
Avoidance of Design Error

Double-blind studies
Placebo and/or positive controls
Parallel group studies preferable, unless washout period
  of drug is clearly established
Pre- and poststudy control periods
Clarity of hypothesis and goal
Adequate sample size (single center and multicenter)
Appropriate statistics
Special considerations for NBAAD
  How long it takes to achieve maximal effect
  Standardized approach to concomitant medications
  Frequency, dose, estimation of response
  Effect on late phase and bronchial hyperresponsiveness

design error. This has been discussed in detail previously. It is important to reiterate that interpretation of data could be made somewhat easier with early attention to these details. Table 11 lists the salient features of avoiding these design errors. For the pharmaceutical industry that would require closer coordination between the clinical research group and regulatory affairs group.

It is expected that in the near future there will be an increased use of aerosol drugs for respiratory pharmacology, with or without the possible discovery of a substitute for freon propellants. It is certain that guidelines and regulations regarding use of aerosol drugs will become more stringent. Therefore, it is in the best interest of the pharmaceutical industry to work with the FDA and design specific guidelines for aerosol drugs.

ACKNOWLEDGMENTS

The author would like to thank Mrs. Annette Bethel for typing the chapter and Dr. Martin Cohn for his critical review of the chapter.

REFERENCES

1. **James, P.,** *The Therapeutics of Respiratory Passages,* William Wood, New York, 1984.
2. **Wood, M.,** Evaluating our new drug regulation system, *Resp. Ther.,* 4, 41, 1974.
3. **Wardell, W. M.,** Introduction of new therapeutic drugs in the United States and Great Britain: an international comparison, *Private Pract.,* 61, 1973.
4. **Ziment, I., Ed.,** *Respiratory Pharmacology and Therapeutics,* W. B. Saunders, Philadelphia, 1978.
5. **Stewart, B. N. and Block, A. J.,** A trial of aerosolized theophylline in relieving bronchospasm, *Chest,* 69, 718, 1976.
6. **Bargar, G. and Dale, H. H.,** Chemical structure and sympathomimetic action of amines, *J. Physiol. (London),* 41, 19, 1910.
7. **Konzett, H.,** Neue broncholytisch hochwirksome Korper der Adrenalinreibe, *Arch. Exp. Pathol. Pharmakol.,* 197, 27, 1940.
8. **Ahlquist, R. P.,** A study of adrenotropic receptors, *Am. J. Physiol.,* 153, 586, 1948.
9. **Lands, A. M., Arnold, A., McAuliff, J. P., Luduena, F. P., and Brown, T. G., Jr.,** Differentiation of receptor systems activated by sympathomimetic amines, *Nature,* 214, 597, 1967.
10. **Svedmyr, N. and Thiringer, G.,** The effects of salbutamol and isoprenaline on β-receptors in patients with COPD, Postgrad. Med. J., 47(Suppl.), 44, 1971.

11. **Brittain, R. T., Dean, C. M., and Jack, D.,** Sympathomimetic bronchodilating drugs, in *Respiratory Pharmacology,* Widdicombe, J., Ed., Pergamon Press, Oxford, 1981, 613.

12. **Svedmyr, N.,** Fenoterol: a b_2-adrenergic agonist for use in asthma. Pharmacology, pharmacokinetics, clinical efficacy and adverse effects, *Pharmacotherapy,* 5, 109, 1985.

13. **Clark, T. J. H.,** The inhaled route as the route of choice in airway disease therapy, in *New Concepts in the Topical Treatment of Asthma and Related Disorders,* Cliggott Publishing, Greenwich, CT, 1982, 15.

14. **Thiringer, G. and Svedmyr, N.,** Evaluation of skeletal muscle tremor due to bronchodilator agents, *Scand. J. Resp. Dis.,* 56, 93, 1975.

15. **Thiringer, G. and Svedmyr, N.,** Comparison of infused and inhaled terbutaline in patients with asthma, *Scand. J. Resp. Dis.,* 57, 17, 1976.

16. **Duncan, D., Paterson, K., Harris, D., and Crompton, G. K.,** Comparison of a bronchodilator effect of salbutamol inhaled as a dry powder and by conventional pressurized aerosol, *Br. J. Pharmacol.,* 4, 669, 1977.

17. **Hetzel, M. R. and Clark, T. J.,** Comparison of salbutamol rotahaler with conventional pressurized aerosol, *Clin. Allergy,* 7, 563, 1977.

18. **Bronsky, E., Bucholtz, G. A., Busse, W. W., Chervinsky, P., Condemi, J., Ghafouri, M. A., Hudson, L., Lakshminarayan, S., Lockey, R., and Reese, M. E.,** Comparison of inhaled albuterol powder and aerosol in asthma, *J. Allergy Clin. Immunol.,* 79, 741, 1987.

19. **Tashkin, D. P.,** Measurement and significance of the bronchodilator response, Jenne, J. W. and Murphy, S., Eds., Marcel Dekker, New York, 1987, 535.

20. **Ahrens, R. C. and Smith, G. D.,** Albuterol: an adrenergic agent for use in the treatment of asthma pharmacology, pharmacokinetics and clinical use, *Pharmacotherapy,* 4, 105, 1984.

21. **Jenne, J. W. and Ahrens, R. C.,** Pharmacokinetics of beta-adrenergic compounds, in Jenne, J. W. and Murphy, S., Eds., Marcel Dekker, New York, 1987, 213.

22. **Choo-Kang, Y. F. J., Simpson, W. T., and Grant, I. W. B.,** Controlled comparison of the bronchodilator effects of three B-adrenergic stimulant drugs administered by inhalation to patients with asthma, *Br. Med. J.,* 2, 287, 1969.

23. **Choo-Kang, Y. F. J., MacDonald, H. L., and Horne, N. W.,** A comparison of salbutamol and terbutaline aerosols in bronchial asthma, *Practitioner,* 211, 801, 1973.

24. **Freedman, B. J.,** Trial of terbutaline aerosol in the treatment of asthma and comparison of its effects with those of salbutamol aerosol, *Br. J. Dis. Chest,* 66, 222, 1972.

25. **Hartnett, B. J. and Marlin, G. E.,** Comparison of terbutaline and salbutamol aerosols, *Aust. N. Z. J. Med.,* 7(1), 13, 1977.

26. **Ahrens, R. C., Bonham, A. C., Maxwell, G. A., and Weinberger, M. M.,** A method for comparing the peak intensity and duration of action of aerosolized bronchodilators using bronchoprovocation with methacholine, *Am. Rev. Resp. Dis.,* 129, 903, 1984.

27. **Salome, C. M., Schoeffel, R. E., Yan, K., and Woolcock, A. J.,** Effect of aerosol fenoterol on the severity of bronchial hyperreactivity in patients with asthma, *Thorax,* 38, 854, 1983.

28. **Ahrens, R. C., Harris, J. B., Milavetz, G., Annis, L., and Ries, R.,** Use of bronchial provocation with histamine to compare pharmacodynamics of inhaled albuterol and metaproterenol in patients with asthma, *J. Allergy Clin. Immunol.,* 79, 876, 1987.

29. **Sly, R. M., Heimlich, E. M., Ginsburg, J., Busser, R. J., and Strick, L.,** Exercise-induced bronchospasm: evaluation of metaproterenol, *Ann. Allergy,* 26, 253, 1968.

30. **Harris, J. B., Ahrens, R. C., and Annis, L.,** Comparison of intervals and duration of effect of albuterol and bitolterol using bronchial provocation with histamine, *Ann. Allergy,* 56, 250, 1986.

31. **Conolly, M. E., Hui, K. K., Borst, S. E., and Jenne, J. W.,** Beta-adrenergic tachyphylaxis (desensitization) and functional antagonism, Jenne, J. W. and Murphy, S., Eds., Marcel Dekker, New York, 1987, 259.

32. **Jenne, J. W., Chick, T. W., Strickland, R. D., and Wall, F. J.,** Subsensitivity of beta responses during therapy with a long acting beta-2 preparation, *J. Allergy Clin. Immunol.,* 59, 383, 1977.

33. **Plummer, A. L.,** Development of drug tolerance to B_2-adrenergic agents in asthmatic patients, *Chest,* 73(Suppl.), 749, 1978.

34. **Weber, R. W., Smith, J. A., and Nelson, H. S.,** Aerosolized terbutaline in asthmatics. Development of subsensitivity with long term administration, *J. Allergy Clin. Immunol.,* 70, 417, 1982.

35. **Repsher, L. H., Anderson, J. A., Bush, R. K., Falliers, C. J., Kass, I. E., Kemp, J. P., Reed, C., Siegel, S., and Webb, D. R.,** Assessment of tachyphylaxis following pro-longed therapy of asthma with inhaled albuterol, *Chest,* 85, 34, 1984.

36. **Larsson, S., Svedmyr, N., and Thiringer, G.,** Lack of bronchial beta-adrenoreceptor resistance in asthmatic during long term treatment with terbutaline, *J. Allergy Clin. Immunol.,* 59, 93, 1977.

37. **Szentivanyi, A.,** The beta adrenergic theory of atopic abnormality in bronchial asthma, *J. Allergy,* 42, 203, 1968.

38. **Conolly, M. E. and Greenacre, J. K.,** The lymphocyte beta-adrenoceptor in normal subjects and patients with bronchial asthma, *J. Clin. Invest.,* 58, 1307, 1976.

39. **Hui, K. K., Conolly, M. E., and Tashkin, D. P.,** Reversal of human lymphocyte B-adrenoceptor desensitization by glucocorticoids, *Clin. Pharmacol. Ther.,* 32, 566, 1982.

40. **Lakshminarayan, S.,** Ipratropium bromide in chronic bronchitis/emphysema: a review of literature, *Am. J. Med.,* 81(Suppl. 5A), 76, 1986.

41. **Pakes, G. E., Brogden, R. N., Heel, R. C., Speight, T. M., and Avery, G. S.,** Ipratropium bromide: a review of its pharmacological properties and therapeutic efficacy in asthma and chronic bronchitis, *Drugs,* 20, 237, 1980.

42. **Gross, N. J. and Skorodin, M. S.,** Anticholinergic, antimuscarinic bronchodilators, *Am. Rev. Resp. Dis.,* 129, 856, 1984.

43. **Mann, J. S. and George, C. F.,** Anticholinergic drugs in the treatment of airways disease, *Br. J. Dis. Chest,* 79, 209, 1985.

44. **Klock, L. E., Miller, T. D., Morris, A. H., Watanalie, S., and Dickman, M.,** A comparative study of atropine sulfate and isoproterenol hydrochloride in chronic bronchitis, *Am. Rev. Resp. Dis.,* 112, 371, 1975.

45. **Pak, C. C., Kradjan, W. A., Lakshminarayan, S., and Marini J. J.,** Inhaled atropine sulfate: dose response characteristics in adult patients with chronic airflow obstruction, *Am. Rev. Resp. Dis.,* 125, 331, 1982.

46. **Allen, C. J. and Campbell, A. H.,** Comparison of inhaled atropine sulfate and atropine methonitrate, *Thorax,* 35, 932, 1980.

47. **Cavanaugh, M. J. and Cooper, D. M.,** Inhaled atropine sulfate: dose response characteristics, *Am. Rev. Resp. Dis.,* 114, 517, 1976.

48. **Botts, L. D., Pingleton, S. K., Schroeder, C. E., Robinson, R. G., and Hurwitz, A.,** Prolongation of gastric emptying by aerosolized atropine, *Am. Rev. Resp. Dis.,* 131, 725, 1985.

49. **Schlueter, D. P.,** Ipratropium bromide in asthma: a review of the literature, *Am. J. Med.,* 81(Suppl. 5A), 55, 1986.

50. **Chervinsky, P.,** Concomitant bronchodilator therapy and ipratropium bromide: a clinical review, *Am. J. Med.,* 81(Suppl. 5A), 67, 1986.

51. **Cugell, D. W.,** Clinical pharmacology and toxicology of ipratropium bromide, *Am. J. Med.,* 81(Suppl. 5A), 18, 1986.

52. **Islam, M. S. and Ulmer, W. T.,** Influence of the inhalative aerosol atrovent on airway resistance and intrathoracic gas volume in healthy volunteers of different ages, *Respiration,* 45, 225, 1984.

53. **Tashkin, D. P., Ashutosh, K., Bleeker, E. R., Britt, E. J., Cugell, D. W., Gross, N. J., Renzetti, A., Sackner, M. A., Skorodin, M. S., Wanner, A., and Watanabe, S.,** Comparison of the anticholinergic bronchodilator ipratropium bromide with metaproterenol in chronic obstructive pulmonary disease: a 90-day multicenter study, *Am. J. Med.,* 81(Suppl. 5A), 81, 1986.

54. **Storms, W. W., Bodman, S. F., Nathan, R. A., Busse, W. W., Bush, R. K., Falliers, C. J., O'Hollaren, J. D., and Weg, J. G.,** Use of ipratropium bromide in asthma: results of a multi-clinic study, *Am. J. Med.,* 81(Suppl. 5A), 61, 1986.

55. **Lefcoe, N. M., Toogood, J. H., Blennerhassett, G., Baskerville, J., and Paterson, N. A.,** The addition of an aerosol anticholinergic to an oral beta agonist plus theophylline in asthma and chronic bronchitis: a double blind single dose study, *Chest,* 82, 300, 1982.

56. **Hoffbrand, B. I. and Phillips, V. J.,** The wheezy patient and duovent, *Postgraduate Med. J.,* 60(Suppl.), 1, 1984.

57. **Beck, R., Robertson, C., Galdes-Sebaldt, M., and Levison, H.,** Combined salbutamol and ipratropium bromide by inhalation on the treatment of severe acute asthma, *J. Pediatr.,* 107, 605, 1985.

58. **Barnes, P. J.,** Airway receptors, Jenne, J. W. and Murphy, S., Eds., Marcel Dekker, New York, 1987, 67.

59. **Ingram, R. H., Wellman, J. J., Mcfadden, E. R., Jr., and Mead, J.,** Relative contribution of large and small airways to flow-limitation in normal subjects before and after atropine and isoproterenol, *J. Clin. Invest.,* 59, 696, 1977.

60. **Douglas, N. J., Sudlow, M. F., and Fenley, D. C.,** Effect of an inhaled atropine-like agent on normal airway function, *J. Appl. Physiol.,* 46, 256, 1979.

61. **Pistelli, R., Potalaro, F., Liberatore, S. M., Patalano, F., Liberatore, S. M., and Incalzi, R. A.,** Selectivity of anticholinergic drugs on central and peripheral airways in normal subjects, *Eur. J. Resp. Dis.,* 128(part 2), 499, 1983.

62. **Storms, W. W., Dopico, G. A., and Reed, C. E.,** Aerosol Sch 1000. An anticholinergic bronchodilator, *Am. Rev. Resp. Dis.,* 111, 419, 1975.

63. **Firstater, E., Mizrachi, E., and Topilsky, M.,** The effect of vagolytic drugs on airway obstruction in patients with bronchial asthma, *Ann. Allergy,* 76, 332, 1981.

64. **Schroeksteihn, D. C., Bush, R. K., Chervinsky, P., and Busse, W. W.,** Twelve-hour bronchodilatation in asthma with a single aerosol dose of the anticholinergic compound glycopyrrolate, *J. Allergy Clin. Immunol.,* 82, 115, 1988.

65. **Chai, H., Farr, R. S., Froehlich, L. A., Mathison, D. A., Mclean, J. A., Rosenthal, R. R., Sheffer, A. L., Spector, S. L., and Townley, R. G.,** Standardization of bronchial inhalation challenge procedure, *J. Allergy Clin. Immunol.,* 56, 323, 1975.

66. **Altounyan, R. E.,** Inhibition of experimental asthma by a new compound, disodium cromoglycate (Intal), *Acta Allergol.,* 22, 487, 1967.

67. **Blumenthal, M. N., Seclow, J., Spector, S., Zeiger, R. S., and Mellon, M.,** A multicenter evaluation of the clinical benefits of cromolyn sodium aerosol by metered-dose inhaler in the treatment of asthma, *J. Allergy Clin. Immunol.,* 81, 681, 1988.

68. **Cox, J. S. G. and Altounyan, R. E. C.,** Nature of mode of action of disodium cromoglycate (Lomudal), *Respiration,* 27(Suppl.), 292, 1970.

69. **Kay, A. B., Walsh, G. M., Moqbel, R., Macdonald, A. J., Nagakura, T., Carroll, M. P., and Richerson, H. B.,** Disodium cromoglycate inhibits activation of human inflammatory cells *in vitro, J. Allergy Clin. Immunol.,* 80, 1, 1987.

70. **Murphy, S.,** Cromolyn sodium, Jenne, J. W. and Murphy, S., Eds., Marcel Dekker, New York, 1987, 669.

71. Intal: Cromolyn Sodium A Monograph, Fisons Corporation, Bedford, MA, 1973.

72. **O'Byrne, P., Dolovich, J., and Hargreave, F. E.,** Late asthmatic responses, *Am. Rev. Resp. Dis.,* 136, 740, 1987.

73. **Cockcroft, D. W. and Murdock, K. Y.,** Comparative effects of inhaled salbutamol, sodium cromoglycate, and beclomethasone dipropionate on allergen-induced early asthmatic responses, late asthmatic responses and increased bronchial responsiveness to histamine, *J. Allergy Clin. Immunol.,* 79, 734, 1987.

74. **Eigen, H., Reid, J. J., Dahl, R., Fasano, L., Gunella, G., Sahlstrom, K. K., Alanko, K. J. L., Greenbaum, J., Hagelung, B., Shapiro, C. G., Sher, N., and Sheffer, A. L.,** Evaluation of the addition of cromolyn sodium to bronchodilator maintenance therapy in the long-term management of asthma, *J. Allergy Clin. Immunol.,* 80, 612, 1987.

75. **Konig, P.,** Inhaled steroids — their present and future role in the management of asthma, *J. Allergy Clin. Immunol.,* 82, 297, 1988.

76. **Wardman, A. S., Simpson, F. G., Knox, A. J., Page, R. L., and Cooke, N. J.,** The use of high dose inhaled beclomethasone dipropionate as a means of assessing steroid responsiveness in obstructive airway disease, *Br. J. Dis. Chest,* 82, 168, 1988.

77. **Tarlo, S. M., Broder, I., Davies, G.. M., Leznoff, A., Mintz, S., and Corey, P. N.,** Six month double-blind, controlled trial of high dose, concentrated beclomethasone dipropionate in the treatment of severe chronic asthma, *Chest,* 93, 998, 1988.

78. **Pepys, J., Davies, R. J., Breslin, A. B., Hendricks, D. J., and Hutchcroft, B. J.,** The effect of inhaled beclomethasone and sodium cromoglycate on asthmatic reactions to provocation tests, *Clin. Allergy,* 4, 13, 1974.

79. **Booij-Noord, H., Orie, N. G., and deVries, K.,** Immediate and late bronchial obstructive reactions to inhalation of house dust and protective effects of sodium cromoglycate and prednisolone, *J. Allergy Clin. Immunol.,* 48, 344, 1971.

80. **Delehunt, J. C., Yerger, L., Ahmed, T., and Abraham, W. M.,** Inhibition of antigen-induced bronchoconstriction by methylprednisolone succinate, *J. Allergy Clin. Immunol.,* 73, 479, 1984.

81. **Burge, P. S., Efthimiou, J., Turner-Warwick, M., and Nelmes, P. T.,** Double-blind trials of inhaled beclomethasone dipropionate and fluocortin butyl ester in allergen-induced immediate and late asthmatic reactions, *Clin. Allergy,* 12, 523, 1982.

82. **Morris, H. G.,** Review of ipratropium bromide in induced bronchospasm in patients with asthma, *Am. J. Med.,* 81(Suppl. 5A), 36, 1986.

83. **Cockcroft, D. W., Ruffin, R. E., and Hargreave, F. E.,** Effect of SCH-1000 in allergen-induced asthma, *Clin. Allergy,* 8, 361, 1978.

84. **Ruffin, R. E., Cockcroft, D. W., and Hargreave, F. E.,** A comparison of the protective effect of fenoterol and SCH-1000 on allergen-induced asthma, *J. Allergy Clin. Immunol.,* 61, 42, 1978.

85. **Howarth, P. H., Durham, S. R., Lee, T. H., Kay, B. A., Church, M. K., and Holgate, S. T.,** Influence of albuterol, cromolyn sodium, and ipratropium bromide on the airway and circulating and mediator responses to allergen bronchial provocation in asthma, *Am. Rev. Resp. Dis.,* 132, 986, 1985.

86. **Clarke, P. S., Jarrett, R. G., and Hall, G. J.,** The protective effect of ipratropium bromide aerosol against bronchospasm induced by hyperventilation and the inhalation of allergen, methacholine and histamine, *Ann. Allergy,* 48, 180, 1982.

87. **Kersten, W.,** Protective effect of metered aerosol SCH-1000 against bronchoconstriction by allergen inhalation, *Respirations,* 31, 412, 1974.

88. **Wolkove, N., Kreisman, H., Frank, H., and Gent, M.,** The effect of ipratropium bromide on exercise-induced bronchoconstriction, *Ann. Allergy,* 47, 311, 1981.

89. **Abraham, W. M.,** The role of leukotrienes in allergen-induced late responses in allergic sheep, in *Biology of the Leukotriene,* Levy, R. and Krell, R. D., Eds., New York Academy of Sciences, New York, 1988, 260.

90. **Barnes, P. J., Chung, K. F., and Page, C. P.,** Platelet activating factor as a mediator of allergic disease, *J. Allergy Clin. Immunol.,* 81, 919, 1988.

91. **Guinot, P., Brambilla, C., Duchier, J., Braquet, P., Bonvoisin, B., and Cournot, A.,** Effect of BN52063, a specific PAF-acether antagonist on bronchial provocation test to allergies in asthmatic patients: a preliminary study, *Prostaglandins,* 34, 723, 1987.
92. **Ahmed, T., D'Brot, J., and Abraham, W.,** The role of calcium antagonists in bronchial hyperreactivity, *J. Allergy Clin. Immunol.,* 81, 133, 1988.
93. **Boushey, H. A., Holtzman, M. J., Sheller, O. R., and Nadel, J. A.,** Bronchial hyperreactivity: state of the art, *Am. Rev. Resp. Dis.,* 121, 389, 1980.
94. **Altounyan, R. E. C.,** Changes in histamine and atropine responsiveness as a guide to diagnosis and evaluation of therapy in obstructive airway disease, in *Disodium Cromoglycate in Allergic Airway Disease,* Pepys, J. and Frankland, A. W., Eds., Butterworths, London, 1970, 47.
95. **Lowhagen, O. and Rak, S.,** Modification of bronchial hyperreactivity after treatment with sodium cromoglycate during pollen season, *J. Allergy Clin. Immunol.,* 75, 460, 1985.
96. **Sotomayer, H., Badier, M., Vervloet, D., and Orehek, J.,** Seasonal increase of carbachol airway responsiveness in patients allergic to grass pollen: reversal by corticosteroids, *Am. Rev. Resp. Dis.,* 130, 56, 1984.
97. **Griffin, M. P., MacDonald, N., and Mcfadden, E. R., Jr.,** Short and long term effects of cromolyn sodium on the airway reactivity of asthmatics, *J. Allergy Clin. Immunol.,* 71, 331, 1983.
98. **D'Brot, J. and Ahmed, T.,** Hypoxia-induced enhancement of non-specific bronchial reactivity: role of leukotrienes, *J. Appl. Physiol.,* 65, 194, 1988.
99. **O'Byrne, P. M., Walters, E. H., Gold, B. D., Aizawa, H. A., Fabri, L. M., Alpert, S. E., Nadel, J. A., and Holtzman, M. J.,** Indomethacin inhibits the airway hyperresponsiveness but not the neutrophil influx induced by ozone in dogs, *Am. Rev. Resp. Dis.,* 130, 220, 1984.
100. **Abraham, W. M., Blinder, L., Wanner, A., Stevenson, J. S., and Tallent, M. W.,** Antigen-induced airway hyperresponsiveness does not contribute to airway late responses, *Am. Rev. Resp. Dis.,* 135, A97, 1987.
101. **Blinder, L., Stevenson, J. S., Tallent, M. W., Jackowski, J. T., Wanner, A., Ahmed, T., and Abraham, W. M.,** Cyclooxygenase products of arachidonate modulate antigen-induced late responses in the airways, *Am. Rev. Resp. Dis.,* 135, A180, 1987.
102. **Steven, D. D.,** Diagnosis, prevention and treatment of adverse reactions to aspirin and non-steroidal anti-inflammatory drugs, *J. Allergy Clin. Immunol.,* 74, 617, 1984.
103. **Diaz, P., Galleguillos, F. R., Gonzalez, M. C., Pantin, C. F., and Kay, B. A.,** Bronchoalveolar lavage in asthma: the effect of disodium cromoglycate (cromolyn) on leukocyte counts, immunoglobulins, and complement, *J. Allergy Clin. Immunol.,* 74, 41, 1984.
104. **Carroll, M., Durham, S. R., Walsh, G. M., and Kay, B. A.,** Activation of neutrophils and monocytes after allergen-induced bronchoconstriction, *J. Allergy Clin. Immunol.,* 75, 290, 1985.
105. **Wanner, A.,** Clinical aspects of mucociliary transport. State of the art, *Am. Rev. Resp. Dis.,* 116, 73, 1977.
106. **Sackner, M. A., Yergin, B. M., Brito, M., and Januskiewicz, A.,** Effect of adrenergic agonists on tracheal mucous velocity, *Bull. Physio-Pathol. Resp.,* 15, 505, 1979.
107. **Weissberger, D., Oliver, W., Jr., Abraham, W. M., and Wanner, A.,** Impaired tracheal mucus transport in allergic bronchoconstriction: effect of terbutaline treatment, *J. Allergy Clin. Immunol.,* 67, 357, 1981.
108. **Wanner, A.,** Effect of ipratropium bromide on airway mucociliary function, *Am. J. Med.,* 81(Suppl. 5A), 23, 1986.
109. **Mezey, R. J., Cohn, M. A., Fernandez, R. J., Januszkiewicz, A. J., and Wanner, A.,** Mucociliary transport in allergic patients with antigen-induced bronchospasm, *Am. Rev. Resp. Dis.,* 118, 677, 1978.
110. **Ahmed, T., Greenblatt, D. W., Birch, S., Marchette, B., and Wanner, A.,** Abnormal mucociliary transport in allergic patients with antigen-induced bronchospasm: role of SRS-A, *Am. Rev. Resp. Dis.,* 124, 110, 1981.
111. **Fazio, F. and Lafortuna, C. L.,** Beclomethasone dipropionate does not affect mucociliary clearance in patients with chronic obstructive lung disease, *Respiration,* 50, 62, 1986.
112. **Goodman, R. M., Yergin, B. M., and Sackner, M. A.,** Effect of S-carboxymethylcysteine on tracheal mucous velocity, *Chest,* 74, 615, 1978.
113. **Jaques, L. B., Mahadoo, J., and Kavanagh, L. W.,** Intrapulmonary heparin: a new procedure for anticoagulant therapy, *Lancet,* 2, 1157, 1976.
114. **Ahmed, T., Oliver, W., Jr., Frank, B. L., Robinson, M. J., and Wanner, A.,** Hypoxic pulmonary vasoconstriction: role of mast cell degranulation, *Am. Rev. Resp. Dis.,* 126, 291, 1982.
115. **Ahmed, T., Oliver, W., Jr., and Marchette, B.,** Modification of hypoxic pulmonary vasoconstriction by aerosolized cromolyn sodium, *Bull. Eur. Physiopathol. Resp.,* 22, 61, 1986.
116. **Waldman, R. H., Pearce, D. E., and Martin, R. A.,** Pentamidine isoethionate levels in lungs, livers, kidneys of rats after aerosol or intramuscular administration, *Am. Rev. Resp. Dis.,* 108, 1004, 1973.
117. **Debs, R. J., Blumenfeld, W., and Brunette, E. N.,** Successful treatment with aerosolized pentamidine of pneumocystis carinii pneumonia in rats, *Antimicrobial Agents Chemother.,* 31, 37, 1987.
118. **Conte, J. E., Jr., Hollander, H., and Golden, J. A.,** Inhaled or reduced-dose intravenous pentamidine for *Pneumocystis carinii* pneumonia, *Ann. Intern. Med.,* 107, 495, 1987.

119. **Montgomery, A. B., Debs, R. J., Luce, J. M., Corkery, K. J., Turner, J., Brunette, E. N., Lin, E. T., and Hopewell, P. C.,** Selective delivery of pentamidine to the lung by aerosol, *Am. Rev. Resp. Dis.,* 137, 477, 1988.

120. **Debs, R. J., Straubinger, R. M., Brunette, E. M., Lin, J. M., Montgomery, B., Friend, D. S., and Papahadjopoulos, D. P.,** Selective enhancement of pentamidine uptake in the lung by aerosolization and delivery in liposomes, *Am. Rev. Resp. Dis.,* 135, 731, 1987.

121. **Southwell, N.,** Inhaled penicillin in bronchial infections, *Lancet,* 2, 225, 1946.

122. **Hodson, M. E., Penketh, A. R. L., and Batten, J. C.,** Aerosol carbenicillin and gentamicin treatment of *Pseudomonas aeruginosa* infection in cystic fibrosis, *Lancet,* 2, 1137, 1981.

123. **Newman, S. P., Woodman, G., and Clarke, S. W.,** Deposition of carbenicillin aerosols in cystic fibrosis: effect of nebulizer system and breathing pattern, *Thorax,* 43, 318, 1988.

124. **Knight, V., McClung, H. W., and Wilson, S. Z.,** Ribavirin small-particle aerosol treatment of influenza, *Lancet,* 2, 945, 1981.

125. **McClung, H. W., Knight, V., Gilbert, V., Gilbert, B. E., Wilson, S. Z., Quarles, J. M., and Devine, G. W.,** Ribavirin aerosol treatment of influenza B virus infection, *JAMA,* 249, 2671, 1983.

126. **Hall, C. B., Walsh, E. E., Hruska, J. F., Betts, B. F., and Hall, W. J.,** Ribavirin treatment of experimental respiratory syncytial virus infection: a controlled double-blind study in young adults, *JAMA,* 249, 2666, 1983.

127. **Hall, C. B., McBride, J. T., Walsh, E. D., Bell, D. M., Gala, C. G., Hildreth, S., and Hall, W. J.,** Aerosolized ribavirin treatment of infants with respiratory syncytial viral infection, *N. Engl. J. Med.,* 308, 1443, 1983.

128. **Liss, H. P. and Bernstein, J.,** Ribavirin aerosol in the elderly, *Chest,* 93, 1239, 1988.

129. **Gadek, J. E., Klein, H. G., Holland, P. V., and Crystal, R. G.,** Replacement therapy with alpha 1-antitrypsin deficiency. Reversal of protease-antiprotease imbalance within the alveolar structure of PiZ subjects, *J. Clin. Invest.,* 68, 1158, 1981.

130. **Robillard, E., Alarie, Y., Dagenais-Perusse, P., Baril, E., and Guilbeault, A.,** Microaerosol administration of synthetic depalmitoyl lecithin in the respiratory distress syndrome: a preliminary report, *Can. Med. Assoc. J.,* 90, 55, 1964.

131. **Chu, J., Cleniats, J. H., Cotton, E. K., Klaus, M. H., Sweet, A. Y., and Tooley, W. H.,** Neonatal pulmonary ischemia: clinical and physiological studies, *Pediatrics,* 40, 709, 1967.

132. **Jobe, A. and Ikegami, M.,** Surfactant for the treatment of respiratory distress syndrome. State of the art, *Am. Rev. Resp. Dis.,* 136, 1256, 1987.

133. **Enhorning, G., Shennan, A., Possmayer, F., Dunn, M., Chen, C. P., and Milligan, J.,** Prevention of neonatal respiratory distress syndrome by tracheal instillation of surfactant: a randomized clinical trial, *Pediatrics,* 76, 145, 1985.

134. **Merritt, T. A., Hallman, M., Bloom, B. T., Berry, C., Benirschke, K., Sahn, D., Key, T., Edwards, D., Jarvenpaa, A., Pohjavuori, M., Kankaanpaa, K., Kunnas, M., Paatero, H., Rapola, J., and Jaaskelainen, J.,** Prophylactic treatment of very premature infants with human surfactant, *N. Engl. J. Med.,* 315, 785, 1986.

135. **Debs, R. J., Straubinger, R. M., Brunette, E. N., Lin, J. M., Lin, E. J., Montgomery, A. B., Friend, D. S., and Papahadjopoulos, D. P.,** Selective enhancement of pentamidine uptake in the lung by aerosolization and delivery in liposomes, *Am. Rev. Resp. Dis.,* 135, 731, 1987.

136. **Frank, R.,** Editorial: are aerosol sprays hazardous?, *Am. Rev. Resp. Dis.,* 112, 485, 1975.

137. **Dollery, C. T., William, F. M., Draffan, G. H., Wise, G., Sahyoun, H., Paterson, J. W., and Walker, S. R.,** Arterial blood levels of fluorocarbons in asthmatic patients following use of pressurized aerosols, *Clin. Pharmacol. Ther.,* 15, 59, 1974.

138. **Sackner, M. A., Epstein, S., and Wanner, A.,** Effect of beta-adrenergic agonists aerosolized by freon propellant on tracheal mucous velocity and cardiac output, *Chest,* 69, 593, 1976.

139. **Sackner, M. A., Friedman, M., Silva, G., and Fernandez, R.,** The pulmonary hemodynamic effects of aerosols of isoproterenol and ipratropium in normal subjects and patients with reversible airway obstruction, *Am. Rev. Resp. Dis.,* 116, 1013, 1977.

140. **Sly, M.,** Adverse effects and complications of treatment with beta-adrenergic agonist drugs, *J. Allergy Clin. Immunol.,* 75, 443, 1985.

141. **Rafferty, P., Beasley, R., and Holgate, S. T.,** Comparison of the efficacy of preservative free ipratropium bromide and atrovent nebuliser solution, *Thorax,* 43, 446, 1988.

142. **Shim, C. S. and Williams, M. H., Jr.,** Cough and wheezing from beclomethasone dipropionate aerosol are absent after triamcinolone acetonide, *Ann. Intern. Med.,* 106, 700, 1987.

143. **Bisgaard, H., Nielsen, M. D., Andersen, B., Andersen, P., Foged, N., Fuglsang, G., Host, A., Leth, C., Pedersen, M., Pelck, I., Stafanger, G., and Osterballe, O.,** Adrenal function in children with bronchial asthma treated with beclomethasone dipropionate or budesonide, *J. Allergy Clin. Immunol.,* 81, 1088, 1988.

144. **Kalra, L. and Bone, M. F.,** The effect of nebulized bronchodilator therapy on intraocular pressures in patients with glaucoma, *Chest,* 93, 739, 1988.

145. Guidelines for the Clinical Evaluation of Bronchodilator Drugs, FDA-79-3073, U.S. Food and Drug Administration, Rockville, MD, 1978.

146. **Anon.,** Guidelines for the evaluation of NBAAD, *J. Allergy Clin. Immunol.,* 78, 489, 1986.

APPENDIX

THE EFFECTS OF WATER IN INHALATION SUSPENSION AEROSOL FORMULATIONS

Nicholas C. Miller

TABLE OF CONTENTS

I. INTRODUCTION

Metered-dose inhalation aerosols are conveniently classified as suspensions or solutions, depending on whether the drug is contained as a separate suspended phase or dissolved in other formulation ingredients. Stability and performance issues are different for the two classes.

Suspension aerosols are often preferred because of chemical stability and improved delivery properties. The drug as a solid is less likely to undergo decomposition. The size of the spray particles emitted from a suspension aerosol is typically smaller because low volatility solvents are not required in the formulation. The size of the aerosol spray is determined to a major extent by the size of the drug particles prior to formulation and can be made fine enough to increase penetration of the spray into deep portions of the lung.

One characteristic of suspension aerosols not shared with solutions is that the stability is often quite sensitive to the presence of trace amounts of water. This phenomenon can limit the possibility of developing suspension aerosols of some compounds, although a knowledge of the mode of water entry and a quantification of the allowable amount of water will often suggest a means of controlling the degradation which is due to the presence of water.

Typically, as long as the concentration is within solubility limits for the formulation, water content is not an important consideration in solution aerosols. The cosolvents ordinarily used in solution formulations are much less volatile than propellant, and this results in a relatively coarse spray. The presence of water up to a few percent of the total formulation does not cause a significantly coarser spray and may increase the effectiveness of the cosolvent. Chemical stability must be considered, although it usually is not adversely affected by the presence of varying amounts of water in the formulation.

II. QUALITATIVE EFFECTS OF WATER ON SUSPENSION AEROSOL FORMULATIONS

Suspension aerosols for inhalation generally contain a mixture of chlorofluorocarbon propellants, a dispersing agent, possibly additional excipients, and the drug in a finely divided form. Almost always, the drug is ground by the process of air micronization or fluid energy milling which results in a powder with a mean size in the range of 2 to 5 μm. The technical literature on the characteristics of pharmaceutical aerosols is not well developed. Product developers who have worked in the area are usually acutely aware that inhalation aerosols are sensitive to the presence of moisture.[1]

Many compounds, including those drugs considered for delivery by inhalation, have some significant interaction with water at the molecular level.[2] The possibilities include passive physically adsorbed water, water contained in a crystal structure, and chemically bound water. In addition, small amounts of water may be dissolved in the liquified propellant. This water may function as a cosolvent to increase the solvent power of the liquid phase. Only a tiny amount of solubility is enough to cause particle growth by the process termed Ostwald ripening.[3] In this process, smaller particles disappear and larger particles grow because the smaller particles are slightly more soluble. A rule of thumb seems to be that if the solubility of the solid in the remainder of the formulation, including propellants, can be measured by the most sensitive method (to the parts per million range), then a suspension will not be stable.

Figure 1 is a photomicrograph[4] (at approximately 450X magnification) of the drug in a freshly prepared aerosol, showing the portion of the drug impacting on a microscope slide when fired through a standard aerosol actuator. The appearance of the particles is distinctive — individual particles are small, well separated, and have a combination of sharp and rounded edges, which is characteristic of micronized powder. A slide prepared directly from the powder would have much the same appearance.

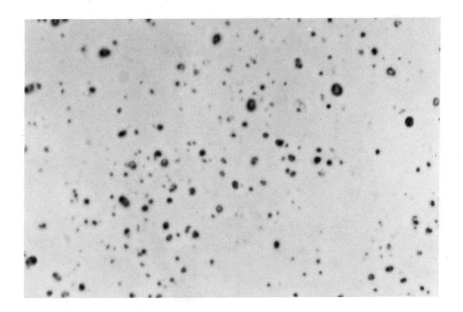

FIGURE 1. Freshly prepared aerosol impacted on glass slide. (Magnification × 450.)

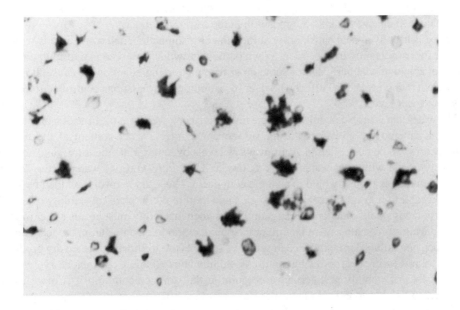

FIGURE 2. Aerosol with slight water contamination.

Figure 2 shows the same aerosol product at the same magnification[4] after it has become contaminated with water. The particles are somewhat larger, and show some alterations in shape. Figure 3 shows the same product at the same magnification[4] somewhat later and with additional water gain, with gross changes in particle size and shape.

Obviously, with the large changes in particle size as depicted in Figures 1 to 3, there is a likelihood that the aerosol valve or the actuator will be physically clogged, which will result in less than the target amount of drug being delivered. Less obviously, but equally unsatisfactory,

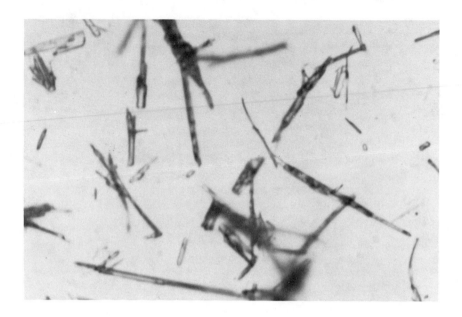

FIGURE 3. Aerosol with severe water contamination.

smaller changes of particle size may result in a product with different aerodynamic characteristics. This will change the site of deposition in the respiratory tract.

Aerosols usually appear satisfactory at the time of manufacture, and some time is required
in order for particle growth to be seen. When particle growth is observed in a formulation, it is
often not apparent whether water or some other formulation ingredient is the cause. It is most
convenient to investigate the effects of water by examining formulations controlled to contain
very low water levels.

The water that is in an aerosol at any time must have been present at the time of manufacture,
or else it entered the container during subsequent storage. Water content at the time of
manufacture can be controlled to arbitrarily low levels by appropriate measures, and aerosols
have been made with total water levels as low as 15 ppm (300 μg of water in the 20 g of
formulation that is typically held in a single container). These dry aerosols can then be stored
in a desiccator to prevent further moisture gain and monitored for physical stability over time.
If the product is stable under anhydrous conditions, then instability must be due either to water
gained during storage after manufacture or to some factor other than water in the formulation.

Suspension failure can be induced in sensitive systems by storing the finished dry product at
high humidities, either at room temperature or slightly above. Failure can then be expressed in
terms of loss of stability at a certain time point at the storage condition. It is more useful,
however, to be able to express the failure as occurring after a certain moisture level in the
formulation is reached, since this can lead to prediction of effects at storage conditions other than
the specific ones studied.

III. ENTRY SITES FOR WATER INTO AEROSOL CONTAINERS

Figure 4 shows a section view of an assembled aerosol in an aluminum vial and Figure 5
shows that for a glass vial. Some other configurations of sealing surfaces are in current use, but
the two shown in the figures describe the placement of gaskets used in the common sealing
techniques.

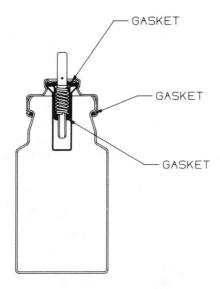

FIGURE 4. Section view of aluminum aerosol container.

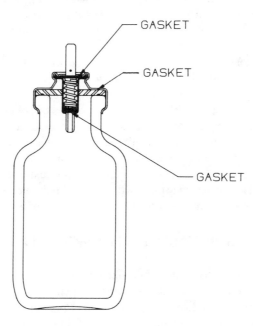

FIGURE 5. Section view of glass aerosol container.

Consider the path a water molecule must take to get from the environment outside the container to the drug particles in suspension. There are two surfaces between inside and outside which are not solid, either metal or glass. These are the gasket around the valve stem and the gasket between the valve body and the vial. It is through these surfaces that water must travel. In addition, water may need to travel through vapor space and through liquid propellant, depending on the orientation of the container, but the gasket is the limiting resistance.

IV. DIFFUSION ANALYSIS

An applicable statement of Fick's law for diffusion through a membrane is[5]

$$Q = 1/R \, (X_o - X_i) \tag{1}$$

where Q is a rate of flow term, R is a resistance to flow, and $X_o - X_i$ is a difference in driving force between points o and i. This equation describes diffusion between any two physical sites defined by o and i, although the resistance term may not be a constant value if there are large changes in X_o or X_i.

The equation can be applied to describe moisture permeation into the aerosol. Q represents the rate of water entry. The driving force for water entering the container, X_o, is the concentration of water in the ambient air, which is conveniently represented as the partial pressure of water. (Note that relative humidity at any temperature is defined as the partial pressure of water divided by the saturation vapor pressure at that temperature.) All the resistance that the water encounters moving between the outside environment and the drug surface is included in the term 1/R.

The driving force for water to move away from the drug surface, X_i, is a complex term. It depends on at least two interacting properties: the total concentration of water in the drug/water system, and the affinity of that water for the drug. The affinity depends on the way in which water is associated with the drug,[2] with physically adsorbed water being held much less tightly than water that becomes incorporated into the crystal structure. In aerosol systems of interest, however, the drug surface is initially very dry and very "eager" to hold onto what little water may be present.

As long as the water content is low, there is essentially no driving force tending to move water away from the drug, so, initially at least, $X_i = 0$. However, as more water becomes associated with the drug, eventually there will be a significant driving force developed which tends to move water away from the drug and out into the environment. A time will be reached when the driving forces are balanced, and the rate of water permeation into the aerosol container will be balanced by water leaving; the net water permeation will reach zero as the system reaches equilibrium.

In summary, it is expected from consideration of the diffusion process that the rate of water pickup by a dry aerosol will be constant initially and will eventually decrease to zero. The rate of decrease will depend on the tendency that the drug has to hold water, with high affinity drugs maintaining a constant rate of water pickup until a higher level of water content is reached.

V. EXPERIMENTAL OBSERVATIONS

The data reported in Figures 6 through 9 were obtained on aerosols prepared in the laboratory[6] under conditions which permitted the water content to be controlled. The same formulation was used for all experiments: a blend of chlorofluorocarbon propellants P11 and P12, sorbitan trioleate as dispersing agent, and less than 1 wt% of a highly hygroscopic drug. The water content was measured after the aerosols were stored in environments controlled for temperature and humidity for varying lengths of time.

Measuring water content at the low levels usually present in aerosols requires special techniques. For the data reported here, an automated Karl Fischer titration instrument was used with a custom sample injection device. The system was demonstrated[7] to detect and resolve 50 μg of water, which represents 2.5 ppm in a typical aerosol.

Figure 6 shows that water pickup rate remains essentially constant for 60 d for this aerosol formulation. The rate depends on the temperature and relative humidity of the storage conditions, with lower temperatures and humidities associated with lower rates of moisture gain.

Figure 7 shows the total amount of water increase in aerosols stored at the same temperature,

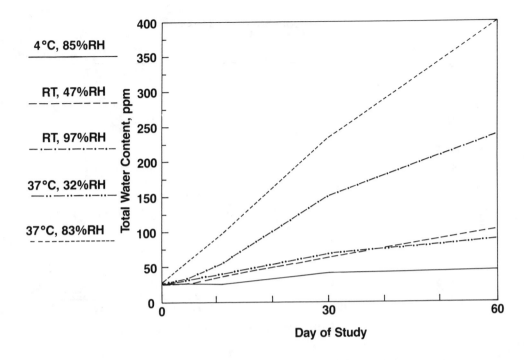

FIGURE 6. Water content after brief storage at various conditions.

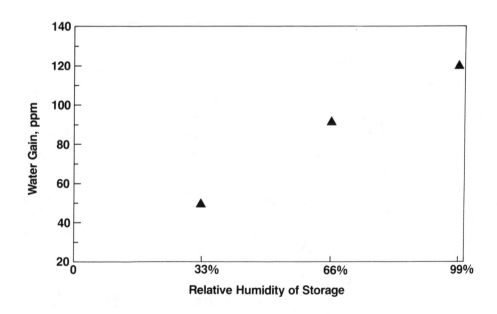

FIGURE 7. Water gain dependence on humidity at room temperature.

but different humidities, for 36 d. Up to the relatively low total water levels considered here, the amount of water uptake was directly proportional to relative humidity, which is the driving force of the water in the environment. Because the same time period was used for all observations, the rate of water uptake was also directly proportional to the driving force of water, as predicted by Equation 1.

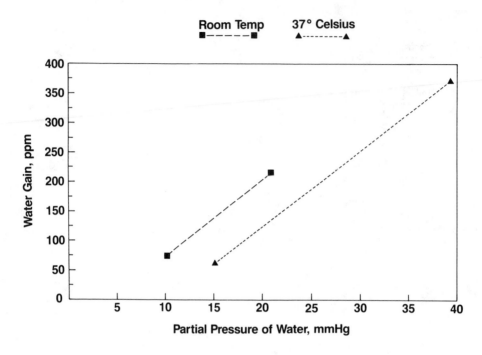

FIGURE 8. Water gain dependence on temperature and humidity.

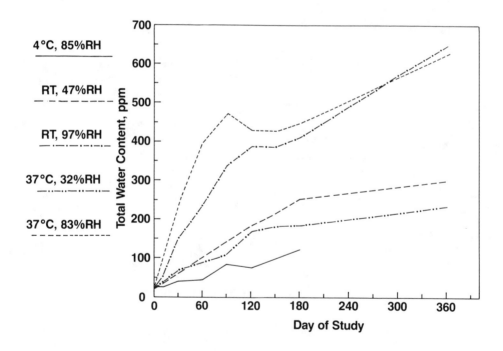

FIGURE 9. Water content after long storage at various conditions.

Figure 8 shows data on the same units as those in Figure 6, plotted as the total amount of water gained in 60 d. This shows the influence of temperature as well as humidity of the storage conditions. Equation 1 predicts that the rate of water gain should depend only upon the driving force in the environment, as measured by the partial pressure of water, but the figure shows a dependence upon temperature as well. This could occur, for example, if the resistance to diffusion were influenced by temperature.

Figure 9 depicts the water gain in the same samples during 1 year. It is not clear from these data whether water entry has reached a plateau, as predicted by Equation 1, or whether it is continuing to increase.

VI. CONCLUSION

Much remains to be done to define completely the mechanism of water entry to aerosols. The fragmentary theory presented here provides a framework for designing experiments to explore possible mechanisms. The data suggest that additional work is needed to define the role of temperature on resistance to water diffusion, as well as to determine the magnitude of the driving force for water away from the surface of the powdered drug when it is incorporated into the formulation.

REFERENCES

1. **Lachman, L., Lieberman, H. A., and Kanig, J. L.,** *The Theory and Practice of Industrial Pharmacy,* 3rd ed., Lea & Febiger, Philadelphia, 1986, chap. 20.
2. **Zografi, G. and Kontny, M. J.,** The interaction of water with cellulose- and starch-derived pharmaceutical excipients, *Pharm. Res.,* 3(4), 187, 1986.
3. **Lachman, L., Lieberman, H. A., and Kanig, J. L.,** *The Theory and Practice of Industrial Pharmacy,* 3rd ed., Lea & Febiger, Philadelphia, 1986, chap. 5.
4. **Gam, V. W.,** personal communication, 1985.
5. **Ansel, H. C.,** *Introduction to Pharmaceutical Dosage Forms,* 4th ed., Lea & Febiger, Philadelphia, 1985, chap. 4.
6. **McNally, R. A.,** unpublished data, 1986.
7. **Schachtner, W. J.,** unpublished data, 1986.

259

INDEX

A

Absorption, 74—76, 150
in lung, see Lung absorption
of peptides, 81—84
Acceptable quality limits (AQLs), 201
Accumulation of drugs, 73—74
ACE, see Angiotensin-converting enzymes
Acinus, 7
Acquired immune deficiency syndrome (AIDS), 209
Active surfaces, 184
Actuation, 176
Actuators, 170, 184
Addition, 48
Adenosine monophosphate (AMP), 219
Adjuvant therapy, 222
Administration techniques, 118—121
β-Adrenergic agonists, 231, see also specific types
testing of, 210—219
β-Adrenergic blockers, 54, 74, see also specific types
Adrenergic bronchodilators, 222, see also specific
types
β-Adrenergic bronchodilators, 152, see also specific
types
α-Adrenoceptor agonists, 75, see also specific types
β$_2$-Adrenoceptor stimulants, 80, see also specific
types
Aerodynamic diameter, 144, 145, 172
Aerodynamic equivalent diameter, 3, 6
Aerodynamic properties, 191
Aerosol generation, 40—45
nonmetered systems and, 150—156
Aggregation, 186
α-Agonists, 235, see also specific types
β-Agonists, 2, 215—217, 235—237, see also specific
types
β$_2$-Agonists, 48, 210, 231, 236, see also specific types
AHR, see Airway hyperreactivity
AIDS, see Acquired immune deficiency syndrome
Air-blast nebulizers, 151, see Jet nebulizers
Airborne contaminants, 40
Airway hyperreactivity (AHR), 229—230
Airway inflammation, 230—231
Airway obstruction, 27
Airway resistance, 32
Albuterol, 169, 210, 212, 215—217, 228
Aldehyde hydrogenase, 68
Allergen-induced bronchoconstriction, 228
Allergic asthma, 229
Allergic disorders, 235, see also specific types
Alveolar airspaces, 8
Alveolar exposure of lungs to drugs, 65
Alveolar fluid, 121
Alveolar macrophages, 40, 127, 128
Alveolar regions, 20, 73, 75
Alveolar zone, 21
AMD, see Area median diameter
Amines, 74, 94, 99, see also specific types

Aminopeptidase, 84
Aminopeptidase inhibitors, 84
AMP, see Adenosine monosphosphate
Analgesics, 74, see also specific types
Anaphylactic reaction, 48
Anesthesia, 67, 74, 77, see also specific types
Angiotensin-converting enzymes (ACE), 83, 84
Anorectics, 74
Antagonists, 48, 209, see also Agonists; specific types
Antazoline, 75
Antiallergenics, 75
Antiarrhythmics, 74
Antiasthmatics, 76, 80, 93, 152, see also Nonbron-
chodilator antiasthmatic drugs (NBAAD)
Antibiotics, 2, 66, 234, see also specific types
Antibodies, 48
Anticholinergic agents, 2, 222, 231, see also specific
types
bronchospasm prevention and, 227—228
side effects of, 237
testing of, 219—223
Antidiuretic agents, 81
Antigen challenge, 227
Antigen-induced bronchoconstriction, 229, 231
Antihistamines, 74, 75
Antimalarials, 74
Antimicrobial agents, see Antibiotics
Antimicrobial preservatives, 157
Antioxidants, 158, see also specific types
α$_1$-Antitrypsin, 235
Antiviral agents, 161, 234, see also specific types
Applied gas pressure, 153
AQLs, see Acceptable quality limits
Arachidonic acid, 228
ARC, see Area under response curve
Area median diameter (AMD), 4
Area under response curve (ARC), 217
Arginine, 83
Asthma, 2, 27, 229, 231, 232
adverse reactions to drugs and, 48
allergic, 229
characterization of, 31
deaths from, 54
exercise-induced, 228
improved treatment of, 168
reversible, 146
treatment of, 168, 209, 221—223
Atomization, 153
Atropine, 124, 219, 220—231

B

BAAD, see Bronchodilator antiasthmatic drugs
Baffles, 156, 158, 173, 199
BAL, 231
Bambuterol, 81, 92, 102
Barium sulfate, 129
Beclomethasone, 80, 225, 227, 229, 235, 237